Surgical Palliative Care

Edited by

Geoffrey P. Dunn

Attending Surgeon, Department of Surgery,
Hamot Medical Center; Medical Director,
Great Lakes Hospice, Erie, USA

and

Alan G. Johnson

Emeritus Professor of Surgery, University of Sheffield, UK

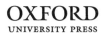
OXFORD
UNIVERSITY PRESS

OXFORD

UNIVERSITY PRESS

Great Clarendon Street, Oxford OX2 6DP

Oxford University Press is a department of the University of Oxford.
It furthers the University's objective of excellence in research, scholarship,
and education by publishing worldwide in

Oxford New York

Auckland Bangkok Buenos Aires Cape Town Chennai
Dar es Salaam Delhi Hong Kong Istanbul Karachi Kolkata
Kuala Lumpur Madrid Melbourne Mexico City Mumbai Nairobi
São Paulo Shanghai Taipei Tokyo Toronto

Oxford is a registered trade mark of Oxford University Press
in the UK and in certain other countries

Published in the United States
by Oxford University Press Inc., New York

British Library Cataloguing in Publication Data

Data available

ISBN 0-19-851000-4

10 9 8 7 6 5 4 3 2 1

Typeset by Integra Software Services Pvt., Ltd, Pondicherry, India
Printed in Great Britain
on acid-free paper by Biddles Ltd., King's Lynn, UK

Contents

Foreword *vii*
John L. Cameron

Preface *ix*
Geoffrey P. Dunn and Alan G. Johnson

List of contributors *xi*

Part I

1 Introduction: is surgical palliative care a paradox? *3*
Geoffrey P. Dunn

2 Selection and preparation of patients for surgical palliation *16*
Alexander Ng and Alexandra M. Easson

3 The ethics of interventional care *33*
Peter Angelos

4 The physiological response to surgical trauma *39*
Matthew D. Barber and Kenneth C.H. Fearon

5 Psychological response to surgery *54*
Laurie Stevens

6 Spirituality and surgery *65*
Peter Ravenscroft and Elizabeth Ravenscroft

7 Interdisciplinary care *85*
Anne Mosenthal, David Price, and Patricia Murphy

8 Quality of life issues in palliative surgery *94*
Michael Koller, Christoph Nies, and Wilfried Lorenz

9 Anaesthesia and perioperative pain management *112*
Karen H. Simpson and Dudley J. Bush

Part II

10 Symptom palliation of diseases of the head and neck (including dentistry) *135*
Simon Rogers

11 The surgical relief of the symptomatic chest *152*
Bill Nelems

12 Surgery for the control of symptoms in the abdomen *159*
Alan G. Johnson

13 Symptom control in urological malignancy *173*
Alan P. Doherty and Joe M. O'Sullivan

14 Wound and reconstructive problems in advanced disease *191*
Thomas J. Krizek

15 Neurosurgical palliation *207*
Dennis L. Johnson

16 The role of the ophthalmologist in advanced disease *227*
David Yorston

17 Perspectives from the developing world and diverse societies *239*
Arjuna Aluwihare

18 Epilogue: a message to all surgeons *248*
Geoffrey P. Dunn and Alan G. Johnson

Index *261*

Supportive Care Series

Volumes in the series:

Supportive care in respiratory disease
Edited by S.H. Ahmedzai and M. Muers

Supportive care for the renal patient
Edited by J. Chambers, M. Germain, and E. Brown

Foreword

From its earliest beginnings, much of surgery has been aimed at palliation. Initially, most early attempts were to relieve pain or stop bleeding. As surgical techniques became more sophisticated, particularly after the introduction of general anaesthesia in 1846, palliation of obstruction also became a common indication for surgery. Today much of surgery can be considered palliative. For example, when a patient with incurable adenocarcinoma of the pancreas presents with obstructive jaundice, obstruction of the duodenum, and severe back pain, the ensuing surgical procedure is obviously palliative. One would perform a hepatico-jejunostomy to relieve the jaundice, a gastrojejunostomy to bypass the obstruction, and a chemical splanchnicecetomy to palliate the pain. However, even patients who present with potentially curable adenocarcinoma of the pancreas, in many ways are merely being palliated. When one performs a pancreaticoduodenectomy in such a patient, one is aware that 20% will survive 5 years, but the remaining 80% will not. Therefore the pancreaticoduodenectomy in the majority of patients upon whom it is performed, could be called a palliative procedure. It relieves biliary and duodenal obstruction as well as pain.

Therefore surgical palliation is certainly not a new field. What is new, however, is the emphasis that is being placed on the palliative role of the surgeon and the palliative function of the surgical procedures that are performed. Now, in many parts of the world a major emphasis is being placed on the importance of appropriate and humane surgical palliative care. This book that Geoffrey Dunn and Alan Johnson have so beautifully edited consists of a series of chapters by contributors from around the world. The first section explains the philosophy and rationale as well as the history of palliative care, with the second part providing a series of surgical examples based on the different anatomical regions of the body.

For too long surgeons have been considered non-caring technicians, interested only in the surgical procedure itself, and the immediate outcome. This book emphasizes that the surgeon has a much broader role in being certain that all of the bothersome and disabling symptoms that the patient has are appropriately addressed. Today we have excellent quality of life tools with which to measure our surgical results. This has allowed surgical palliation to be quantitative, and we are now better able to evaluate our success in our attempts at surgical palliation. Hopefully this book will be read not only by surgeons, but also by non-surgeons participating in the care of patients who require some form of palliation. Surgeons need to be fully aware of the importance of surgical palliation, but our colleagues also need to be aware of our role, and what we are capable of delivering. This book is a pioneering contribution in an old area of surgery that finally has had the spotlight placed on it, and for the first time is receiving the visibility and attention that it richly deserves. Dr Dunn and Professor Johnson have done a marvellous job in bringing this topic to the forefront.

John L. Cameron, MD, FACS
The Alfred Blalock Distinguished Professor of Surgery
The Johns Hopkins Hospital

Preface

A 42 year old woman with a diagnosis of widely metastatic cancer of the breast sustains a pathological fracture of the femur. An elderly man develops malignant obstructive jaundice. A young man undergoes personality changes due to a solitary frontal lobe metastasis from a melanoma. Surgical expertise may be of considerable value in each of these scenarios, so familiar to palliative care clinicians, even if no operation is undertaken. Unfortunately, the opportunity for effective intervention by surgeons may be missed in these instances due to lack of patients' and health care professionals' knowledge about what surgery can offer and, sometimes, the reluctance of surgeons to participate in the care of patients facing inevitable and imminent decline. Symptoms that might readily yield to surgical intervention frequently occur in settings where there may be no surgical expertise at hand; or conversely, if they occur in a surgical setting, the surgeon may not understand the value of the interdisciplinary approach to palliative intervention.

This book brings the domains of surgery and palliative (supportive) care together. Both of these disciplines are dedicated to relieve suffering, though this may not be so obvious in the practice of surgery because surgical care has become increasingly, often dramatically, successful in prolonging life. Ironically, it was this success that created the need for surgeons to address the quality of life issues as patients lived longer but not necessarily better. The success of the hospice movement and its derivative, palliative care, buttressed as they are by cross-cultural public acceptance and the contributions of many disciplines, have challenged the assumption that prolongation of life or cure were surgery's only legitimate goals. The incorporation of surgery into the spectrum of supportive care has offered surgeons a new opportunity to reclaim the ancient and noble surgical tradition of responding decisively and effectively to the problem of physical suffering. This goal of surgery is understandably overlooked in light of the dizzy 'curative' successes of cardiac surgery, transplantation, and trauma care. The reader will see that, even in these areas, the twin imperatives of responding to suffering and promoting well being actually provided the basis of these successes.

This volume, divided into two sections, is written by individuals representing an interdisciplinary and global perspective. The editors readily admit that not all national, cultural, and spiritual viewpoints have been represented but it is our hope that the book provides a sufficiently broad foundation for the development of a comprehensive philosophy of palliative care. The first section addresses issues relevant to all surgical encounters and provides the philosophical framework for the second section which addresses problems seen in selected surgical subspecialties. We have particularly included a perspective from the developing world where diseases are usually first seen at an advanced stage and where financial constraints are enormous. We demonstrate that surgery in palliative care is more than a repertoire of operations for the relief of symptoms: It is a comprehensive approach to palliation by surgeons and surgical means. This relief of suffering and promotion of quality of life, need not be limited to those with incurable, life-threatening disease but involves the supportive care of all other surgical patients. To paraphrase a comment made by a well known expert in palliative medicine: 'If I have a wrist fracture, I still want good pain relief, and I don't want the news from someone who doesn't seem to care even if there is every prospect of the fracture healing'.

The book concludes with a message from the editors, to all surgeons, surgical institutions and carers encouraging them to participate more broadly in palliative care. Suggestions are given about how to do this with the reassurance that these efforts are completely consistent with the standards of Surgical Colleges and Certifying Boards. It is our belief that the fusion of the two great traditions of surgery and palliative care will result in the enhancement of both for the better service of our patients.

Geoffrey P. Dunn, MD, FACS
Alan G. Johnson, MChir, FRCS

The publishers would like to thank Kjersti Hjelmeland Brakstad for designing the covers for the Supportive Care series.

List of contributors

Arjuna Aluwihare, Professor of Surgery, University of Peradeniya, Kandy, Sri Lanka

Peter Angelos, Associate Professor of Surgery and Associate Professor of Medical Humanities and Bioethics, Northwestern University Medical School, Chicago, USA

Matthew D. Barber, Specialist Registrar in Surgery, Department of Clinical and Surgical Sciences (Surgery), Royal Infirmary of Edinburgh, Edinburgh, UK

Dudley J. Bush, Consultant in Pain Medicine, Pain Management Service, St James' University Hospital, Leeds, UK

Alan P. Doherty, Consultant Urological Surgeon, Queen Elizabeth Medical Centre, Birmingham, UK

Geoffrey P. Dunn, Attending Surgeon, Department of Surgery, Hamot Medical Center; Medical Director Great Lakes Hospice, Erie, Pennsylvania, USA

Alexandra M. Easson, Assistant Professor of Surgery, Department of Surgical Oncology, Princess Margaret Hospital, Toronto, Ontario, Canada

Kenneth C.H. Fearon, Professor of Surgical Oncology, Department of Clinical and Surgical Sciences (Surgery), Royal Infirmary of Edinburgh, Edinburgh, UK

Alan G. Johnson, Emeritus Professor of Surgery, University of Sheffield, Sheffield, UK

Dennis L. Johnson, Professor of Medicine, Surgery and Pediatrics, Department of Medicine, Penn State College of Medicine, Hershey, PA, USA

Michael Koller, Institute of Theoretical Surgery, Philipps-University Marburg, Marburg, Germany

Thomas J. Krizek, Courtesy Professor of Religious Studies and Professor of Surgery and Medicine (Ethics), University of South Florida, Tampa, Florida, USA

Wilfried Lorenz, Professor, Institute of Theoretical Surgery, Philipps-University Marburg, Marburg, Germany

Anne Mosenthal, Associate Professor of Surgery, UMDNJ New Jersey Medical School, Newark, New Jersey, USA

Patricia Murphy, Advanced Practice Nurse for Ethics and Bereavement, UMDNJ New Jersey Medical School, Newark, New Jersey, USA

Bill Nelems, Professor of Surgery, University of British Columbia; Thoracic Surgeon, Interior Health Authority, Kelowna General Hospital, British Columbia, Canada

Christoph Nies, Professor of Surgery, Department of Surgery, Marien Hospital, Osnabrück, Germany

Alexander Ng, Surgical Oncology Fellow, Department of Surgical Oncology, Princess Margaret Hospital, Toronto, Ontario, Canada

Joe M. O'Sullivan, Senior Clinical Research Fellow, Academic Unit of Radiotherapy and Clinical Oncology, Institute of Cancer Research and the Royal Marsden NHS Trust, Sutton, UK

David Price, Clinical Bioethicist, UMDNJ New Jersey Medical School, Newark, New Jersey, USA

Elizabeth Ravenscroft, Pastoral Care Associate, Department of Pastoral Care, Newcastle Mater Hospital, Newcastle, New South Wales, Australia

Peter Ravenscroft, Professor of Palliative Care, University of Newcastle and Director of Palliative Care, Newcastle Mater Hospital and Hunter Area Health Service, Newcastle, New South Wales, Australia

Simon Rogers, Consultant and Hon. Reader, Regional Maxillofacial Unit, University Hospital Aintree, Liverpool, UK

Karen H. Simpson, Consultant in Pain Medicine, Pain Management Service, St James' University Hospital, Leeds, UK

Laurie Stevens, Associate Clinical Professor of Psychiatry, Columbia University College of Physicians and Surgeons, New York, USA

David Yorston, Specialist Registrar, Moorfields Eye Hospital, London, UK

Part I

Chapter 1

Introduction: is surgical palliative care a paradox?

Geoffrey P. Dunn

Surgeons and palliative care: cultural conflict?

During my hospice team's discussion about a patient not long ago, one of the team members exclaimed, 'Don't let the surgeons get their hands on him, all they want to do is operate!' Despite the fact I was considered a 'friendly' surgeon by the team – no longer operating, unarmed as it were, and one who was trusted not to take such a comment personally – my blood began to boil. The case under discussion, an individual with hip pain and an impending pathological fracture, was actually one in which operative intervention promised not only relief but also protection from impending disaster. Yet, there were reasons for the comment, some trivial and entertaining and others profound and troubling. I sensed a cultural conflict occurring on a much deeper level than one of debate on optimum pain management. Adding to the difficulty in understanding cultural differences between surgery and non-surgical medical care was the fact that the philosophy of all medical interventions on behalf of individuals with advanced disease was in a process of change. Experience with interdisciplinary teamwork had already convinced me that some of the most intractable problems we had had with patients and care-givers were rooted in cultural differences.

The greatest barrier to introducing surgical means for the relief of suffering is not the unavailability of surgical expertise or repertoire but the stereotypes surgeons, non-surgical practitioners, and patients/families have of each other and the conditions they treat. The concern shared by all of these parties is the compatibility of surgery and surgeons with the vision of palliative care. The increasing reach of palliative care has raised important questions regarding the place of surgery and surgeons in the continuum of this type of care, not only for non-surgeons but also among surgeons themselves. To many the image of the surgeon is one who is 'frequently right, never in doubt'. If this stereotype is true, how can this personality be incorporated in the practice of palliative care where empathy and consensus are such vital elements of success? Some surgeons may freely admit their discomfort with advanced, incurable illness and cringe at the degree of empathy and introspection required to respond appropriately to the words of a dying patient, 'I'm frightened, doctor. Can you help me?'

There are undoubtedly surgeons who feel they are unsuited to provide palliative care despite the fact its importance to surgeons has been demonstrated.[1] Limited expectations regarding the surgeon's capability to respond sensitively and adroitly in these instances overlook the richness of surgical history and letters, some of the positive aspects of surgical character, the unique nature of the surgical encounter, and changing perceptions by patients and practitioners regarding the meaning of chronic and life-limiting illness.

A brief history of palliation in surgery: innovations and personalities

The concept of palliation, the relief of suffering, is not new to surgery and may well have had its origins in a 'surgical' procedure, such as reducing a markedly angulated fracture or extraction of a missile from a mortal wound. Ancient skulls showing partially healed trephination sites may be evidence of attempts to relieve some form of spiritual, psychological, or social anguish rather than attempts to reverse a physical condition. One may go so far as to say that the surgical encounter is as old as humanity itself: humanity may have had its first moment when a hominid used a tool on another hominid to help rather than to harm. There may be more than a grain of truth to the cliché well known to surgeons, 'I can teach any gorilla to operate, but not how to be a surgeon.'

In more recent history, surgery and its closest companion, anaesthesia, have provided the means to reduce the suffering brought on by what ultimately proved to be fatal illness. Following are examples of innovations, all with palliative intent, that not only changed surgery dramatically, but changed surgeons and their patients as well.

Anaesthesia, first practised by dentists and surgeons in the 1840s, not only provided one of the most definitive and broadly applicable innovations for the palliation of pain, but also made the subsequent growth of surgery possible. It also made the advent of a gentler, more cognitive and reflective surgeon possible. The temperament of an individual who prided himself in the amputation of a leg of an unanaesthetized patient in 27 seconds is different from one who would resect a deep, highly vascular tumour from the brain of a child. The most skilful and gentle surgeons always seemed the most aware of their patients' sensibilities, whether the response to physical pain or the response to less localized perceptions.

Sherwin Nuland, a surgeon and author of the book *How we die*,[2] points out in another writing[3] that innovation helped open the field to different talents and qualities in surgeons with the result that the modern surgeon has little resemblance to the surgeons of the nineteenth century or even much of the twentieth.

He gives an earlier example of surgeons' resistance to an idea that represented a fundamental departure from the prevailing view of the physical world. The idea was the 'germ' theory and it required surgeons to look beyond the observable physical world in such a way that drove them into the laboratory and to become scientists. This led to the progressive replacement of the showy and the swift of hand by the intellectual and the thoughtful. Now, once again, the surgeon's practise must adjust to an unseen world, only this time it is not the invisible physical world of microbes but the invisible realms of the psyche and the spirit. Belief in the presence of this new unseen world by surgeons has as much potential to radically change surgery and surgeons as their acceptance of the germ theory did in the late nineteenth century. Surgeons are already becoming aware that fundamental guidance exclusively sought in the laboratory will once again come from the patient's bed. Following this leap of faith in things unseen, the isolation of the laboratory will be replaced by the communality of the clinical team. The previous irrelevance of the non-physical outcomes to surgeons was reflected by their absence from earlier clinical trials. Hopefully, it won't be long before any surgical investigator will not consider a prospective trial without measuring social, psychological, financial, and spiritual outcomes.

One wonders what the selection pressure of current innovation such as robotics or increased cross-cultural awareness will do to shape the personality of future surgeons. A look into the past about how surgeons responded to the immediate challenge of suffering will renew hope about what they could do in the future. Ironically, our current expectation of cure or prolonged survival began after we succeeded in the decisive relief of suffering and hopelessness.

Cancer surgery as we recognize it today began with the treatment of highly symptomatic patients who were usually those most unlikely to be cured. The fact that some of these procedures later *did* cure was the result of improvement in technique, earlier detection of disease, and the luckier patients with less aggressive disease. There was no screen for early detection of gastric carcinoma in 1881 when Theodor Billroth, a close friend of composer Johannes Brahms, performed the first 'successful' gastrectomy for this disease. How did the operation succeed? The procedure that removed an obstructing cancer of the pylorus exchanged an imminent death associated with vomiting with a more peaceful demise from anorexia and cachexia due to liver metastases four months later.[4] We now take for granted immediate operative survival following elective procedures, though this was not at all the case in the time of Billroth. This case represents a historic example of the willingness to test the principle of double effect: the bad (death) may be the result, not the intention, of doing the good (operation for the relief of suffering).

The foundation for the modern treatment of cancer of the breast, the most common malignancy in women encountered by surgeons, was laid by William Stewart Halstead. His impact on the world of surgery, particularly in the United States, is as profound as it is wide, and it would be hard to imagine how different surgery would be without his influence, for better and for worse. His work and life also had some interesting features that resonate with our current interest and concept of palliative care. He did seminal work in the use of cocaine, which led not only to an increased understanding of the use of local anaesthesia but also was the agent of his own substance abuse disorder. He also suffered other forms of chronic pain, most notably pain due to common duct calculi from which he ultimately expired. This quasi-tragic figure metamorphosed from an advantaged, socially extroverted, ambitious young surgeon with a darkening future to a reclusive, relentless worker, always under the shadow of previous and possible future cocaine addiction, who managed to introduce one of the great ideas in the history of surgery, the concept of 'safe surgery'. The pillars of this safe surgery were atraumatic tissue handling and haemostasis, convenient metaphors for the gentleness and respect that characterize the best palliative care. His reclusive nature did not prevent him from demonstrating his concern for co-workers. Because of the skin-irritating effect of antiseptic solutions used by his scrub nurse (later to become his wife), he introduced the use of rubber gloves at the operating table. As in the other examples that are given, this gesture of concern for immediate distress had the unintended consequence of prolonging life by protecting both patient and surgeon from microbes.

In the current era of lumpectomy and sentinel node biopsy, we easily forget what prayers were answered in Halstead's time by his introduction of the radical mastectomy for the treatment of breast cancer, now seen as an outdated, draconian remedy. Not unlike his contemporary, Freud, who also indulged in risky self-experimentation, his lasting contribution lay much more in his clinical technique (atraumatic, haemostatic) and his mentoring than his specific theories regarding pathology. Another parallel between these two medical Prometheans has been the degree that their own distress provided them insight and direction in the relief of others. It could be argued that both of these men rarely cured a major, chronic illness but certainly left a bounty of means for us to adapt to them.

Another example of surgical innovation for the relief of severe symptoms with doubtful expectations of prolonging survival was the treatment of angina. Initially this was accomplished by indirect coronary revascularization by techniques such as omentopexy and talc poudrage introduced in the 1930s and 1940s. These procedures provided circulation and stimulated collateral capillary circulation: a support system for the heart's isolated, pained myocardium. This operation provides a metaphor that should be useful for those working in palliative care. These earlier procedures were replaced by direct surgery on the coronary vessels in the 1960s, made possible by improved techniques of myocardial preservation, including the heart bypass pump. As it turned out, these procedures *did* prolong survival and certainly contributed to the rising tide of technical operative and periopertive care innovation that also improved survival for all surgical patients. The same pattern could be observed in the development of cardiac valvular surgery. The poignant descriptions of children and young women with congenital and acquired valvular lesions presenting with cyanosis, dyspnoea, and cachexia give a hint of the stimulus that made surgeons try what was considered a desperate intervention: quite literally, a stab wound to the heart, to relieve the dyspnoea due to a completely obstructed mitral valve. Even with the limited survival following these earlier procedures, the dramatic relief of symptoms resuscitated hope enough to allow opportunities for subsequent more enduring success.

A final category of illness for which surgical innovation provided relief of symptoms long before life prolongation could be assumed was the treatment of organ failure by transplantation. Ironically, the first successful human kidney transplant owed some of its success to the fact that the immunological conditions were very close to what someday could be achieved by cloning: the donor was the identical twin of the recipient with whom a common placenta was shared at birth. The idea of organ transplant as a form of palliation may not readily come to mind because of the invasiveness of the procedure until one realizes that the transplanted state is not at this time a cure, but a long-term respite. Despite advances made in more selective immunosuppression, the recipient of an organ transplant replaces the more rapidly fatal disease of organ failure with the generally mild or asymptomatic chronic 'diseases' of immunosuppression and procedure-related sequelae and complications. However, transplantation has created a whole new category of chronic illness, chronic rejection, that has its own specific needs for palliative care. The transplanted patient is in more ways than one a chimera: the patient is both a 'cure' and a chronic disease.

An unanticipated but valuable contribution transplantation made to surgery was the degree of ethical insight and discourse that transplantation necessitated. Although many would not cavil about proceeding with a major resection for a neoplasm in a healthy patient or debate attempting the first ever correction of a previously untreated lethal vascular condition such as aortic coarctation, the ethical justification for a living donor nephrectomy or termination of life support in a potential organ donor might seem more precarious. Innovation was not only selecting out new characteristics in surgeons but also new ethical dilemmas. These new ethical questions addressed not only the rights of the patient but the social, spiritual, and economic right of others as well. As the age of genetic engineering is dawning, the experience surgeons and others have had in transplant-related ethical debate will increasingly show its importance.

The historical pattern of innovation in surgery has broadly demonstrated repeated dramatic attempts to respond to previously hopeless situations despite the slim promise of survival. It was the need to respond decisively to the immediate distress of overwhelming symptoms, disability, and hopelessness itself that was the driving factor for surgeons, which suggests that surgery was always a palliative calling even after the introduction of operations that actually saved or prolonged lives.

In addition to technical innovation surgeons have made literary and social contributions to palliative care. One of the most notable examples of this was J. Englebert Dunphey's 1976

Annual Oration to the Massachusetts Medical Society entitled 'On Caring for the Patient With Cancer'.[5] A revered surgeon and educator who had widely disseminated prostate cancer at the time of his oration, he concluded, 'Death holds no fearful threat. Living without life is Hell. Death is natural; it may be just; it is often easeful and merciful; it ought always to be dignified. Who knows, it may be Paradise.' At approximately the same time, another surgeon, Balfour Mount, who introduced the term 'palliative care', was among those introducing the hospice concept to North America. Another surgeon, J.M. Zimmerman, published a book in 1980 (early in the experience of the United States) entitled *Hospice – complete care for the terminally ill*.[6] A number of surgeons were among the early supporters, and in some cases providers, of hospice care in the United Kingdom and the United States.

Burn care: the ultimate surgical metaphor for palliative care

It is in burn care that surgeons have historically most clearly demonstrated their ability to address comprehensively the multidimensional nature of 'total pain' as described by Cicely Saunders.[7] Our capacity to feel, interpret, and respond to pain of all kinds is dependent upon our perceptual apparatus consisting of our neurological and immunological systems. Though the activity of this apparatus has a unique signature for each individual, it is the means of establishing each individual's connection and homeostasis with the external world and all who inhabit it. Few diseases demonstrate as broad and profound an impact upon the perceptual apparatus as a burn injury. This devastating injury provides the opportunity for profound insight into what palliative care means and what it asks of us. The necessity of the team approach and its gratifying results have been more evident in burn care than anywhere else in surgery except in the operating theatre where patient contact is far more brief and generally limited to physical interventions. One famous burn surgeon described the 'covenant' as opposed to a 'contract' that exists between the doctor and patient.[8] This kind of terminology reflects a level of shared experience one would expect in a setting which witnesses such intense suffering.

The burn injury and its treatment are compelling metaphors for the problem of suffering and our response to it. When the civilized world watched in horror at the persons jumping to their deaths from the inferno of the World Trade Center it is viscerally excruciating to imagine what they were fleeing from as well as what they were jumping to. A leitmotif of many popular illness narratives is the transformation of the self necessary to complete the individual's journey to wholeness, and nowhere is that more evident than in the process of re-epithelialization of the skin, recovery of function, and the restoration of spirit and purpose that is observable in burn patients.

Resuscitation of a patient with a major burn begins with a collective 'facing of the fire' followed swiftly by intravenous analgesia for pain relief, often administered before direct involvement of a physician. It could be further argued that survival itself would be far less likely without expert attention to pain control in these patients due to the detrimental effects of unopposed massive sympathetic nervous system activity due to untreated pain. How often do we see the order of priorities of relief of suffering and the promotion of survival reversed? As the burn patient comes into the scope of medical care, the rehabilitation begins even as early as performance of escharotomies to prevent later loss of function due to ischaemic nerve injury, though other compelling reasons exist for this simple surgical manoeuvre. I recall in vivid detail a young woman, massively burned, with a completely circumferential, full-thickness chest burn who was cyanosed and quite dyspnoeic for several reasons, one of which was the strangulating effect of the inelastic burned tissue squeezing her like a vice around her chest. Several quick cuts through the tissue allowing it to gap apart provided her instant relief, though tracheostomy was also necessary to lessen her dyspnoea from massive swelling in her upper airway prohibiting oro-tracheal or naso-tracheal intubation. It was obvious at the outset that her burn would be lethal within hours due to its size and the limitations of care at that time and place, but that fact did not lessen the need for surgical attention and skill in her last hours of need. Intravenous access, necessary for the provision of reliable analgesia as well as resuscitative fluids, required the skill of a surgeon or at least an individual capable of establishing deep venous access through toughened, burned tissue in a writhing, moaning patient. Following these interventions, she became more peaceful and lapsed into coma and succumbed several hours later. Without the added distraction and burden of uncontrolled physical suffering, her family and attendants were better prepared for the impending loss of this person's life and potential future spiritual repercussions related to a death in needless agony.

The surgical character and the problem of suffering

Although history may demonstrate that surgeons have been invaluable contributors to the relief of suffering based on their propensity to act decisively and invasively, did this require callousness or a deliberate suppression of sensitivity? The stereotype of the calloused, lout-like surgeon seems simplistic given the evidence of cultivated sensitivity in many of the most well-known surgeons. Halstead's sensitivity has already been acknowledged. Harvey Cushing, who provided much of the foundation of neurological surgery, wrote a Pulitzer Prize-winning book about a fellow physician, Sir William Osler. Cushing was also a very accomplished draughtsman. Billroth's friendship with Brahms, which was based in part on his interest in music, has also been noted. Not only does every surgeon find his own equilibrium of reflection and action, but also every era of surgery finds its balance between these poles. In the nineteenth century, life and disease were even more brutish and short than in the present. Then, the quick and decisive response to acute and fulminant disease may have been more adaptive than the more reflective and deliberate response needed now to address complex chronic illness.

Joan Cassell notes in her anthropological study of surgeons, *Expected miracles*, '... the surgical ethos stresses decisiveness, control, confidence, and certitude, and that these characteristics are selected for in surgical training programs and reinforced during that training ... these are necessary, that a person who is insufficiently decisive, certain, and in control is likely to make a poor surgeon.'[9] The benefit of this ethos is clear when confronting a well-defined enemy or problem, but what about more ambiguous situations or situations where the emphasis on control and the need for certainty can be counter-productive? There are three possible responses by the surgeon:

1 leave the problem to someone else;
2 solve the problem decisively as it is defined by the surgeon; or
3 allow redefinition of the problem in league with others and then solve it decisively.

Surgeons are frequently compared to test pilots, warriors, and athletes, all of whom would agree that hesitation is loss. The third option requires an 'interior distancing', the capacity to gain perspective on a problem yet unsolved in the face of strong emotion such as fear or anger. Although the capacity of interior distancing and skilled communication prerequisite for palliative care are not readily accomplished by surgeons working long hours attempting to meet excessive external expectations (patients, colleagues, plaintiff attorneys, and payers), the more profound impediment may be the fear of introspection, not unlike the tight-rope walker who dares not look down at his feet for fear of losing his balance.

The image of the surgeon as the emotionally and socially detached individual with a high degree of over-external events is the ultimate human expression of the classic scientific model that has evolved since the time of Descartes, who among other things was a student of anatomy, the basic science historically most dear to surgeons. For Descartes, mechanics was the basis of his medicine, or physiology, which in turn was the basis of his moral psychology. Descartes believed that all material bodies, including the human body, are machines that operate by mechanical principles. In his physiological studies, he pioneered vivisection with the dissection of animal bodies to show how their parts move. He argued that because animals have no souls, they do not think or feel, thus justifying vivisection.

The unfortunate result of this vision of science has been the deconstruction of suffering where only physical pain is real. Other manifestations of this view are:

1 the devaluation of the non-physical components of personhood;

2 over-reliance on what is referred to as 'objective' data (x-rays, electrocardiograms, etc.) coupled with scepticism towards subjective data provided by the patient;

3 limitation of the surgeon's interest to the patient's body, body part, or body molecules.[10]

The metabolic response to surgery,[11] a landmark book written in 1952 by the esteemed surgeon and educator Francis D. Moore, is representative of the increasingly scientific domination science had over surgery after the Second World War, offering an orientation that made it possible to conjure up a patient dying in 'perfect electrolyte balance'. His initial studies demonstrated the distribution of ions in the various body compartments by the use of radioactive tracers. Of great interest in light of the impact burns care has had on the development of palliative philosophy was the fact that much of the impetus for Moore's work with fluid and electrolytes was the result of his work with victims of the Coconut Grove fire in 1942 in which several hundred perished. Even now in Boston, USA there are still a few surgeons living who recall the overwhelming challenge that fire posed that evening. Little did they realize that what they learned from this catastrophe would later save countless lives from physical demise, but at the cost of reinforcing a conceptual framework that would later blind surgeons and physicians to non-physical forms of distress and demise.

Surgeons have always been proud of the ironic relationship between war, catastrophe, and surgery. Both catastrophe and war have always been boons to surgical innovation no matter what the motives for the war or the surgery. My father, a surgeon who served in the European Theatre during World War II, recalls how astonished he and others were when they saw a steel hip fixation nail, discovered on an x-ray of a wounded Wehrmacht soldier. Nothing comparable had been done by the better-resourced Allies. In this case, desperation was the mother of innovation. For the purpose of continued capacity for war-making, not relief of individual suffering, a new orthopaedic technique had a trial sooner than may have occurred in the absence of war. Since then operative fixation of fractures has offered thousands a speedy and durable remedy for fractures. The surgeon's tendency to fight rather than lament has led them to find in war exactly what the palliative care practitioner searches for in peace: a blessing (*ex malo bonum*).

The advent of the quantum model of physics has provided a new opportunity (or crisis) to surgeons who have limited their vision to the classical scientific model. The derivative language of quantum physics – 'continuum', 'space-time', 'energy field' – poses a conceptual and psychological challenge to those who require the maintenance of boundaries between patient and surgeon, individual and society, disease and nature, organ and body, body and mind. For those working in palliative care it may be helpful to understand that the surgeon typically is more at home with the earlier Cartesian world view, while the more recent quantum perspective may be more evident in the non-surgical members (social workers, chaplains) of the interdisciplinary team.

In order to remain unflappable in the face of a patient's anguish, distancing behaviours by surgeons are not unexpected whether in their interaction with their patients or their own inner feelings. Often patients themselves will be apologetic for the brusque, aloof surgeon, explaining, 'They have to be that way in order to do what they have to do' or 'They got that way because of what they have to do.' Examples of this type of behaviour include bypassing the terminally ill patient on rounds and moving along quickly to the next patient, and 'signing off' a case even when it is obvious that the patient's trust in the surgeon may be the only indication of the patient's sustained hope. Krizek[12] describes this distancing behaviour as a 'psychological death' that protects [surgeons] in dealing with suffering and death. The result of this form of 'death' hampers the surgeon's capacity to be an effective care-giver when the demands are palliation rather than cure. The popular television series, *MASH*, showed the world, accurately, the importance of humour even in the operating room as an alternative adjustment.

'Captain of the ship': is it the right metaphor for the palliating surgeon?

Both the interdisciplinary model of care and patient-defined success criteria, central principles to palliative care, challenge the surgeon's historical notion of authority. The concept of 'captain of the ship' is deeply entrenched in the social, legal, and ethical experience of surgeons and has only more recently been challenged on the basis of individual autonomy, whether referring to the patient or other non-surgeons entrusted with the patient's care. The images of authority and isolation implicit in this metaphor suggest two potential barriers to helpful participation by surgeons in the interdisciplinary model of palliative care.

The ascent to a position of authority in surgery is a very steep one and is referred to as the 'pyramid' system of surgical training. It developed in the late nineteenth century in Germany, Great Britain, United States, and other countries in their leading surgical centres. In this system, the surgeon in training is granted progressively more responsibility and authority in exchange for demonstrated competence and reliability. This ascendency culminates in the ultimate responsibility and recognition: operating unsupervised. Completion of this ascendency results in the surgeon's exaggerated sense of personal responsibility for outcomes even when an outcome is predetermined. Bosk noted in his landmark anthropological study of surgeons, *Forgive and remember*, the question asked of a surgeon by surgical colleagues following the death of a patient reveals this sense of complete accountability for a patient's outcome: 'What did you (or didn't you) do?' Other members of the medical profession, he adds, typically ask, 'What happened?'[13]

Mortality and morbidity rounds ('M and M' rounds) are an important part of the surgical apprenticeship and one of the central rituals of surgical culture. In these gatherings where the wisest (usually the oldest!) speak last, disclosure is given to the assembly of surgeons about mortality and complications following surgical procedures and admissions. Typically, a resident or intern will present the case in question followed by commentary or explanations by the patient's attending surgeon. Usually, representatives of other disciplines such as radiology or pathology are present for their portion of the presentations. The case presentation is followed by questions and comments that run the spectrum of censure to forgiveness. Occasionally, approval and even a heightened respect may result from this ceremony.

Many reputations are made and lost in these sessions, role models are demonstrated, invaluable information is passed on, and the opportunities are given for the sense of belonging so critical to counterbalance the dangerous impulse the surgeon may have to act in isolation. A potential barrier to the success of the interdisciplinary approach that best exemplifies palliative care is the continuous reinforcement of the 'captain of the ship' standard of conduct in the context of disease-directed treatment that still occurs in the surgical mortality and morbidity ceremony.

Redefining surgical success in advanced illness

Although the loftiest goal of the mortality and morbidity conference is improved patient care, the measure of success up until now has been physical survival and morbidity. Recently there has been increased recognition of the importance of other parameters of 'success' in the surgical literature,[14] though measurement of these parameters has been both inconsistent and incomplete[15] and remains the work of the future. In a symposium given at the 2001 Clinical Congress of the American College of Surgeons (ACS), 'Palliative Care by the Surgeon: how to do it', revision of the mortality and morbidity institution to reflect quality-of-life outcomes was identified as a prerequisite to improving surgical palliative care.[16] If improved patient comfort or satisfaction is to become the new standard of success, then consistent outcome measurement of these goals will be necessary to harness the potential power of the mortality and morbidity conference.

Cassel[17] pointed out that the salient feature of the surgical character has been *decisiveness*, an 'action-oriented' approach to problem solving in contradistinction to a reflective and contemplative response. Many surgeons would agree that the most significant problem they are called upon to solve is the rescue of patients from life-threatening disease. However, it was not until the past century that this expectation was routinely realized, and when it was, the technical and cognitive skill required was rudimentary when compared to many procedures routinely performed today. What hasn't changed over the several centuries of identifiable surgical specialization is the decisiveness of the surgeon's response to 'the enemy', but perhaps the nature of 'the enemy' has.

Mismatched perceptions by the surgeon, the patient, and other involved parties of what 'the enemy' is becomes more likely when quality of life, a multidimensional concept, and not survival is the barometer of success. These mismatches created much of the gulf of distrust between surgeons and their patients as well as surgeons and their colleagues. An example of this trap a consulting surgeon may fall prey to is a request to perform an amputation for gangrene from advanced systemic vascular disease suffering multiple co-morbidities. If the surgeons are dependent on referrals, they may be more likely to yield to the rationale that the disease and not the distress is sufficient justification for recommending operation. The surgeon may not be aware of alternative choices of management in this scenario such as the use of communication as a procedure and pharmacotherapy for the relief of pain. In a survey of oncologic surgeons presented at the ACS 2001 Clinical Congress'[18] fear of taking away hope was identified as the biggest barrier to offering palliative surgery. Occasionally I have seen surgeons reluctantly perform operations they felt were 'futile' based on their own experience with outcomes and their intuitive sense that the operation would somehow 'miss the mark' for other reasons.

An example of this was a patient I recently saw who underwent laparotomy and colectomy for a carcinoma of the colon with diffuse liver metastases identified during preoperative staging. This patient had no symptoms referable to his primary site of disease but he presented with right upper quadrant pain due to stretching of the hepatic capsule from secondary disease – a symptom normally quite responsive to pharmacotherapy. The purpose of the resection was 'to prevent problems in the future', though the 'future' had never been discussed by the surgeon since 'that was the oncologist's job'. The consulting oncologist completed the vicious circle by deferring discussion about prognosis to the surgeon since 'he would be in the best position to know once the operation was done'. Four days after the operation the patient developed a large wound dehiscence requiring operative closure. His abdominal dehiscence, only partly closed, stood as a vivid metaphor for the lack of closure during his last days as precious time, energy, and resources were diverted to its care.

In this instance, the surgeon had succeeded in creating an enormous physical distraction from all other aspects of the illness. The temptation to surgeons to create these distractions exists in other settings of advanced illness, especially if the emotionally charged issues of nutrition and hydration are at stake. A study of 1446 physicians and nurses found that 45% of the surgical attending physicians who responded, as opposed to 34% of the medical attending physicians, believed that even if all forms of function support are stopped, nutrition and hydration should always be continued.[19] Given the opportunity and the means to redefine 'success', the surgeon, the patient, and others entrusted with the patient's care can avoid the trap of performing 'reasonable' operations without a good reason.

The interdisciplinary team engaging surgical expertise must be aware of the reasons, conscious and unconscious, why a surgeon may recommend an operative procedure. Sometimes the rationale is based on the surgeon's own fear of addressing the latent issues related to the patient's (and their own) vulnerability and mortality, sometimes it is based on misinformation or lack of information concerning effective non-operative approaches for symptom management such as medical management of malignant bowel obstruction, and sometimes the surgeon's rationale is based on sound communication with the patient and experience with the utility of the procedure for the problem identified.

The tenets of palliative or supportive care do not identify disease or death as adversaries. This deeply challenges the surgeon's traditional conceptualization of 'success' (conquering the disease) and 'failure' (disease conquering the patient). As one well-known and respected surgeon reflecting on the surgeon's suitability for providing palliative care put it, '. . . no surgeon or nurse would work in a burn unit that treated only lethal burns.'[20] Despite this belief, surgeons are routinely involved in the care of patients who routinely die of their disease, whether from an advanced lung cancer or massive head injury. It has been the ability to save or prolong lives, such as repair of congenital cardiac defects or resuscitation of gunshot wound victims, that has provided surgeons their most visible acclaim. One is much less likely to hear about the quiet accomplishments of pain relief or restored psychological function. By redefining success, the traditional notions of surgical authority and responsibility will also need to be redefined.

At this time the vast amount of data that has accumulated about operative interventions that purposefully or inadvertently served palliative purposes has not provided much direction for surgeons or anyone else beyond matters of operative technique because outcome has been defined by length of survival and presence of morbidity. Identifying successful palliation by surgical means has been confounded by conflicting definitions of 'palliative' in the surgical literature. Easson[21] identified three definitions of palliative surgery in the surgical literature:

1 surgery to relieve symptoms, knowing in advance that all of the tumour left *in situ* could not be removed;
2 resection with microscopic or gross residual tumour left *in situ* at the end of the procedure;
3 resection for recurrent or persistent disease after primary treatment failure.

Only one of these definitions, the first one, addresses symptoms which, by definition, are relevant to the patient. The others are framed in terms of disease control (or lack of it) which can only be assumed to be relevant to the patient. Success in symptom control affirms the fact that true contact has been made with the individual – that the signal transmitted by the individual's perceptual apparatus has been heard and responded to.

Until quite recently there has been very little written specifically about the role of surgery and even less about the role of the surgeon working within the paradigm of palliative care as it has evolved in the United Kingdom since Palliative Medicine was accorded speciality status in 1987. In the 1998 edition of the *Oxford Textbook of Palliative Medicine*, surgical palliation is discussed in terms of five essential roles the surgeon has in the palliation of advanced cancer.[22] These roles include:

1 the initial evaluation of the disease;
2 local control of the disease;
3 control of discharge and haemorrhage;
4 control of pain;
5 reconstruction and rehabilitation.

Palliative surgery is not limited to the surgical management of stage IV oncologic disease but it is the intervention by surgeons and surgery for the relief of problems associated with all incurable illness. Staging advanced illness for purposes of palliation is different than disease staging since it must incorporate non-physical dimensions to comprehend the meaning of the illness. New success criteria for palliative surgical care when compared to traditional standards of success might look like this:

Pathocentric model	*Palliative model*
Diagnosis and staging of disease	Characterization and staging of illness
Eradication or control of disease	Eradication or control of suffering
Increased physical survival	Survival or reintegration of personhood regardless of physical status. Improved survival secondary to control of suffering
Minimal physical morbidity	Minimal distress, whether related to physical or non-physical complications
Restored or improved physical function	All functional realms (physical, psychological, social, and spiritual) protected, restored, or improved if possible
Improved patient outcome	Improved patient/family/care-giver outcome

Redefining surgical ethics in advanced illness

It is impossible for surgeons to redefine success and failure without stirring their ethical concerns since ethical (normative) errors are one of the two categories of error acknowledged by surgeons,[23] the other being technical error. A potential barrier to surgeons accepting the philosophy of palliative care is their deeply held belief that not 'fighting' disease is a form of abandonment, which is not only the deepest fear of patients but also the most unforgiveable of sins in surgical culture.

Elsewhere in this volume it will be argued that surgical palliative care is totally consistent with traditional medical ethics encompassing all domains of medical care. Recently, a surgeon, based on his experience as a surgeon and as a patient, proposed a distinctively surgical ethic[24] that clearly demonstrates the fundamental compatibility of current palliative philosophy with an ethical framework unique to surgeons and surgical experiences. The language he uses to identify five categories within the moral domain of the surgeon – patient relationship resonates with that from patient testimony and anecdote so familiar to palliative care. Rescue, proximity (similar to intimacy in describing the surgeon's closeness to the patient), ordeal, and aftermath are the first four of these categories reflecting the ethical, the relational, the existential, and the experiential. These describe the patient's experience while the fifth category, *presence*, is the surgeon's ethical response to these experiences.

In the context of Little's surgical ethic, it is difficult to ignore the potential value of a relationship between surgeon and patient in any advanced illness. The surgeon's presence, which demonstrates their response to the experience shared with their patient, so obviously necessary at the operating table is equally necessary at the other table, the interdisciplinary team conference table, since the surgeon's proximity to the patient brings a perspective no one else could duplicate. In spite of the aloofness of the surgeon and the scepticism of non-surgeons, surgery and surgeons are not only needed in palliative care but represent one of its most heroic and positive expressions of this noble idea. In reciprocating, surgery and surgeons have always been and always will be rejuvenated and redeemed by the call to arms against all forms of suffering.

References

1. McCahill, L.E., Krouse, R.S., Chu, D.Z.J., Juarez, G., Uman, G.C., Ferrell, B.R., *et al.* (2002). Indications and utilization of palliative surgery: results of Society of Surgical Oncology survey. *Ann. Surg. Oncol.*, **9** (1).

2. Nuland, S.B. (1997). *How we die: reflections on life's final chapter.* Alfred A. Knopf, New York.

3. Nuland, S.B. (1998). The past is prologue: surgeons then and now. *J.A.M.A.*, **186** (4), 457–65.

4. Ellis, H. (2001). *A history of surgery*, p. 104. Greenwich Medical Media, Inc., London.

5. Dunphey, J.E. (1976). Annual discourse: On caring for the patient with cancer. *N. Engl. J. Med.*, **295**, 313–19.

6. Zimmerman, J.M. (1981). *Hospice – complete care for the terminally ill.* Urban and Schwarzenberg, Baltimore.

7. Saunders, C., and Sykes, N. (1993). *The management of terminal malignant disease* (3rd edn). Edward Arnold, London.

8. Regier, H. (1998). *Family divided in requests for father's terminal care.* 1997 Clinical Congress of the American College of Surgeons. *Gen. Surg. News*, June.

9. Cassell, J. (1991). *Expected miracles. Surgeons at work*, p. 37. Temple University Press, Philadelphia.

10. Storey, P., and Knight, C. (1997). *Alleviating psychological and spiritual pain in the terminally ill*, p. 11. UNIPAC Two. American College of Hospice and Palliative Medicine, Gainesville, Florida.

11. Moore, F.D., and Ball, M.R. (1952). *The metabolic response to surgery*, pp. 1–156. Thomas, Springfield, Illinois.

12. Krizek, T. (2001). Spiritual dimensions of surgical palliative care. *Surg. Oncol. Clin. North Am.*, **10** 1(1), 45–6.

13. Bosk, C. (1979). *Forgive and remember: managing medical failure*, pp. 29–30. University of Chicago Press, Chicago.

14. Wood-Dauphinee, S. (1996). Quality of life assessment: recent trends in surgery. *Can. J. Surg.*, **36**, 368–72.

15. Velanovich, V. (2001). Quality of life studies in general surgical journals. *J. Am. Coll. Surg.*, **193** (3), 288–96.

16. Dunn, G.P., Milch, R.A., Mosenthal, A.C., Lee, K.F., Easson, A.M., and Huffman, J.L. (2002). Palliative care by the surgeon: how to do it. *J. Am. Coll. Surg.*, **194** (4), 508–37.

17. Cassell, J. (1991). *Expected miracles. Surgeons at work*, p. 35. Temple University Press, Philadelphia.

18. McCahill, L.E., Krouse, R.S., Chu, D.Z.J., Juarez, G., Uman, G.C., Ferrell, B.R., *et al. Decision making in palliative surgery*. Paper presentation at the 87th Clinical Congress of the American College of Surgeons, 9 October 2001.

19. Solomon, M.Z., O'Donnell, L., Jennings, B., Guilfoy, V., Wolf, S.M., Nolan, K., *et al.* (1993). Decisions near the end of life: professional views on life sustaining treatments. *Am. J. Pub. Hlth*, **83**, 14–23.

20. Krizek, T. (2001). Spiritual dimensions of surgical palliative care. *Surg. Oncol. Clin. N. Am.*, **10** (1), 54.

21. Easson, A.M. (2001). Palliative general surgical procedures. *Surg. Oncol. Clin. N. Am.*, **10** (1), 161.

22. Ball, A.B.S., Baum, M., Breach, N.M., Shepherd, J.H., Shearer, J., Thomas, J.M., *et al.* (1998). Surgical palliation. In: *Oxford textbook of palliative medicine* (3rd edn) (ed. D. Doyle, G.W.C. Hanks, and N. MacDonald), pp. 282–4. Oxford University Press, Oxford.

23. Bosk, C. (1979). *Forgive and remember: managing medical failure*, pp. 36–70. University of Chicago Press, Chicago.

24. Little, M. (2001). Invited commentary: Is there a distinctively surgical ethic? *Surgery*, **129** (6), 668–71.

Chapter 2

Selection and preparation of patients for surgical palliation

Alexander Ng and Alexandra M. Easson

Introduction

I will keep 'the sick' from harm.

Hippocrates[1]

The decision to offer any surgical procedure to a patient must balance the potential benefits of the expected outcome of the intervention with the inevitable risks of pain and complications. This is particularly important for the patient who is suffering from a terminal illness. For the surgeon, trained to intervene, a decision to operate is often the easiest one to make. The true skill of the surgeon as physician, however, lies in the careful selection and preparation of those patients who will benefit from a surgical procedure, as well as a continued commitment to the care of patients for whom surgery is not selected. The question that must be answered is not 'Can this operation be done?', rather 'Should this operation be done for this patient at this time?'

Palliation means 'affording relief, not cure . . . to reduce the severity of'.[2] Palliative surgery may therefore be defined as 'procedures where the major goal is the relief of symptoms and suffering, not the prolongation of life, for patients for whom there is no chance of cure'.[3] Surgical interventions may be used to treat a wide variety of symptoms which may occur as part of the natural course of an eventually terminal disease (Box 2.1). These can be broadly described as:

1 palliative, in which the goal of the intervention is the relief of symptoms;
2 supportive, in which the procedure is a technical intervention done as part of a multidisciplinary treatment plan.[3]

Palliative procedures may be beneficial for terminal patients where death may be imminent, but the definition also includes patients with, chronic disease where death may be months or years away. Like conventional surgery, palliative surgery encompasses a wide spectrum of procedures, all with differing levels of invasiveness, requirements for anaesthesia, inherent technical difficulty, and attendant risks. While the final decision to proceed with a palliative surgical procedure must be individualized to each patient, a careful process of selection and preparation will assist in surgical decision making and maximise the number of patients who will benefit from an improvement in quality of life and low procedural morbidity.

Box 2.1 Examples of palliative surgical procedures

Palliative *(intervention as treatment)*

- Drainage of effusions (ascites, pleural, pericardial):
  - percutaneous drainage
  - peritoneal or pleural catheters +/− sclerotherapy
  - open drainage: pericardial window, pleural decortication
- Relief of obstruction (respiratory, gastrointestinal, biliary, vascular, urologic):
  - placement of stents (percutaneous, endoscopic)
  - surgical bypass
  - tumour resection
- Control of fistulas (tracheo-oesophageal, intestinal, perineal)
- Control of bleeding (stomach, rectum, bladder, kidney, gynaecological):
  - tumour resection
  - tumour embolization
- Control of pain:
  - coeliac plexus block, thorascopic splanchnicectomy

Supportive *(part of a treatment plan)*

- Tissue sampling
- Vascular access
- Enteral nutritional support

Selection of patients

An approach to the selection of patients who will benefit from palliative surgery considers the following:

- disease factors, which requires knowledge of the diagnosis and natural history of the disease, including expected preterminal and terminal symptoms specific to the disease
- patient factors, which includes an understanding of the patient's prognosis and medical status, and also the patient's personality, expectations, and social supports
- technical factors, which requires knowledge of the full spectrum of available modalities, surgical as well as non-surgical, and their level of invasiveness, effectiveness, and potential morbidity
- societal factors, which considers the cultural, ethical, legal, and economic context.

For the purposes of this discussion, the terminal cancer patient is the main emphasis, but similar principles may be applied to any patient with advanced incurable disease.

Disease factors

A rational consideration of the benefits and timing of a surgical intervention requires an understanding of the patient's underlying terminal disease. In particular, knowledge of its natural history, its treatment, and the symptoms it produces will assist in deciding the most appropriate method of palliation.

Natural history

An understanding of the time course of the patient's disease, as well as how it is altered by anti-disease therapy, is essential. Patients with cancers known to follow an aggressive course may not benefit from radical surgery because the attendant morbidity may worsen the quality of the remaining life. Anaplastic thyroid cancer, for example, causes death in most patients within four to five months of diagnosis due to mechanical upper airway obstruction.[4] While resection is often technically feasible at presentation, the disease's natural history is not altered by aggressive surgical or other therapy. In contrast, aggressive local resection of metastatic medullary thyroid cancer, also a terminal disease, may result in effective and long-term palliation.[5] Surgical decision making is more difficult when the underlying diagnosis is unknown and the tendency is to offer aggressive therapy.

Knowledge of the natural history of the disease may also allow the anticipation of expected disease complications, leading to earlier and potentially less morbid surgical palliation. Operative morbidity and mortality rates are significantly higher after emergency rather than elective procedures.[6] Colonic resection in metastatic colorectal cancer, for example, is often offered to patients with obstructive symptoms to prevent acute obstruction, while recognizing that this will not alter the progression of disease.

Advances in medical therapy may significantly alter the natural history of the disease. The dramatic improvement in survival and performance status for Acquired Immune Deficiency Syndrome (AIDS) patients with the use of retroviral medication is a recent example. Palliative surgical procedures may now be contemplated where it was not rational to do so in the past. Surgeons must keep aware of such advances in therapy.

Local and regional symptoms

Locally advanced, recurrent or metastatic tumours can cause a number of local and regional symptoms, which may be palliated by a surgical procedure (Box 2.1). These include effusions, uncontrolled tumour growth, obstruction of vital structures, bleeding, and pain.

Effusions The accumulation of fluid in the abdomen, pleural space, or pericardium is common in terminal patients with and without malignancy. In the palliative setting, surgical drainage is not necessary unless it causes significant symptoms that are relieved by drainage of the fluid. Fluid compression of nearby organs may cause shortness of breath, pain, and in the abdomen, ascites, early satiety, abdominal distention, and decreased mobility. Pericardial effusions may be acutely life threatening.

Percutaneous fluid drainage is the simplest intervention, and offers rapid but temporary relief as the effusion will recur unless the underlying cause is treated. More definitive surgical procedures vary in their degree of invasiveness. An external drainage catheter with or without a sclerosing agent is commonly used for pleural and pericardial effusions,[7–9] and may be used (without sclerosis) for malignant ascites.[10] Internal drainage shunts are also described,[11,12] but are infrequently used in malignant ascites due to high complication rates.[13] Thorascopic or open drainage with decortication, pericardiectomy, or creation of a pericardial window are effective but require general anaesthesia. The degree of invasiveness chosen is determined by the severity of the symptoms, the underlying disease, and the patient's condition.

Uncontrolled soft tissue tumour growth Locally advanced primary or metastatic soft tissue tumours may result in difficult wound problems because of pain, ulceration, or fistula formation causing odour, discharge, or bleeding. Social interactions may be affected because the symptoms are often apparent. Examples include fungating and ulcerating breast tumours, eroding head and neck tumours, enterocutaneous and perineal fistulas draining bile, stool, or urine, and bulky axillary or inguinal nodes causing progressive lymphoedema. Surgical resection, with or without radiation therapy, may result in significantly improved quality of life. Radical resection with extensive reconstruction is usually not indicated. Consideration for surgery should balance the magnitude of the required procedure against the potential morbidity.

Obstruction Mechanical obstruction of an organ or viscus is common in palliative patients. Extrinsic compression or intrinsic tumour growth may obstruct the respiratory, gastrointestinal, biliary, vascular, and urologic systems partially or completely, acutely or chronically. Recognition of the symptoms of impending obstruction may prevent an acute life-threatening event. Knowledge of the disease's natural history may predict the risk of obstruction, and preventative measures may be indicated, as in the case of impending duodenal obstruction from pancreatic carcinoma.[14] Relief from obstruction may allow many months of symptom-free survival and is most successful when there is a single rather than multiple sites of obstruction.

The resultant symptoms depend on the site of obstruction and the organ involved. It is important to note however that these symptoms may require confirmation of the obstructive aetiology. For example, bronchial obstruction is only one of many causes of shortness of breath. The anatomic location and mechanism of the obstruction must be identified and treated only if it contributes to the symptom. A number of investigative modalities are available to achieve this and include radiological imaging (angiography, fluoroscopy, ultrasound, or computed tomography [CT] scanning), and endoscopy, which may also be therapeutic.

A variety of procedures may be used to relieve obstructive symptoms.[3] Local ablative techniques using laser, electrocautery, cryotherapy, or photodynamic therapy are available for easily accessed areas such as the trachea and rectum. Percutaneous gastric, biliary, or urinary drains may effectively decompress obstructed viscera, but require the additional care of an external drainage catheter. Endoscopic and fluoroscopic placement of stents through an obstructed lumen may also provide effective relief. Such internal stents, long used in the biliary tree, oesophagus, bronchus, and ureters, are now available for the stomach, duodenum, colorectum, and major blood vessels. More invasive management includes surgical bypass and/or tumour resection, by either minimally invasive or open techniques. These often provide the best long-term relief of obstruction, but require a general anaesthetic and are accompanied by the attendant risk of morbidity and mortality.

Bleeding Tumour haemorrhage can present acutely or chronically in a variety of malignancies. Treatment options range from transfusion for symptomatic relief to active intervention for more severe and/or acute haemorrhage: these include local fulguration, arterial embolization, and palliative resection.

Pain Pain is the most feared and one of the commonest symptoms in cancer patients, regardless of the tumour site.[15] Often undertreated, cancer pain requires prompt recognition, treatment, and referral to a pain service when appropriate. Postoperative pain must be effectively treated as a part of the operative care of the patient. Neuropathic pain secondary to tumour or to surgical procedures, such as post-thoracotomy or phantom limb pain, are treated by early pharmacological intervention.[16] Neurolytic coeliac plexus blockade has been shown to prevent or significantly relieve severe pain in 70–90% of patients with pancreatic cancer and should be considered for all patients whose tumours are considered incurable.[17,18] Tumour resection may be considered if the mechanism of the pain is such that this is felt to be beneficial.

Systemic symptoms

Asthenia, anorexia, and cachexia are common systemic symptoms which occur in many illnesses. Although reversible by successful treatment of the underlying disease, they are generally considered preterminal symptoms in palliative patients due to progression of disease. Asthenia is characterized by generalized weakness and profound physical and mental fatigue. Asthenia and anorexia were found in 90% and 85%, respectively, of patients admitted to a palliative care unit.[19] Cachexia is a catabolic process seen in many advanced illnesses, including end-stage organ failure (cardiac, lung, renal, and liver), AIDS, and lung and gastrointestinal cancer. Its effects are patient dependent, varying even among patients with similar tumour types and size. While anorexia-induced malnutrition is a factor in this condition, the weight loss and muscle wasting in cachexia is a result of a complex metabolic change different from simple starvation. When a healthy person is deprived of food, the body's metabolism slows to conserve energy and reduce protein breakdown. In cachectic patients, the catabolic process continues at a progressive rate, actively breaking down glucose and protein, particularly skeletal muscle, with reduced protein and fat synthesis.[20] Metabolic studies have suggested a number of responsible factors, including cytokines, neurotransmitters and acute phase proteins, tumour or disease products, and hormonal changes. Asthenia, anorexia, and cachexia are interrelated processes and all may contribute to the weakness and weight loss seen with advanced illness.

Patients with these symptoms have significantly higher complication and mortality rates after surgical intervention. Decreased mobility from asthenia results in increased postoperative pulmonary complications. Anorexia leads to decreased oral intake, and the resultant malnutrition affects healing and immune function. If cachexia is present, the anabolism required for healing and immune function is further impaired. The presence of these symptoms has a profound impact on the choice of surgical intervention.

Patient Factors (Box 2.2)

Medical factors

As with any operation, the patient's overall medical and physical status is an important consideration when deciding on the magnitude of the intervention and the patient's operative risk. Operative morbidity and mortality are those events occurring within 30 days of a procedure. In palliative patients the patient's disease process is the major determinant of operative mortality.

Prognosis An assessment of prognosis is essential to determine a risk–benefit ratio for the proposed surgical intervention, or whether the anticipated benefits of the intervention are worth the risks. It is often helpful to discuss the anticipated disease course with the primary physician caring for the patient, wanting especially to know about a history of previous response to and future eligibility for anti-disease therapy.

Studies of the ability to predict prognosis have yielded mixed results. A prospective study found that clinicians estimated prognosis quite accurately when asked whether or not a patient with terminal cancer was expected to live six months.[21] In another study of terminal cancer patients, however, treating physicians tended to overestimate the survival of patients, and in particular failed to predict those who died early (within two months).[22] Several clinical prognostic indices have been

Box 2.2 Patient factors

Medical factors

- Prognosis
- Age: biological, physiological
- Performance status
- Co-morbidities: cardiac, respiratory, hepatic, renal, diabetes, psychiatric
- Concurrent illness: sepsis, anaemia, metabolic abnormalities
- Malnutrition and/or cachexia

Psychosocial

- The patient:
  - knowledge of disease, natural history, and prognosis
  - expectations of treatment
  - values and beliefs
  - attitude towards their own mortality
  - personality and past experience
- Family and friends:
  - relationship to the patient
  - cultural/religious beliefs
- Social:
  - finances
  - community support

developed for terminal patients which combine objective clinical criteria such as weight loss and performance status (patient function) with clinician estimates.[23–26] The simplest and best known performance status scale is the Karnofsky Performance Scale, as it has been widely used in the selection of patients for medical oncology trials.[27,28] Objective clinical criteria perform as well (or as poorly) as clinician estimates.[26,29] The Study to Understand Prognoses and Preferences for Outcomes and Risks of Treatment (SUPPORT) found that recommended clinical prediction criteria were not effective in identifying patients with a survival prognosis of six months or less in seriously ill hospitalized patients with advanced chronic obstructive pulmonary disease, congestive heart failure, or end-stage liver disease.[30] A meta-analysis of 24 studies found a small association between clinicians' estimation of survival and actual survival.[29] Other less well defined factors also impact on prognosis. Extent of disease and quality of life together predicted survival better than each parameter alone in patients with breast cancer.[31] Symptom distress alone predicted survival in lung cancer patients.[32] Patients with a low quality of life score were more likely to die within six months than those with higher scores, but low scores were not strong predictors of survival in individual patients.[33] Clinician predictions and objective indices of prognosis should be considered as only one of many criteria by which to choose therapeutic interventions.

An early example of a surgical prognostic index was the Child – Turcotte classification of portal hypertension.[34] It used five clinical and laboratory values to categorize patients prior to undergoing surgery for portal hypertension by a portosystemic shunt. Widely used, it proved to reliably estimate early preoperative mortality.[35] No similar index has been developed for the risk of surgical morbidity and mortality in advanced cancer patients. Difficulty in predicting time to death makes an assessment of the risk – benefit ratio of a procedure more difficult and a clearer understanding of the actual operative risk for patients with advanced disease is necessary. In cases where the prognosis is unknown, the approach is generally to attempt intervention to 'give the patient the benefit of the doubt', recognizing the generally poor ability of the clinician to predict the future. Most often, the assessment of prognosis comes down to a 'gut' feeling in the clinician, guided by the patient's performance status and appearance, and clinical experience.

Other As with any intervention, the patient's preoperative general health status will influence the choice of procedure. Factors known to increase operative risk include: increased age; the presence of underlying cardiac,[36] renal, hepatic, and respiratory disease;[37] performance status; and concurrent illness, such as sepsis, anaemia, and uncontrolled metabolic abnormalities. The presence of ascites increases the operative risk for open abdominal operations.[38] Operative risk is always increased if the procedure is done as an emergency procedure.[6] A preoperative assessment using the American Society of Anesthesiologists (ASA) Classification of Physical Status correlates well with postoperative mortality.[39]

Psychosocial factors

Since the goals of the procedure are the relief of suffering and improvement in quality of life, the patient's own perceptions and wishes are perhaps the most crucial determinants in procedure selection. A surgical intervention is generally proposed to address a specific symptom, often one among many that the patient is experiencing. It is particularly important in this population to understand how the procedure will relate to the patient as a whole and unique individual. Patient decisions will be shaped by their personality, education, social situation, finances, religious beliefs, culture, employment, and personal relationships. Some time must be spent getting to know that is important for the patient. A few directed questions may be very helpful, such as 'Of all the symptoms that you have, which one bothers you the most?' and 'If I were able to fix this symptom for you, would this significantly improve your life?' Since every procedure carries with it potential morbidity and patient suffering, only those procedures which will potentially improve problems that are important to the patient should be performed.

Patient treatment choices are also determined by what the patient and family understands about their disease and prognosis. Weeks *et al.* found that the decision about whether or not cancer patients should have aggressive therapy related to their perception of their own survival.[21] Cancer patients tended to overestimate their survival; those who thought that there was at least a 10% chance that they would die within six months were more likely to favour less aggressive therapies. The patient's acceptance (or not) of their own mortality will shape the tone of the discussion. Psychiatric conditions must also be kept in mind; Chochinov found that patients who did not acknowledge their prognosis (9.5% of 200 advanced cancer patients) were almost three times more likely to be clinically depressed.[40]

Technical factors

The surgeon may select from a wide spectrum of procedures, with differing levels of invasiveness, anaesthetic requirements, technical complexity, and attendant risk (Box 2.3). The decision

Box 2.3 Technical factors

- ◆ Degree of invasiveness:
  - – interventional radiology
  - – endoscopy
  - – laparoscopic surgery
  - – open surgery
- ◆ Anaesthetic requirements:
  - – local/regional
  - – general
- ◆ Location of intervention:
  - – patient home
  - – doctor's office
  - – day surgery or overnight stay
  - – hospital inpatient
- ◆ Postoperative complications:
  - – bleeding, infection
  - – wound problems
  - – pain
  - – hospital stay
  - – mortality of intervention (30-day mortality)

of which option to recommend is dependent on the disease process, the anatomy of the region of interest (guided by imaging studies), the risk – benefit ratio for the procedure, and the available technical expertise. Ongoing developments in the fields of minimally invasive surgery and interventional radiology are particularly important in surgical palliation as these procedures are often associated with lower morbidity.[41] It should be noted that laparoscopy in the abdomen still requires a general and paralysing anaesthetic, which may be a major contributor to morbidity. Generally, the most minimally invasive effective procedure is chosen so as to result in the least discomfort, morbidity, and time in hospital. However, this should not result in the withholding of more invasive procedures in appropriately selected patients when they are more effective for the relief of symptoms.

As much information as possible should be obtained prior to recommending and embarking on a procedure. This will provide the best estimate of what the procedure can accomplish, as well as the likelihood of success. It will minimise intraoperative surprises, and allow the procedure to proceed as safely as possible. Preoperative imaging with plain x-rays, ultrasonography (US), CT or Magnetic Resonance Imaging (MRI) scans, angiography, or contrast studies provides the knowledge of the relevant anatomy, essential to guide decision making. Plain films may have a role in the reassessment of effusions or bowel obstructions. Ultrasound scanning is a non-invasive modality useful in guiding percutaneous drainage of deeply located fluid collections, or the placement of percutaneous catheters. CT or MRI scanning is especially helpful because it can help stage disease as well as provides precise anatomical information. Preoperative abdominal CT scans with oral contrast, for example, are critical in assessing the underlying nature of malignant bowel obstruction.[42] Endoscopy to further delineate the anatomy is often helpful, especially when combined with imaging, as in the case of endoscopic retrograde cholangiopancreatography (ERCP). Used to image the biliary tree, ERCP can diagnose and locate sites of malignant biliary obstruction and at the same time provide palliation in the form of stent placement. This, in conjunction with anatomical confirmation from CT that a tumour is incurable, may spare a pancreatic cancer patient an exploratory laparotomy.

An assessment of the risk of operative mortality is of major importance. The incidence of operative mortality is a function of the basic disease process that includes surgery, choice of anaesthetic, technical complexity of the procedure, degree to which the surgery disrupts normal physiological function, and the general health status of the patient and their ability to withstand operative trauma. Operative risk increases when surgery is performed on an emergency versus an elective basis.[6]

Anaesthetic options include either regional or general anaesthesia. Regional anaesthesia involves the reversible blockade of pain perception by the application of local anaesthetic drugs. When injected around a major nerve trunk, local anaesthesia can provide anaesthesia to entire anatomical areas. Major surgical procedures in the lower portion of the body can be done using epidural or spinal anaesthesia. The patient remains awake and breathing spontaneously during the procedure, useful for patients with cardio-respiratory compromise. A general anaesthetic is required for most abdominal and thoracic procedures, and is usually tolerated by all except the very ill palliative patients. Anaesthesia related mortality is extremely low, although difficult to separate out from the other contributors to the patient's mortality.

A thorough knowledge of effective alternatives to surgery may avoid an operation. Examples of this include the use of photodynamic therapy to treat recurrent chest wall tumours,[43] laser therapy for recurrent head and neck therapy,[44] and stenting or laser ablation for intraluminal tumours causing obstruction.[3] While stents are often not as durable in their ability to maintain patency and may be prone to blockage and subsequent infection, experience with biliary stenting has shown that more frequent hospital admissions for stent replacement and infection management does not decrease quality of life when compared to the morbidity of open surgical bypass. The judicious use of palliative radiation therapy must be considered. Aggressive medical management of malignant bowel obstruction or the placement of a venting gastrostomy tube may allow patients with carcinomatosis to live without a nasogastric tube.[45] The use of less aggressive interventions must be considered where appropriate; however, depending on the patient's performance status, a patient should not be denied the most effective intervention just because they are not curable.

Societal factors

Treatment options are influenced by the economic, cultural, socio-economic, ethical, and legal environment in which the patient, their family, and the physician reside. The choice of procedure will be affected by the available community and personal resources available. These factors include the location where the patient is cared for after the procedure (hospital, hospice, or at home), the expertise of the care-givers (nurse, family, palliative care physicians, home care), and the equipment available (portable pain pumps, ostomy care). Patients living in remote communities may not have easy access to a health care facility. An intervention may be a significant financial burden for some families. A procedure should make ongoing care as easy as possible for the patient and the care-givers. For example, an external drainage tube may be less invasive but will require management of a drainage bag; an internal stent placement may be more invasive but may require less care.

Defining the goals of care

Palliative surgery aims to achieve the best quality of life by the management of symptoms and the relief of suffering. The degree of relief of symptoms that a single intervention will achieve will often fall along a continuum of complete to partial achievement of this aim. The surgeon and patient should therefore try to define clearly and agree upon the exact goals of the intended intervention. This must involve input from the patient and family, as well as relying on the expertise and experience of the surgeon and other members of the health care team.

The patient's individual goals of care and expectations of treatment should be articulated and understood. This may be the first time during the course of the illness that such a discussion has taken place. Education about normal disease progression and a realistic discussion about prognosis are important. Whether or not a patient has accepted their own mortality is an important topic for discussion; unrealistic expectations of cure may be present. A family meeting is often helpful to explore patient and family expectations. If patient preferences about the trade-offs between the risks and benefits associated with alternative treatment strategies are based on inaccurate perceptions of prognosis, then treatment choices may not reflect each patient's true values.[21] It is not the role of the surgeon to remove hope from a patient. However, the decision to undertake a procedure is a contract with the surgeon and the patient (and ideally family) to achieve shared goals. The patient's attitude and acceptance of the achievable goals must be realistic and clearly defined preoperatively in order to avoid disappointment. The patient must be able to understand and take responsibility for the possible negative consequences if complications occur. This is especially true if radical surgery is contemplated for palliation, such as pelvic exenterations. A survey of surgical oncologists within our institution revealed that the inability of the patient to understand what is being contemplated was the single most common reason for surgeon refusal to perform a radical procedure. Once such a procedure is done, the primary care of all surgical complications falls to the operating surgeon. Successful care as the patient approaches the end of life depends on trust and communication, and is especially difficult if patients are not comfortable with the steps that have been taken to date.

This is often easier said than done. The surgeon, patient, and family may have widely different goals preoperatively (Miner et al., unpublished work, 2000). SUPPORT documents that physicians and surrogates are often unaware of seriously ill patients' preferences. The care provided to patients is often not consistent with their preferences and is often associated with factors other than preferences or prognoses.[46] Part of the problem is that there is little data in the current surgical literature on which to base sound palliative surgical choices.[47] Improvement in quality of life and symptom relief should be the best measure of any therapy in cancer.[48] These outcomes have not been a large part of traditional surgical thinking, which has tended to focus on quantity, rather than quality, of life, although this is slowly beginning to change.[49] Reports of outcomes after palliative surgery currently reveal conflicting results about the quality of life and survival after palliative surgery, but very little prospective data are available.[47,50–52]

The situation is more difficult if patients are unable to articulate their goals. Has an advance directive been prepared which states the patient's preference in this situation? Such a document provides patients with the opportunity to express their own values and preferences. Unfortunately, vague nomenclature and changing circumstances may make advanced directives difficult to apply and limit their usefulness in practice.[53] Has a surrogate decision maker (power of attorney for health care) been identified who can clearly speak about the patient's wishes? Surgeons often find themselves in the middle of the night dealing with an emergency operation on a patient and family that they have never met before. This common and difficult situation highlights the need to anticipate emergency events and the preparation of a living will while the patient is able to articulate one.

The decision to operate is often the easiest decision. This allows the surgeon and family to feel that 'something is being done'. This may be the appropriate first step which will allow time for the patient to come to terms with the terminal nature of their illness when they are ready to do so. However, a surgeon or any physician is not required to perform futile procedures. Futile treatments violate the ethical principles of justice, beneficence, and nonmaleficence. Real problems occur when patients or their families demand treatments that they feel are of value but the clinician considers no longer beneficial to the patient.[54] In this situation, colleagues may be consulted for a second opinion. In cases of doubt, it is often helpful to agree upon a trial of therapy with the patient. For example, a laparotomy may be undertaken to see if a repairable point of obstruction can be found, with the express understanding that this may not be helpful. Alternatives to a procedure may be found which will satisfy the patient's goals of care. An important principle to remember is that the decision not to operate does not mean that the patient will be abandoned and will not receive good care.

Tools such as decision aids have been developed to try and improve knowledge, reduce decisional conflict, and stimulate patients to be more active in decision making.[55] Unfortunately, these tools have not led to a decrease in anxiety, and did not improve patient satisfaction with care.[56]

Because the outcome may be uncertain, it is wise to discuss all possible outcomes with the patient and family preoperatively in order to prepare them for the worst should it occur, as well as to provide some guidance should that situation occur. The patient's and family's wishes should be articulated, and it is often helpful to identify someone who will be able to speak for the patient about their wishes should the patient not be able to speak for themselves. For example, we operated on a patient with unresectable lung cancer who was bleeding from an isolated metastasis in the gastrointestinal tract. Because of her poor lung function, we felt that long-term postoperative intubation was a possibility as she had a high risk of developing pulmonary complications. Preoperatively it was decided that she would have aggressive respiratory intervention, including ventilator support should it be necessary, for two postoperative weeks. Should there be no improvement in her condition after that period of time, she did not wish further aggressive intervention. This discussion made her postoperative management much easier. Although extubated within 48 hours of her surgery, she required reintubation on the fifth postoperative day. Fortunately, she improved quickly, and was discharged home with the help of the palliative care service on the 15th postoperative day.

Preparation of patients

Medical factors

General preparation

Once the decision to perform a procedure is made, the patient's medical status must be optimized prior to surgery. Underlying cardiac, renal, hepatic, and respiratory dysfunction must be identified and their function maximized. Anaemia and electrolyte or metabolic abnormalities must be identified and corrected. Fluid resuscitation and antibiotics must be given as appropriate to treat any concurrent illness. As with any patient with a higher than average operative risk, preoperative involvement of the anaesthetist and internist may be very helpful.[57] Postoperative care planning is initiated at this time by other health care workers such as social workers and home care nurses; preparation for hospice or palliative home placement is begun. Education about normal disease progression and an exploration of sources of distress for both patients and families will allow for successful advance planning around the terminal phase of the illness. It may be appropriate to discuss the need for funeral arrangements and the preparation of a will preoperatively. Though the surgeon may balk at the scope of this counselling, it is time well spent considering the future time and opportunities lost when these things are not discussed.

Nutrition

Studies of perioperative nutritional support have shown that only the most malnourished patients may benefit (Table 2.1), but they can be difficult to identify.[58] Clinical assessment is as effective as objective measurements such as weight loss, serum concentration of proteins manufactured in the liver, immune function, energy and strength.[59,60] An attempt to distinguish between the weight loss from malnutrition and that from cachexia should be made as the chronic catabolic process of cachexia cannot be reversed with short-term nutritional supplementation, and these patients will do poorly. Patients with malnutrition due to mechanical causes of weight loss, such as in patients with oral cancer who are unable to swallow, or with a resectable site causing bowel obstruction, should be offered short-term perioperative nutrition. Other reversible causes of reduced food intake should be identified and treated. These include inadequately treated pain, nausea, malabsorption, gastroparesis due to autonomic dysfunction (common in advanced malignancy), and clinical depression.[20,61,62] The diagnosis of cachexia

Table 2.1 Key clinical trials evaluating the use of perioperative total parenteral nutrition (TPN) in surgical patients

Study/author	Patients	Conclusion	Comment
Bozzetti[66]	Gastric and colorectal cancer with >10% weight loss	Perioperative TPN ↓ complications 57% to 37%,but ↑ length of hospital stay	% of operative procedure with curative or palliative intent unknown
Muller[67]	Gastrointestinal cancer	Preoperative TPN ↓ major complications and mortality rate	% of operative procedure with curative or palliative intent unknown
Brennan[68]	Major pancreatic resection	Postoperative TPN ↑ major complications rate	Curative intent
Fan[69]	Hepatocellular cancer	Perioperative TPN ↓ pneumonia, less ascites	Curative intent
Buzby[70]	Meta-analysis	Preoperative TPN beneficial only for severely malnourished elective surgical patients	All surgical patients
Veterans Affairs Cooperative Trial[71]	All surgical patients	TPN beneficial only for severely malnourished elective surgical patients	Definition of severely malnourished unclear
Detsky et al.[72]	Meta-analysis	Preoperative TPN beneficial only for severely malnourished elective surgical patients	All surgical patients

is made by clinical history, which includes a history of substantial weight loss and a physical examination which demonstrates muscle wasting. Anaemia, decreased serum albumin, and an elevated C-reactive protein, an acute phase protein, may reflect the severity of the condition.[63] More recently, a protein excreted in the urine of cachexic patients that induces cachexia in mice has been discovered, offering promise as a diagnostic tool.[64,65] Malabsorption from pancreatic insufficiency due to pancreatic cancer or upper abdominal radiation therapy should be treated with enzyme supplementation. The intake of preoperative, protein-rich, oral nutritional supplementation should be encouraged and provided.

A management approach (Box 2.4)

Ultimately, the decision on whether or not to offer a surgical procedure to a patient for palliative purposes is based upon the same considerations that would apply to any other patient. The risks and benefits are weighed, and the ultimate decision is a mutual one between surgeon and patient. Unfortunately, at this point in time, there is little guidance in the literature to help in surgical decision making. Often the surgical decision comes down to a gestalt feeling on considering the patient and the surgeon's own personal experience. Hopefully better research in the future will allow a more rational preparation and selection of patients for palliative surgery.

Box 2.4 An approach to the selection and preparation of patients for palliative surgery

Information gathering

- Disease factors:
  - diagnosis, knowledge of natural history
  - presence/absence of expected symptoms
- Patient factors:
  - prognosis
  - history and physical examination, imaging studies
  - the patient as an individual
- Societal factors:
  - family and community resources
- Technical factors:
  - feasibility, choice of modality
  - morbidity and mortality

Goals of care

- A contract with the patient
- Advance directives
- Family meetings

Box 2.4 An approach to the selection and preparation of patients for palliative surgery *(continued)*

General principles

- ◆ Anticipation and prevention of impending symptoms
- ◆ Thorough preoperative evaluation to avoid intraoperative surprises
- ◆ Avoid emergency situations
- ◆ Communication with the patient and family about the goals of care
- ◆ Commitment to continue to provide care despite outcome of surgery

References

1. Edelstein, L. (1943). Hippocratic oath – classical version. *The Hippocratic oath: text, translation, and interpretation.* Johns Hopkins Press, Baltimore.
2. Friel, J.P. (ed.) (1985). *Dorland's illustrated medical dictionary*, p. 1023. W.B. Saunders, Philadelphia.
3. Easson, A.M., Asch, M., and Swallow, C.J. (2001). Palliative general surgical procedures. *Surg. Oncol. Clin. North Am.*, **10**, 161–84.
4. Fraker, D.L., Skarulis, M., and Livolsi, V. (1997). Thyroid tumors. In: *Cancer: principles and practice of oncology* (ed. V.T. Devita, S. Hellman, and S.A. Rosenberg), p. 1643. Lippincott-Raven, Philadelphia.
5. Chen, H., Roberts, J., Ball, D.W., Eisele, D.W., Baylin, S.B., Udelsman, R., *et al.* (1998). Effective long-term palliation of symptomatic, incurable metastatic medullary thyroid cancer by operative resection. *Ann. Surg.*, **227**, 887–95.
6. Cohen, M.M., Duncan, P.G., and Tate, R.B. (1988). Does anaesthesia contribute to operative mortality? *J.A.M.A.*, **260**, 2859–63.
7. Patz, E.F., Jr. (1998). Malignant pleural effusions: recent advances and ambulatory sclerotherapy. *Chest*, **113**, S74–S7.
8. Robinson, R.D., Fullerton, D.A., Albert, J.D., Sorensen, J., and Johnston, M.R. (1994). Use of pleural Tenckhoff catheter to palliate malignant pleural effusion. *Ann. Thorac. Surg.*, **57**, 286–8.
9. Tsang, T.S., Seward, J.B., Barnes, M.E., Bailey, K.R., Sinak, L.J., Urban, L.H., *et al.* (2000). Outcomes of primary and secondary treatment of pericardial effusion in patients with malignancy. *Mayo. Clin. Proc.*, **75**, 248–53.
10. Belfort, M.A., Stevens, P.J., DeHaek, K., Soeters, R., and Krige, J.E. (1990). A new approach to the management of malignant ascites: a permanently implanted abdominal drain. *Eur. J. Surg. Oncol.*, **16**, 47–53.
11. Petrou, M., Kaplan, D., and Goldstraw, P. (1995). The management of recurrent malignant pleural effusion: the complementary role of talc pleurodesis and pleuroperitoneal shunting. *Cancer*, **75**, 801–5.
12. Fiocco, M., and Krasna, M.J. (1997). The management of malignant pleural and pericardial effusions. *Hematol. Oncol. Clin. North Am.*, **11**, 253–65.
13. Parsons, S.L., Watson, S.A., and Steele, R.J.C. (1996). Malignant ascites. *Br. J. Surg.*, **83**, 6–14.
14. Lillemoe, K.D., Cameron, J.L., Hardacre, J.M., Sohn, T.A., Sauter, P.K., Coleman, J., *et al.* (1999). Is prophylactic gastrojejunostomy indicated for unresectable periampullary cancer? A prospective randomized trial. *Ann. Surg.*, **230**, 322–8.
15. Donnelly, S., and Walsh, D. (1995). The symptoms of advanced cancer. *Semin. Oncol.*, **22**, 67–72.
16. Martin, L.A., and Hagen, N.A. (1997). Neuropathic pain in cancer patients: mechanisms, syndromes, and clinical controversies. *J. Pain Sympt. Manage.*, **14**, 99–117.

17. Eisenberg, E., Carr, D.B., and Chalmers, T.C. (1995). Neurolytic celiac plexus block for treatment of cancer pain: a meta-analysis. *Anesth. Analg.*, **80**, 290–5.

18. Lillemoe, K.D., Cameron, J.L., Kaufman, H.S., Yeo, C.J., Pitt, H.A., and Sauter, P.K. (1993). Chemical splanchnicectomy in patients with unresectable pancreatic cancer. A prospective randomized trial. *Ann. Surg.*, **217**, 447–55.

19. Bruera, E., and Beattie-Palmer, L.N. (2001). Pharmacologic management of non-pain symptoms in surgical patients. *Surg. Oncol. Clin. North Am.*, **10**, 89–107.

20. Bruera, E. (1997). ABC of, palliative care: anorexia, cachexia, and nutrition. *B.M.J.*, **315**, 1219–22.

21. Weeks, J.C., Cook, E.F., and O'Day, S.J. (1998). Relationship between cancer patients prediction of prognosis and their treatment preferences. *J.A.M.A.*, **279**, 1709–14.

22. Vigano, A., Bruera, E., Jhangri, G.S., Newman, S.C., Fields, A.L., and Suarez-Almazor, M.E. (2000). Clinical survival predictors in patients with advanced cancer. *Arch. Intern. Med.*, **160**, 861–8.

23. Sloan, J.A., Loprinzi, C.L., Laurine, J.A., Novotny, P.J., Vargas-Chanes, D., Krook, J.E., *et al.* (2001). A simple stratification factor prognostic for survival in advanced cancer: the good/bad/uncertain index. *J. Clin. Oncol.*, **19**, 3539–46.

24. Morita, T., Tsunoda, J., Inoue, S., and Chihara, S. (1999). The Palliative Prognostic Index: a scoring system for survival prediction of terminally ill cancer patients. *Support Care Cancer*, **7**, 128–33.

25. Maltoni, M., Nanni, O., Pirovano, M., Scarpi, E., Indelli, M., Martini, C., *et al.* (1999). Successful validation of the palliative prognostic score in terminally ill cancer patients. *J. Pain Sympt. Manage.*, **17**, 240–7.

26. Knaus, W.A., Harrell, F.E., Jr., Lynn, J., Goldman, L., Phillips, R.S., Connors, A.F., Jr., *et al.* (1995). The SUPPORT prognostic model. Objective estimates of survival for seriously ill hospitalized adults. *Ann. Intern. Med.*, **122**, 191–203.

27. Yates, J.W., Chalmer, B., and McKegney, F.P. (1980). Evaluation of patients with advanced cancer using the Karnofsky Performance Status. *Cancer*, **40**, 2222–4.

28. Cubiella, J., Castells, A., Fondevila, C., Sans, M., Sabater, L., Navarro, S., *et al.* (1999). Prognostic factors in nonresectable pancreatic adenocarcinoma: a rationale to design therapeutic trials. *Am. J. Gastroenterol.*, **94**, 1271–8.

29. Vigano, A., Dorgan, M., Buckingham, J., Bruera, E., and Suarez-Almazor, M.E. (2000). Survival prediction in terminal cancer patients: a systematic review of the medical literature. *Pall. Med.*, **14**, 363–74.

30. Fox, E., Landrum-McNiff, K., Zhong, Z., Dawson, N.V., Wu, A.W., and Lynn, J. (1999). Evaluation of prognostic criteria for determining hospice eligibility in patients with advanced lung, heart, or liver disease. *J.A.M.A.*, **282**, 1638–45.

31. Seidman, A.D., Portenoy, R., Yao, T.J., Lepore, J., Mont, E.K., Kortmansky, J., *et al.* (1995). Quality of life in phase II trials: a study of methodology and predictive value in patients with advanced breast cancer treated with paclitaxel plus granulocyte colony-stimulating factor. *J. Natl. Cancer Inst.*, **87**, 1316–22.

32. Degner, L.F., and Sloan, J.A. (1995). Symptom distress in newly diagnosed ambulatory cancer patients and as a predictor of survival in lung cancer. *J. Pain Sympt. Manage.*, **10**, 423–31.

33. Addington-Hall, J.M., MacDonald, L.D., and Anderson, H.R. (1990). Can the Spitzer Quality of Life Index help to reduce prognostic uncertainty in terminal care? *Br. J. Cancer*, **62**, 695–9.

34. Child, C.G., and Turcotte, J.C. (1964). Surgery and portal hypertension. In: *Major problems in clinical surgery: the liver and portal hypertension* (ed. C.G.I. Child), pp. 1–85. W.B. Saunders, Philadelphia.

35. Turcotte, J.G., Raper, S.E., and Eckhauser, F.E. (1996). Portal hypertension. In: *Surgery, scientific principles and practice* (ed. L.J. Greenfield, M.W. Mulholland, K.T. Oldham, and G.B. Zenelock), pp. 887–908. J.B. Lippincott Co, Philadelphia.

36. Goldman, L., Caldera, D.L., Nussbaum, S.R., Southwick, F.S., Krogstad, D., Murray, B., *et al.* (1977). Multifactorial index of cardiac risk in non-cardiac surgical procedures. *N. Engl. J. Med.*, **297**, 845–50.

37. Rosenberg, S.A. (1997). Principles of cancer management: surgical oncology. In: *Cancer principles and practice of oncology* (ed. V.T. Devita, S. Hellman, and S.A. Rosenberg), pp. 295–305. Lippincott-Raven, Philadelphia.

38. Yazdi, G.P., Miedema, B.W., and Humphrey, L.J. (1996). High mortality after abdominal operation in patients with large-volume malignant ascites. *J. Surg. Oncol.*, **62**, 93–6.

39. Dripps, R.D., Eckenhoff, J.E., and Vandam, L.D. (1988). *Introduction to anaesthesia: the principles of safe practice.* W.B. Saunders, Philadelphia.

40. Chochinov, H.M., Tataryn, D., Wilson, K.G., Enns, M., and Lander, S. (2000). Prognostic awareness and the terminally ill. *Psychosomatics*, **41**, 500–4.

41. Croce, E., Olmi, S., Azzola, M., Russo, R., and Golia, M. (1999). Surgical palliation in pancreatic head carcinoma and gastric cancer: the role of laparoscopy. *Hepato-Gastroenterology*, **46**, 2606–11.

42. Krouse, R.S., McCahill, L.E., Easson, A.M., and Dunn, G.P. (2002). When the sun *can* set on an unoperated bowel obstruction: management of malignant bowel obstruction. *J. Am. Coll. Surg.* In press.

43. Taber, S.W., Fingar, V.H., and Wieman, T.J. (1998). Photodynamic therapy for palliation of chest wall recurrence in patients with breast cancer. *J. Surg. Oncol.*, **68**, 209–14.

44. Paiva, M.B., Blackwell, K.E., Saxton, R.E., Calcaterra, T.C., Ward, P.H., Soudant, J., *et al.* (1998). Palliative laser therapy for recurrent head and neck cancer: a phase II clinical study. *Laryngoscope*, **108**, 1277–83.

45. Easson, A.M., Hinshaw, D.B., and Johnson, D.L. (2002). The role of tube feeding and total parenteral nutrition in advanced illness. *J. Am. Coll. Surg.*, **194**, 225–8.

46. Covinsky, K.E., Fuller, J.D., Yaffe, K., Johnston, C.B., Hamel, M.B., Lynn, J., *et al.* (2000). Communication and decision-making in seriously ill patients: findings of the SUPPORT project. The Study to Understand Prognoses and Preferences for Outcomes and Risks of Treatments. *J. Am. Geriatr. Soc.*, **48**, S187–S193.

47. Miner, T.J., Jaques, D.P., Tavaf-Motamen, H., and Shriver, C.D. (1999). Decision making on surgical palliation based on patient outcome data. *Am. J. Surg.*, **177**, 150–4.

48. Michael, M., and Tannock, I.F. (1998). Measuring health-related quality of life in clinical trials that evaluate the role of chemotherapy in cancer treatment. *C.M.A.J.*, **158**, 1727–34.

49. McLeod, R.S. (1999). Quality of life measurement in the assessment of surgical outcome. *Adv. Surg.*, **33**, 1–17.

50. Feuer, D.J., and Broadley, K.E. (1999). Systematic review and meta-analysis of corticosteroids for the resolution of malignant bowel obstruction in advanced gynaecological and gastrointestinal cancers. Systematic Review Steering Committee. *Ann. Oncol.*, **10**, 1035–41.

51. Averbach, A.M., and Sugarbaker, P.H. (1996). Recurrent intra-abdominal cancer causing intestinal obstruction: Washington Hospital Center experience with 42 patients managed by surgery and intraperitoneal chemotherapy. *Cancer Treat. Research*, **81**, 133–47.

52. Shekarriz, B., Shekarriz, H., Upadhyay, J., Banerjee, M., Becker, H., Pontes, J.E., *et al.* (1999). Outcome of palliative urinary diversion in the treatment of advanced malignancies. *Cancer*, **85**, 998–1003.

53. SUPPORT Principal Investigators (2000). A controlled trial to improve care for seriously ill hospitalized patients. The study to understand prognoses and preferences for outcomes and risks of treatments (SUPPORT). *J.A.M.A.*, **274**, 1591–8.

54. Brescia, F. (1999) Supportive care and the quality of life. In: *Oxford textbook of palliative medicine* (ed. D. Doyle, G. Hanks, and N. MacDonald), pp. 2905–11. Oxford University Press, Oxford.

55. Fiset, V., O'Connor, A.M., Evans, W., Graham, I., DeGrasse, C., and Logan, J. (2000). Development and evaluation of a decision aid for patients with stage IV non-small cell lung cancer. *Health Expect.*, **3**, 125–36.

56. O'Connor, A.M., Rostom, A., Fiset, V., Tetroe, J., Entwhistle, V., Llewellyn-Thomas, H., *et al.* (1999). Decision aids for patients facing health treatment or screening decision: a systematic review. *B.M.J.*, **319**, 731–4.

57. Griffith, R.S. (1992). Preoperative evaluation. Medical obstacles to surgery. *Cancer*, **70**, 1333–41.

58. Easson, A.M., and Souba, W.W. (1999). Total parenteral nutrition in surgical patients. *Contemp. Surg.*, **54**, 218–26.

59. Baker, J.P., Detsky, A.S., Whitwell, J., Langer, B., and Jeejeebhoy, K.N. (1982). A comparison of the predictive value of nutritional assessment techniques. *Hum. Nutr. Clin. Nutr.*, **36**, 233–41.

60. Detsky, A.S., Baker, J.P., Mendelson, R.A., Wolman, S.L., Wesson, D.E., and Jeejeebhoy, K.N. (1984). Evaluating the accuracy of nutritional assessment techniques applied to hospitalized patients: methodology and comparisons. *J. Parenter. Enteral Nutr.*, **8**, 153–9.

61. Bruera, E., and Fainsinger, R.L. (1999). Clinical management of cachexia and anorexia. In: *Oxford textbook of palliative medicine*, (ed. D. Doyle, G. Hanks, and N. MacDonald), pp. 534–45.

62. Fearon, K.C., Barber, M.D., and Moses, A.G. (2001). The cancer cachexia syndrome. *Surg. Oncol. Clin. North Am.*, **10**, 109–26.

63. Barber, M.D, Ross, J.A., and Fearon, K.C. (1999). Changes in nutritional, functional, and inflammatory markers in advanced pancreatic cancer. *Nutr. Cancer*, **35**, 106–10.

64. Cariuk, P., Lorite, M.J., Todorov, P.T., Field, W.N., Wigmore, S.J., and Tisdale, M.J. (1997). Induction of cachexia in mice by a product isolated from the urine of cachectic cancer patients. *Br. J. Cancer*, **76**, 606–13.

65. Tisdale, M.J. (2000). Metabolic abnormalities in cachexia and anorexia. *Nutrition*, **16**, 1013–14.

66. Bozzetti, F., Gavazzi, C., Miceli, R., Rossi, N., Mariani, L., Cozzaglio, L., *et al.* (2000). Perioperative total parenteral nutrition in malnourished, gastrointestinal cancer patients: a randomized, clinical trial. *J. Parenter. Enteral Nutr.*, **24**, 7–14.

67. Muller, J.M., Brenner, U., Dienst, C., and Pichlmaier, H. (1982). Preoperative parenteral feeding in patients with gastrointestinal carcinoma. *Lancet*, **1**, 68–71.

68. Brennan, M.F., Pisters, P.W., Posner, M., Quesada, O., and Shike, M. (1994). A prospective randomized trial of total parenteral nutrition after major pancreatic resection for malignancy. *Ann. Surg.*, **220**, 436–41.

69. Fan, S.T., Lo, C.M., Lai, E.C., Chu, K.M., Liu, C.L., and Wong, J. (1994). Perioperative nutritional support in patients undergoing hepatectomy for hepatocellular carcinoma. *N. Engl. J. Med.*, **331**, 1547–52.

70. Buzby, G.P. (1993). Overview of randomized clinical trials of total parenteral nutrition for malnourished surgical patients. *World J. Surg.*, **17**, 173–7.

71. The Veterans Affairs Total Parenteral Nutrition Cooperative Study Group (1991). Perioperative total parenteral nutrition in surgical patients. *N. Engl. J. Med.*, **325**, 525–32.

72. Detsky, A.S., Baker, J.P., O'Rourke, K., and Goel, V. (1987). Perioperative parenteral nutrition: a meta-analysis. *Ann. Intern. Med.*, **107**, 195–203.

Chapter 3

The ethics of interventional care

Peter Angelos

Introduction

In the following pages, we will consider the ethical basis of interventional care. Interventional care is a broad topic that includes many aspects of medical care. Certainly, all surgery is an intervention – it is invasive care. Yet not all interventions are surgery. For example, a fine-needle aspiration of the thyroid is an intervention and is invasive, but it is not surgery. When considering the general topic of surgical palliative care, one must carefully consider the underlying ethical assumptions and principles that ground the decision to proceed with surgery on a particular patient. When the goal of surgery is cure, the principles grounding the decision seem obvious. However, when the goal of surgery is to palliate symptoms, the decision must be carefully considered in light of the risks. In the following pages, we will examine the philosophical basis for recommending surgery in general terms. We will consider similarities and differences between palliative and curative surgery. We will consider how risks and benefits are analysed in the different situations. Finally, we will consider the similarities and differences between surgical interventions and other types of medical interventions and the important role that surgeons often occupy for their patients.

Philosophical basis of surgical intervention

Every surgical intervention is grounded in the assumption that the benefits of the procedure outweigh the risks. Although every medical treatment is undertaken with the goal that the benefits outweigh the risks, in surgery this analysis must be more explicitly considered. Every surgical procedure involves a deliberate infliction of pain and potentially permanent disfigurement upon the patient. In order to legitimately consider offering a surgical procedure to a patient, the expectations of benefit from the procedure must clearly outweigh the known risks of the procedure. This assumption is more fundamental even than is the principle of informed consent. Surgeons ought not perform every operation that a patient may have freely consented to. Some patients will have such high risks associated with an operation that the expected benefits do not rise to a high enough level to warrant proceeding with the operation. In those cases, even if the patient may consent to the surgery, or even desire the surgery, the risks may be too high for the surgeon to offer the operation as a possibility.

By way of illustration, consider a patient with widely metastatic recurrent colon cancer who develops acute cholecystitis. At the time of the patient's previous surgery, he was noted to have extensive peritoneal spread of the cancer and malignant ascites. The options for treating his newly diagnosed acute cholecystitis include non-operatively with antibiotics, surgically by performing a cholecystectomy, or by percutaneous cholecystostomy tube. Even if this patient might prefer to have surgery and alleviate the potential for further problems with acute cholecystitis, the surgeon must determine an appropriate risk–benefit ratio prior to even offering surgery. Depending on the patient and the extent of malignant disease, one might argue that the patient is unlikely to live long enough to develop complications from the acute cholecystitis. In this case, if the risks of developing complications outweigh the benefits of the operation, the surgeon should not offer a cholecystectomy as an option, even if the patient is willing to give consent for the surgery.

Curative operation versus palliative operation

Much in contemporary surgical care is directed toward curing the patient. This emphasis on cure is reflective of the broad influence of the curative model in contemporary medicine. The curative model of medicine is narrowly focused on the goal of curing disease. According to this understanding of the goal of medicine, 'cure' is taken to be 'the eradication of the cause of an illness or disease [or] the . . . interruption and reversal of the natural history of the disorder'.[1] The curative model pushes physicians to focus on a specific set of questions and approaches to patients. In the curative model, a patient with an illness becomes a disease to be diagnosed and eradicated rather than a patient to be treated. The curative model pushes physicians into analytic and rationalistic thinking in which objective facts and empirical knowledge are favoured over subjective or unverifiable issues.[2] By focusing on the curative model, contemporary medicine minimizes non-objective concerns such as pain control. The underlying assumption of the curative model is that pursuit of a goal other than cure is less valuable to patients and less worthy of a physician's concern.

As is readily evident, the curative model of medicine is too narrow a view for much of medical care. The alternative view, the palliative model, focuses on broader issues including control of symptoms, relief of suffering, and re-establishment of functional capacity. Rather than being a less important set of issues, the goals of the palliative model are different, but equally important goals. Treatment of any chronic disease must be understood as grounded in the palliative model of medicine. Instead of thinking of medicine in terms of the dichotomy between curative and palliative models, physicians could have a greater and more lasting effect on patients if the goals of medicine addressed the issues of both the curative and the palliative models of medicine.

Closely paralleling the artificial dichotomy between curative and palliative models of medicine has been the artificial dichotomy between a curative operation and a palliative operation. A curative operation is one that is designed to cure the patient of the disease or illness. The benefits of a curative operation are readily apparent, objective, and measurable. If the possibility of cure from the operation outweighs the risks of harm from the surgical procedure, then the operation will likely be seen as desirable.

In order to understand how a palliative operation should be assessed, we must carefully consider what is meant by a palliative operation. The *Oxford English Dictionary* places the contemporary usage of 'palliate' in the context of cloaking, disguising, or patching up. To palliate something was 'to disguise or colour the real enormity of (an offense) by favourable representations or excuses; to represent (an evil) as less than it really is; to cause to appear less guilty or offensive by urging extenuating circumstances'.[3] Thus, a palliative operation is one that is designed to cover up symptoms. In contrast to a curative operation that is directed at cure, a palliative operation is one that is often seen as an alternative goal only if cure is not possible. Surgeons often plan an operation with the goal being to resect the tumour for cure. If such a complete resection is not possible, the surgeon often settles for a palliative procedure only as a second choice.[4] This view of palliative operations is, however, short-sighted.

From the patient's perspective, when cure is not a possibility, the option of surgery to significantly diminish symptoms is an excellent choice. Even if such a procedure is a second choice, the palliative operation may have tremendous benefits to the patient. As such, the risk–benefit analysis for palliative surgery must more directly focus on the symptoms that will be alleviated by the surgery relative to the risks of the operation itself. This type of risk–benefit analysis is more complicated because in contrast to survival rates that are widely known for most conditions, rates of *adequate palliation* of symptoms are extremely difficult to predict. Many of the symptoms may be subjective (e.g. pain). Even the concept of 'adequate palliation' depends on the subjective assessment by the patient of what is 'adequate'. In order to assess the risk–benefit ratio for a palliative operation, the surgeon must carefully and thoughtfully assess the patient's complaints and how the surgery might impact each of these complaints. Such decisions cannot be made unilaterally by the surgeon, but require joint decision making with the patient.

Even though both surgeons and patients would prefer a curative operation if the option presents itself, undertaking a palliative operation can be just as important for a patient. However, a palliative operation will lose appeal to the patient if the trauma of the procedure itself is too great. Any palliative operation, therefore, requires the surgeon to honestly consider the pain, suffering, etc. associated with the operation. In contrast to a curative operation for which patients would be willing to go through much pain to achieve, a palliative operation loses all value if the patient must trade the pain of the disease for the postoperative pain of the procedure.

Consider a case to illustrate the issues involved in palliative operations. A 42-year-old man was diagnosed with adenocarcinoma of the cecum with spread through the serosa with multiple sites of peritoneal studding of tumour. Despite resection of the primary tumour and treatment with chemotherapy, the patient developed bulky intraperitoneal disease and lung metastases. Approximately four months after his initial operation, the patient was admitted with signs and symptoms of a complete bowel obstruction. Despite nasogastric tube decompression, the patient continued to have nausea, vomiting, and abdominal pain. In considering a palliative procedure to try to alleviate the obstruction, the surgeon and patient must consider the expected postoperative pain, the likelihood of success in alleviating the obstruction, the patient's life expectancy with and without surgery, the risks of intra-abdominal infection, and other issues. These considerations make the assessment of whether to proceed with surgery much more complicated than if the operation being considered was planned as curative.

'Too sick for surgery'

Based on the previous discussion of palliative operations, one must consider in what situations a patient might not be a good candidate for any surgical intervention. In other words, when faced with a critically ill patient who needs a high-risk surgical intervention to possibly prolong life or alleviate suffering, must the surgeon operate on the patient if there is even a possibility of benefit to the patient? Most surgeons would answer the preceding question with a resounding 'no'. If this answer is to be defensible, how is this situation different from performing cardiopulmonary resuscitation (CPR) on a patient with a very poor prognosis, which is widely considered a mandatory intervention?

As discussed previously, any surgical intervention requires the deliberate infliction of bodily injury by the surgeon on a patient with the expectation that the benefits of the operation will outweigh the pain and suffering caused by the surgery itself. If the possible benefits of the surgery to the patient are extremely low, the surgeon might draw the conclusion that the procedure should not be performed. In order to come to this conclusion appropriately, the surgeon must determine that there is a small chance that the intervention will change the patient's status or when the patient is so critically ill that the intervention itself is likely to lead to death. This situation is raised when the surgeon makes the assessment that a patient is 'too sick for surgery'. Therefore, even if a patient or family wants surgery for a critically ill patient, the surgeon may decline to offer an operation to the patient.

Consider how the previous situation is different from that faced by an internist whose patient needs CPR.[5] Even if the physician believes that the patient's chances of surviving CPR are minimal, a cardiopulmonary arrest in virtually any patient provides a strong argument for CPR. At the point that a patient's heart has stopped beating, the risk–benefit analysis of attempting to start the patient's heart again strongly favours providing CPR. However, despite the apparent differences between CPR and offering surgery, important similarities remain. In specific cases, a do-not-resuscitate (DNR) order may be written against the wishes of a patient's surrogate decision makers.[6] Such an order would be justifiable if CPR offers no chance of significant benefit and a great chance of harm to the patient.[7] Thus, the same principle applies to CPR as to surgical interventions. If the risks of operating on a patient are just too great considering the few potential benefits, the patient may be 'too sick for surgery' and surgery should be appropriately withheld from the patient.

Should there be limits to palliative surgery?

When considering whether a palliative operation is justifiable for a specific patient, the physician must consider more than whether the benefits of the intervention outweigh the risks to the patient. Consideration must also be given to whether there are broader risks to be considered beyond those of the patient. If the surgical intervention necessary to palliate the patient requires that significant risks be taken by the surgical team, those risks need to be carefully considered. Although no exact calculation of risks to surgical team compared to potential benefits to patient can be uniformly applied, the surgeon must at least ensure that no procedure be undertaken where the benefits to the patient are very low while the risks to the surgical team are very high.

A second potential limit to palliative interventions is of more theoretical concern. If the context of care is one of absolute scarcity of resources, the physician must consider the resources necessary to provide palliative care. If providing palliative interventions for one patient requires many other patients to be lacking in more basic medical interventions, rules for the system as a whole should be set down so that individual decisions are being made in the context of an equitable distribution of resources.

Are surgical interventions different from other interventions?

We began this chapter considering surgery as an example of interventional care. Although all surgery is interventional care, not all interventional care is surgery. Surgical interventions are, however, a special type of intervention that necessitate a more critical analysis of risks and benefits than do almost any other type of intervention. Even though other types of interventional care may prove to be as dangerous to patients as surgery, the psychological considerations that bind surgeons to their patients are different from those of other physicians. Any consideration of whether to put a patient through the risks of surgery in order to alleviate symptoms must address the bond between surgeon and patient. The psychological burden is different on a physician whose patient dies after receiving a medical treatment as compared with a surgeon whose patient dies after being operated upon. As medical sociologist Charles Bosk has said, 'The specific nature of surgical treatment links the action of the physician and the response of the patient more intimately than in other areas of medicine. When the patient of an internist dies, the natural question his colleagues ask is "What happened?" When the patient of a surgeon dies, his colleagues ask "What did you do?".'[8] In other words, undertaking an operation that leads to a patient's death is different from undertaking other medical interventions that lead to the patient's death.

In some ways, the 'connection' between a surgeon and patient is different from that between, for example, the internist and patient. Although many surgeons feel that they have a 'special' relationship with their patients by virtue of having operated on the patient, defining what is different in this relationship has been difficult. Dr Miles Little has provided some insights into the special nature of the surgeon–patient relationship when he has tried to define a 'distinctively surgical ethics'.[9] Although all of Little's analysis is not relevant for our purposes, he accurately identifies 'proximity' as a central difference in the surgeon–patient relationship. In the act of operating upon a patient, the surgeon gains access to the patient beyond even what the patient has access to. As Little states, '[The relationship] achieves a unique intimacy after the operation, when the surgeon knows so much about aspects of the bodily identity that the patient can never know.'[9] Such intimacy is a major component in the unique nature of the relationship between surgeon and patient.

The proximity that Little has identified in the relationship leads to the importance of 'presence' as both a virtue and a duty for the surgeon.[9] Patients expect the presence of their surgeons after surgery. One of the central expectations of surgeons is that they will continue to care for patients even after the operation is over. This expectation is codified in the 'Statement on Principles' of the American College of Surgeons that proscribes itinerant surgery.[10] Despite the numerous physicians that many patients have involved in their care in a modern medical centre, the patient often identifies the surgeon most clearly as 'my doctor'.

This situation can be both a gift and a burden to surgeons. When patients near the end of life, they often look to their surgeon for assistance. When palliation becomes the major emphasis in a patient's care, the surgeon must diligently maintain the presence with the patient that the patient has come to expect. Although surgeons may not be the experts in all aspects of palliative care, surgeons should not readily turn the care of a patient over to a palliative care expert without maintaining presence. In addition to control of symptoms, when patients are dying they often need the attention of a trusted physician. The presence of the surgeon continuing to maintain contact with a dying patient often is as important to the patient as was the performance of the earlier operation.[11] Surgeons must realize that the bond with a patient and the presence demanded by that bond can have great therapeutic benefits to patients even when another operation is not indicated. Surgeons should be empowered by the significant positive role that they can have for their patients even at the ends of life.

Conclusions

In the preceding pages, we have closely examined the ethical considerations involved in decisions to proceed with surgical palliative care. The overriding concern in each case is the analysis of risks and benefits for the specific situation being considered. Since every surgical intervention necessitates the infliction of some pain and suffering upon the patient, only those interventions that result in improvements in symptoms are justifiable. Even though there are differences between curative and palliative surgery, the differences are minimized when we identify the goals of surgery to include those of the palliative care model. We have identified the unique bond between the surgeon and patient that pushes so many patients to identify their surgeon as their 'primary doctor'. Surgeons must realize the critical role that they play with patients and maintain their presence with patients after surgery and even at the ends of life.

References

1. Pellegrino, E.D. and Thomasma, D.C. (1997). *Helping and healing*, p. 27. Georgetown University Press, Washington, DC.
2. Fox, E. (1997) Predominance of the curative model of medical care: a residual problem. *J.A.M.A.*, **278**, 761–3.
3. *Oxford English Dictionary* (online version). Available at www.oed.com.
4. Angelos, P. (2001). Palliative philosophy. *Surg. Oncol. Clin. North Am.*, **10**, 31–8.
5. Blackhall, L.J. (1987). Must we always use CPR? *N. Engl. J. Med.*, **317**, 1281–5.
6. Casarett, D. and Siegler, M. (1999). Unilateral DNR orders and ethics consultation: a case series. *Crit. Care Med.*, **27**, 1116–20.
7. Luce, J. (1995). Physicians do not have a responsibility to provide futile or unreasonable care if a patient or family insists. *Crit. Care Med.*, **23**, 760–6.
8. Bosk, C. (1979). *Forgive and remember*, pp. 29–30. University of Chicago Press, Chicago, IL.
9. Little, M. (2001). Invited commentary: is there a distinctively surgical ethics? *Surgery*, **129**, 668–71.
10. American College of Surgeons, Statement on Principles available online at www.facs.org.
11. Angelos, P. (2000). A lesson in doctoring. *Focus on Surg. Educ.*, **17**.

Chapter 4

The physiological response to surgical trauma

Matthew D. Barber and Kenneth C.H. Fearon

There is a circumstance attending accidental injury which does not belong to disease, namely that the injury done, has in all cases a tendency to produce, both the disposition and means of cure.

John Hunter (1794)

Following surgical trauma a series of metabolic changes occur locally and systemically with the intention of restoring the *status quo*. The local response of inflammation and wound healing is supported by a generalized response to provide an optimal infrastructure for homeostasis by conserving fluid and providing energy and amino acids for repair.

The father of the modern study of the metabolic response to injury was the Scottish physiologist Sir David Cuthbertson. Working with patients who had sustained long bone fractures, in the 1930s he described changes in urine biochemistry, energy expenditure, and protein metabolism in injured patients not seen in healthy individuals confined to bed. This led to his description of the classical ebb and flow phases of the response to injury.[1,2] The initial brief 'ebb' phase of reduced peripheral perfusion, hypometabolism, and low urine output and the 'flow' phase with hypermetabolism, fat and protein mobilization, urinary nitrogen excretion, and weight loss. Following this was the longer anabolic period with replenishment of body stores and ultimate restoration of normality (Figure 4.1).

In practical terms, it is management of the postoperative catabolic period of the flow phase which has concerned surgeons and physiologists, but recognition and attention to the other phases of injury response forms a part of optimal patient management and may speed the homeostatic process and thus prompt recovery.

In patients with terminal illness, limited life expectancy, and reduced metabolic reserves, it is important to recognise the nature of the metabolic response likely to be generated by surgery as any delay in recovery has a profound effect on the palliative nature of a procedure.

Initiation of the metabolic response to surgery

During surgery, a number of stimuli may occur which help induce a metabolic response. These include:

- volume depletion with loss of circulating volume through bleeding, evaporation from exposed viscera, weeping from raw surfaces and local oedema and inflammation at the diseased site, and dehydration, producing stimulation of arterial pressure receptors and cardiac volume receptors
- nerve stimulation at the site of surgery, notably from pain impulses transmitted to the hypothalamus and other parts of the brain

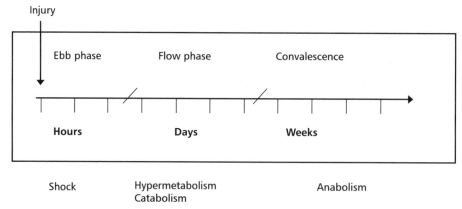

Fig. 4.1 Phases of the physiological response to injury.[1]

- the release of bacteria or their products from infected tissue, from gut spillage, or from translocation across an ischaemic or damaged gut leading to secondary mediator release
- direct damage caused by surgery causing the local release of inflammatory mediators at the site of surgical injury, including prostaglandins, cytokines, and kinins, and exposing tissues to inflammatory cells from the circulation
- relative tissue underperfusion as a result of volume loss or initial sympathetic pressor responses.

The importance of these agents in stimulating the metabolic response lies in the fact that they may be manipulated, reduced, or even abolished, producing a profound effect on the resultant response and therefore the recovery of the patient.

Mediators of the metabolic response to surgery

The stimuli outlined above result in the production of a cascade of mediators producing broad metabolic changes. A variety of insults, including non-surgical trauma, infection, cancer, and inflammatory diseases, result in the production of similar mediators and a similar stereotyped response. The mediators of the metabolic response are divided into complementary neuroendocrine and cytokine groups (Figure 4.2). Prominent neuroendocrine mediators whose circulating concentrations increase include cortisol, epinephrine, glucagon, aldosterone, and vasopressin/antidiuretic hormone (ADH). These catabolic hormones are referred to as 'counter-regulatory'. Meanwhile, the concentration of insulin, the main anabolic hormone, falls.

Neural stimulation from the site of injury acts via the hypothalamus, resulting in release of adrenocorticotrophic hormone (ACTH) which simulates cortisol release from the adrenal cortex.[3] Neuronal stimulation of the hypothalmus from both arterial pressure sensors in the carotid artery and volume sensors in the right atrium also add to the release of ACTH.

ADH release from the posterior pituitary is stimulated by atrial volume receptors as a result of the fall in circulating volume, neuronal pain stimuli via the hypothalamus, and anterior hypothalamic osmoreceptors. ADH acts on the collecting tubules of the kidneys and to a lesser extent on the distal tubule to promote the reabsorption of water. Aldosterone is produced from the adrenal cortex largely in response to the renin–angiotensin system. Renin is released from the juxtaglomerular cells of the kidney due to a reduction in arteriolar inflow pressure detected by these cells, reduction in sodium concentration in the distal tubule detected by the macula densa adjacent to the juxtaglomerular cells, and by increased sympathetic nervous activity. Renin initiates the cleavage of a cascade of angiotensins, the primary active molecule thought to be angiotensin II. In addition to vasopressor activity, angiotensin II acts on the adrenal cortex to produce aldosterone. Aldosterone acts principally on the distal renal tubules to promote reabsorption of sodium and bicarbonate, with resultant increase in the excretion of potassium and hydrogen ions.

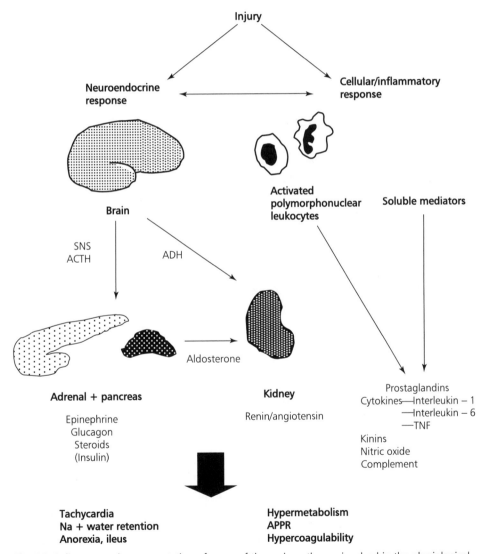

Fig. 4.2 A diagrammatic representation of some of the main pathways involved in the physiological response to injury. (TNF – tumour necrosis factor; ADH – antidiuretic hormone; ACTH – adrenocorticotrophic hormone; SNS – sympathetic nervous system; APPR – acute phase protein response.)

Experimental infusion of hormone combinations such as hydrocortisone (or cortisol), glucagon, and adrenaline in healthy volunteers will produce features of the metabolic response such as protein loss, an acute phase protein response, increased energy expenditure, and glucose intolerance.[4,5]

Many cytokines are involved in the inflammatory metabolic response and, indeed, in its resolution. The main pro-inflammatory cytokines include interleukin-1, interleukin-6, and tumour necrosis factor. Administration of these cytokines leads to features of the metabolic response to surgery, including anorexia, weight loss, an acute phase protein response, protein and fat breakdown, a rise in levels of cortisol and glucagon, and a fall in insulin concentration accompanied by insulin resistance.[6–12]

The importance attached to different mediators has waxed and waned over decades. Studies of blockade of single or small groups of mediators have demonstrated that no single mediator has predominance over any other. Rather there appears to be a web of overlap, redundancy, and mutual amplification (Figure 4.2).

Characteristics of the metabolic response to surgery

Changes in vital signs and symptoms

In response to surgery there is often an increase in pulse rate. This occurs due to catecholamine release (mainly epinephrine via cardiac β receptors) and may be accompanied by a widening in pulse pressure due to loss of circulating volume. The sympathetic response to fluid loss, involving mediators such as catecholamines, vasopressin/antidiuretic hormone, and angiotensin II, results in a constriction in arteriolar beds in muscle and skin, reducing peripheral perfusion (classically a norepinephrine effect via α receptors). This will result in the patient appearing cold and clammy with poor capillary refill. This corresponds to Cuthbertson's initial ebb phase of the metabolic response to injury. With fluid resuscitation the patient often becomes oedematous.

Later, as the patient enters the flow phase, they may appear warm and pink with an increase in body temperature. This reflects an increase in metabolic rate (see below) and a degree of resetting of the hypothalamic temperature regulation centre. Interleukin-1 has been implicated in this response.

With major surgery or the development of serious complications, patients may progress into the systemic inflammatory response syndrome with tachycardia, hypotension, and pyrexia with loss of the normal contractile ability of vascular smooth muscle. The latter is due to the synthesis of the potent vasodilator nitric oxide by endothelial cells.

Gastrointestinal effects

After surgery patients often become anorexic. While this may not be important if food consumption is to be delayed for a few days after bowel surgery, it may be important if the metabolic response to surgery is prolonged by complications, particularly in a patient who may already be nutritionally depleted or frankly cachectic. This anorexia is probably due in part to interleukin-1 acting at the level of the appetite control centre in the hypothalamus.

Abdominal surgery is often associated with a loss of gastrointestinal function in the form of a paralytic ileus. The small bowel often recovers within 24 hours, but effective gastrointestinal function depends on the recovery of the stomach and colon which may take several days longer.[13] Ileus is partly a local neurological response to handling of the bowel with somatovisceral and viscerovisceral reflex components. It is also part of the systemic response to surgery as mediated by catecholamines and cortisol. Gastrointestinal function is also suppressed by the administration of opioid drugs.

Water and salt retention

A reduction in urine output and retention of sodium occur as a response to surgical trauma. The kidneys are the primary route of excretion of sodium and potassium. Approximately 50–80 mmol of each ion are excreted in urine every 24 hours. In response to surgery, daily urinary sodium losses may fall to 10–20 mmol while potassium excretion may rise to 100–200 mmol. Primary mediators of this response include ADH, aldosterone, and cortisol.

Energy metabolism and substrate cycling

In simple starvation there is a compensatory fall in resting energy expenditure. However, in the palliative care patient, starvation is rarely simple. Surgery is often required for an acute event such as obstruction or occurs on a background of a chronic problem such as cancer. In these circumstances, and in response to a traumatic injury such as surgery, there is a metabolic response to injury resulting in increased energy expenditure.[14,15] This occurs due to increases in protein synthesis, mobilization of energy stores, and cycling of substrates as outlined below. The importance of this increased resting energy expenditure on overall energy balance during a metabolic response is unclear as it may be accompanied by a reduction in the other components of total energy expenditure, namely dietary thermogenesis and physical activity.[16]

Carbohydrate metabolism

The body's store of carbohydrate consists of liver and muscle glycogen totalling around 300 g. In the absence of food intake this store lasts less than a day. Despite this, following surgery there is a period of hyperglycaemia due to breakdown of stored glycogen, gluconeogenesis from amino acids, and insulin resistance. Glucose is also recycled in the liver from lactate (derived from anaerobic metabolism) in the energy-requiring Cori cycle.

Catecholamines increase directly glycogenolysis and also suppress insulin release and stimulate glucagon production. Patients also become relatively insulin-resistant. This hormonal balance promotes amino acid release from muscle for gluconeogenesis.

Protein metabolism

Skeletal muscle provides the body's major labile protein reserve. In the perioperative period, amino acids are generally not available from dietary sources. Thus during the metabolic response to surgery, skeletal muscle is broken down to provide amino acids for gluconeogenesis in the liver and to act as both substrate for protein synthesis for healing the wound and for the synthesis of defensive 'acute phase' proteins in the liver.[14,15,17,18] Thus overall protein synthesis may be increased but there is a greater increase in catabolism, resulting in negative nitrogen balance.

After surgery, urinary nitrogen excretion increases as protein is broken down for gluconeogenesis. In normal starvation the body adapts rapidly to preserve protein by utilizing ketone bodies and free fatty acids derived from fat for energy.[19,20] If the metabolic response to surgery is prolonged by factors such as infection then this adaptation may be impaired and protein breakdown prolonged. About a fifth of the body's protein may be lost over a three-week recovery from a traumatic insult.[14,15]

Fat metabolism

Fat in the form of triglyceride in adipose tissue provides a large, relatively dense store of energy. Fat oxidation is increased during a metabolic response to provide energy.[14] Triglyceride is broken down by lipase whose activity is stimulated by catecholamines, glucagon, and cortisol.

The acute phase protein response

The acute phase protein response is a reprioritization of liver protein synthesis often seen in trauma (including surgery), cancer, inflammation, and infection.[21,22] The acute phase protein response is stimulated by pro-inflammatory cytokines, notably interleukin-6.[23] It is characterized by a fall in the concentration of negative acute phase proteins such as albumin and transferrin and a rise in positive acute phase proteins including C-reactive protein and fibrinogen. In general, acute phase proteins aid tissue repair, blood clotting, the prevention of ongoing tissue damage, and the destruction of infective organisms.[22] While the concentrations of proteins such as albumin may fall, this does not appear to result in metabolic sparing as synthesis continues at the same rate.[24,25]

It has been suggested that the breakdown of muscle protein to support acute phase protein synthesis may be exaggerated as there is an imbalance between the amino acid composition of skeletal muscle and acute phase proteins.[26] It has been assumed that the provision of nutrients during the metabolic response may reduce the need for skeletal muscle breakdown, however there is some evidence that feeding in the presence of a metabolic response may actually further stimulate the synthesis of acute phase proteins.[25] This may account, in part, for the suboptimal anabolic response to nutritional support during ongoing inflammation (Figure 4.3).

Changes in blood coagulation

After surgery, patients become hypercoagulable. This occurs as a result of increased platelet number and adhesiveness, and increased concentrations of fibrinogen and complement activation. These are stimulated by catecholamines, cortisol, and cytokines. Hypercoagulability is exacerbated by malignancy and immobility.

The anabolic phase

With uncomplicated recovery from surgery, continued catabolism to mobilize body stores becomes no longer necessary and the patient reaches a 'turning point'. It is often obvious clinically as the patient begins to feel better, regains their appetite, and has a diuresis. Concentrations of catabolic mediators fall and insulin concentrations increase. With time, stores of protein and fat are restored. In the palliative care patient a prompt turning point is a crucial factor in the palliative intent of any surgical procedure. Unfortunately, palliative care patients are often susceptible to a number of factors which may prolong the metabolic response to surgery as outlined below.

Appropriateness of the metabolic response to surgery

Water and sodium retention have evolved to preserve circulating volume while excess potassium released from damaged cells is excreted. Changes in carbohydrate, protein, and fat metabolism, including the acute phase response, occur to provide fuel and raw materials for inflammation, defence, and repair. Hypercoagulability should ensure prompt arrest of traumatic bleeding. These changes have evolved over thousands of years as an appropriate

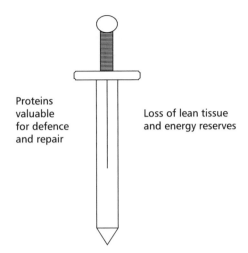

Proteins
valuable
for defence
and repair

Loss of lean tissue
and energy reserves

Fig. 4.3 The acute phase protein response. A double-edged sword?

defence to preserve life and promote recovery following injury. However, they evolved in an environment without hospital availability and without planned surgical intervention. They also evolved in an environment where those with depleted metabolic reserves and terminal illness were not likely to survive. In the circumstances of modern, hospital-based, surgical care where the trauma of surgery is relatively controlled and fluid and nutritional support may be given, the metabolic response to surgery may be a double-edged sword causing catabolism without perceptible benefit (Figure 4.3). In palliative care patients these factors are of profound importance in effect-ing the palliative outcome of surgery and therefore any decision to operate.

Perioperative factors modifying the metabolic response to surgery

The magnitude and duration of the metabolic response following surgery is modified by a variety of factors. These include:

- *The magnitude of surgery.* In general, the greater the extent and duration of surgery the greater the response. With longer operations, loss of heat and fluid by evaporation during surgery are added to loss of blood, more extensive tissue dissection (and therefore damage), and more prolonged artificial ventilation. Mild hypothermia due to surgery is associated with increased blood loss, wound infection, and protein loss.[27]

- *Co-existing disease.* Patients requiring surgery for palliation, usually for advanced cancer, often already have a demonstrable metabolic response. This may disguise or potentiate some of the changes attributable to surgery but will also have depleted the metabolic reserves of the patient prior to any surgical intervention. Such patients may also have disease of other systems potentially affecting respiratory, cardiac, or renal function, therefore influencing any metabolic response and also the safety of surgery.

- *Infection* also produces a metabolic response of its own, potentiating the catabolic phase until it has resolved.

- *Surgical complications*, including bleeding, infection, haematoma, deep venous thrombosis, pressure sores, and myocardial infarction, will prolong the metabolic response and, ironically, some may be made more likely by the metabolic response.[28,29]

- *Nutritional status.* The majority of patients requiring palliative surgery are nutritionally depleted. Frequently contributing to this is a pre-existing metabolic response to cancer such that the reserve of metabolic substrates of malnourished patients is already depleted, leading to potentially more severe repercussions from the ensuing additive effects of the metabolic response to surgery. Surgical patients with over 10% weight loss have been shown to be at increased risk of complications, particularly of respiratory tract infection, with longer hospital stay.[28,29] The depth of the metabolic deficit to be refilled in recovery is greater and so takes a larger proportion of the patient's limited lifespan.

- *Anaesthesia and drugs* have the potential to affect the metabolic response to surgery, for example morphine stimulates ADH release and prolongs paralytic ileus. However, the particular importance of these factors is their potential to attenuate the metabolic response by measures such as fluid replacement and regional anaesthesia.

Planning surgery, patient understanding, and consent

As outlined above, palliative care patients coming to surgery are often nutritionally depleted, may be immunosuppressed after oncological treatment, and may have a pre-existing metabolic response to their illness which will not abate even after apparent recovery from surgery. While a gastrointestinal obstruction may be physically bypassed, this will not provide benefit for the patient if full gastrointestinal function does not return due to the metabolic response to surgery or disease. The extent and nature of surgery must be clearly thought out by the surgeon, bearing in mind the likely metabolic effects the surgery will produce and how this will affect the recovery of a patient with a limited lifespan. Non-surgical or less invasive options may be explored, including endoscopic stenting of colonic and oesophageal obstructions and medical treatment of small bowel obstructions.[30] These issues should be discussed with oncology, radiology, and anaesthetic colleagues and explored with the patient and their relatives in simple terms to allow them to participate in the decision-making process and provide true informed consent.

Modulation of the metabolic response to surgery

While every effort must be made to prevent complications in a group of patients who may be especially prone to such problems, the key to minimising the metabolic response to surgery appears to be in its prevention rather than cure. The extent of the metabolic response to surgery is extremely variable and dependent on many factors previously discussed. By controlling these factors as much as possible it should be feasible to reduce the extent of the response.

Thromboembolic prophylaxis

Palliative care patients, usually with poor mobility and advanced cancer, are at high risk of thromboembolic complications which will produce their own metabolic response, prolonging recovery. Local guidelines for prophylaxis should be followed, usually involving the wearing of compression stockings and the administration of subcutaneous heparin with consideration of intermittent calf compression during surgery.[31]

Preoperative carbohydrate loading

It has been suggested that traditional preoperative fasting exacerbates the metabolic effects of surgery, particularly increased insulin resistance. In an attempt to minimize this effect, studies have been performed of the provision of carbohydrate-rich drinks two hours prior to surgery. These have resulted in no additional anaesthetic problems and substantial attenuation of the decrease in insulin sensitivity normally seen following surgery. These patients still exhibit other features of the metabolic response to surgery such as increased energy expenditure and increased cortisol and glucagon concentrations.[32,33]

Fluid resuscitation

Adequate fluid resuscitation prior to and during surgery will help attenuate the stimulation of the ebb phase of the metabolic response and so should reduce the severity and duration of catabolism. However, inappropriate overprescription of fluids, particularly saline, can lead to significant fluid retention, gut dysfunction, and prolongation of hospital stay.[34]

Regional anaesthesia

Afferent neural stimuli are a potent stimulator of the metabolic response to surgery. This has led to interest in the effects of blockade of these signals. Epidural local anaesthetic blockade during abdominal procedures appears to reduce the release of a variety of metabolic mediators, including catecholamines and cortisol. While it may complicate fluid balance by causing lower body vasodilatation, prolonged epidural blockade for 24–48 hours after surgery reduces protein catabolism, lipolysis, and hypermetabolism.[35,36] A recent meta-analysis has suggested a substantial reduction in morbidity in patients undergoing regional rather than general anaesthesia.[37] It has been shown to be possible to discharge patients about two days after colonic cancer resection after maintaining epidural anaesthesia until the second morning after surgery.[38] Postoperative paralytic ileus may also be reduced by prolonged epidural blockade.[13] In contrast, epidural opioid administration appears to have minimal influence on the metabolic response.

Appropriate surgery

Repeated operations or the incomplete surgical eradication of sepsis are recipes for metabolic disaster, exacerbating and prolonging the metabolic response and increasing mortality. This is particularly important in the palliative care patient with limited reserves and finite survival. If the decision is made to operate, every attempt should be made to do one operation and do it right.

Minimal access surgery

Consideration should be given to a laparoscopic approach to abdominal surgery. As long as it does not unduly prolong surgery and bearing in mind that a pneumoperitoneum may increase the risk of lower body venous thrombosis, laparoscopic surgery may reduce the metabolic impact of surgery probably by reducing the size of the wound. Comparing laparoscopic with open elective gallbladder surgery, reduction in postoperative interleukin-6 concentrations has been noted after laparoscopic cholecystectomy with a corresponding reduction in the acute phase response as measured by C-reactive protein concentration.[39,40] A similar reduction in postoperative interleukin-6 concentrations has also been shown after laparoscopic colonic resection.[41]

Laparoscopic surgery in malignancy was thought to have some specific detrimental effects, in particular the appearance of metastases at port sites.[42] However, this is now thought to be less of a problem and this is unlikely to be a major concern in the palliative care setting.

Alternative anaesthetic and analgesic drugs

Newer volatile and intravenous anaesthetics such as desflurane, sevoflurane, and propofol and short-acting analgesics such as remifentanyl may allow rapid recovery with a reduction in the hangover effect of traditional anaesthetics and a reduced incidence of postoperative nausea and vomiting.

Non-steroidal anti-inflammatory drugs (NSAIDs) should in theory suppress some of the mediators of the metabolic response to surgery. A reduction in ACTH and cortisol release and interleukin-6 concentrations has been documented following cholecystectomy after pretreatment with ibuprofen.[43] Clinical benefits of this have been more difficult to demonstrate but the use of NSAIDs may allow reduced doses of opioids with their suppressant effect on gastrointestinal function. However, care should be taken with the side-effects of NSAIDs such as gastrointestinal bleeding and platelet dysfunction.

Specific pharmacological intervention

While a network of cytokines appears to play an important role in the metabolic response to injury, specific anti-cytokine treatments have not been shown to affect the inflammatory process in septic patients. Antibodies to tumour necrosis factor and interleukin-1 receptor antagonist have been studied in large groups of patients.[44–46] It is likely that the redundancy and overlap of the cytokine network limits the value of such specific treatments.

Steroids are also known for their anti-inflammatory effects and a reduction in inflammatory mediators and improved outcome have been demonstrated following oesophageal resection with a single, high dose of methylprednisolone.[47] However, steroids have numerous side-effects, including immunosuppression, and their use is not routine following major surgery.

Growth hormone has been administered to patients undergoing major surgery in an attempt to promote anabolism, although concentrations are often normal or high following surgery. On its own it appears to have little effect but in combination with nutritional support, usually via the parenteral route, it may be of some benefit, resulting in less loss of weight and protein than providing nutrition alone (with some studies managing to abolish negative nitrogen balance).[48–51] However, once a systemic inflammatory response has developed, administration of growth hormone has been shown to increase mortality.[52,53]

Insulin has also been administered perioperatively and following trauma in an attempt to attenuate the catabolic response. Following surgery there appears to be some normalisation of glucose metabolism and a reduction in concentrations of cortisol and glucagon.[54] Following trauma, insulin infusion does stimulate protein synthesis and so reduces net protein loss, but only in severely catabolic patients.[55,56] The place of these hormonal interventions in palliative surgery is not clear, but it is only likely to be appropriate in those with a moderate life expectancy undergoing very major surgery. Recently, a study of surgical patients in intensive care has suggested that tight control of glucose concentrations by insulin infusion may reduce mortality.[57]

Early mobilization

Bed rest produces a degree of protein catabolism and predisposes to surgical complications, including venous thromboembolism, chest infection, urinary tract infection, and pressure sores.[58] While there is no evidence that mobilization helps gastrointestinal function or attenuates the metabolic response, it is a crucial part of rehabilitating the palliative care patient.

Postoperative nutrition

The early resumption of food intake (as early as six hours after colonic surgery) seems to have a small but significant effect on the return of gastrointestinal activity, in some cases hastening hospital discharge.[13,38,59]

A positive nitrogen balance can probably not be achieved in the catabolic phase of the metabolic response to injury by the provision of nutrients by any means. It has been shown that the anabolic response to nutrition is absent in cancer patients in contrast with healthy individuals as a result of the metabolic response to cancer producing a block to the repletion of lean tissue.[60] However, net protein loss may be reduced by parenteral nutrition.[61] The provision of parenteral nutrition has significant complications and is only of value if given for at least 7–10 days. Thus parenteral nutrition has only a limited role in the perioperative palliative care patient. In patients with advanced cancer, a pre-existing metabolic response to the malignancy may reduce any potential benefit of conventional nutritional support.[62] The potential benefit of nutritional supplementation in combination with growth hormone is discussed above.

A number of modified oral nutritional supplements enriched with specific fuels, such as glutamine or arginine, or anti-inflammatory agents such as fish oil, have been studied in the perioperative and palliative care setting. Reductions in infective complications and hospital stay have been shown in patients with upper gastrointestinal cancer undergoing surgery given oral nutritional supplementation containing a combination of the above nutrients,[63,64] although the benefit appears to be largely in more depleted patients undergoing more major surgery. A study of a nutritional supplement enriched with fish oil in advanced pancreatic cancer has shown a gain in weight, lean body mass, and performance status in patients losing weight as a result of the metabolic response to their tumour.[65] Measures of inflammation suggested some down-regulation of the metabolic response. This preparation has not been studied in the perioperative setting.

Summary of management options

The surgical management of individual palliative care patients must be tailored to their individual case. It seems sensible that simple measures such as thromboembolic prophylaxis, fluid resuscitation, and prompt mobilization be used in every case. Consideration of regional anaesthesia is appropriate for the majority of cases and minimal access surgery for some. The place of more specific interventions such as hormone infusions and modified nutrition remains unclear and will probably only be appropriate for a few more severely catabolic patients undergoing more major surgery. Clearly the appropriateness of such surgery in such an unwell palliative care patient must be carefully considered.

Conclusion

In surgery with palliative intent it is crucial that the metabolic response, in particular the catabolic phase, is as minimal in extent and as short in duration as possible so that a normal metabolic environment is restored as promptly as possible. While the metabolic response to surgery in particular and injury in general has evolved to preserve circulating volume, promote haemostasis, and mobilise body stores for healing, its value in a modern surgical setting is questionable, particularly in the palliative care patient in whom speedy recovery is vital. Various measures exist to minimise the extent of the metabolic response to surgery and these should be heeded as part of the management of the palliative care patient.

References

1. Cuthbertson, D.P. (1935). Further observations on the disturbance of metabolism caused by injury, with particular reference to the dietary requirements of fracture cases. *Br. J. Surg.*, **23**, 505–20.
2. Cuthbertson, D.P. (1942). Post-shock metabolic response. *Lancet.*, **I**, 433–7.
3. Hume, D.M., and Egdahl, R.H. (1959). Importance of the brain in the endocrine response to injury. *Ann. Surg.*, **150**, 697–712.
4. Bessey, P.Q., Watters, J.M., Aoki, T.T., and Wilmore, D.W. (1984). Combined hormonal infusion simulates the metabolic response to injury. *Ann. Surg.*, **200**, 264–81.
5. Watters, J.M., Bessey, P.Q., Dinarello, C.A., Wolff, S.M., and Wilmore, D.W. (1986). Both inflammatory and endocrine mediators stimulate host responses to sepsis. *Arch. Surg.*, **121**, 179–90.
6. Selby, P., Hobbs, S., Viner, C., Jackson, E., Jones, A., Newall, D. *et al.* (1987). Tumour necrosis factor in man: clinical and biological observations. *Br. J. Cancer*, **56**, 803–8.
7. Michie, H.R., Spriggs, D.R., Manogue, K.R., Sherman, M.L., Revhaug, A., O'Dwyer, S.T., *et al.* (1988). Tumor necrosis factor and endotoxin induce similar metabolic responses in human beings. *Surgery*, **104**, 280–6.
8. Moldawer, L.L., Andersson, C., Gelin, J., and Lundholm, K.G. (1988). Regulation of food intake and hepatic protein synthesis by recombinant-derived cytokines. *Am. J. Physiol.*, **254**, G450–G456.
9. Morrone, G., Ciliberto, G., Oliviero, S., Arcone, R., Dente, L., Content, J., *et al.* Recombinant interleukin-6 regulates the transcriptional activation of a set of human acute phase genes. *J. Biol. Chem.*, **263**, 12554–8.
10. Starnes, H.F., Warren, R.S., Jeevanandam, M., Gabrilove, J.L., Larchian, W., Oettgen, H.F., *et al.* (1988). Tumor necrosis factor and the acute metabolic response to tissue injury in man. *J. Clin. Invest.*, **82**, 1321–5.
11. Ballmer, P.E., McNurlan, M.A., Southorn, B.G., Grant, I., and Garlick, P.J. (1991). Effects of human recombinant interleukin-1β on protein synthesis in rat tissues compared with a classical acute-phase reaction induced by turpentine. *Biochem. J.*, **279**, 683–8.
12. Stouthard, J.M.L., Romijn, J.A., van der Poll, T., Endert, E., Klein, S., Bakker, P.J.M., *et al.* (1995). Endocrinologic and metabolic effects of interleukin-6 in humans. *Am. J. Physiol.*, **268**, E813–E819.
13. Holte, K., and Kehlet, H. (2000). Postoperative ileus: a preventable event. *Br. J. Surg.*, **87**, 1480–93.
14. Monk, D.N., Plank, L.D., Franch-Arcas, G., Finn, P.J., Streat, S.J., and Hill, G.L. (1996). Sequential changes in the metabolic response in critically injured patients during the first 25 days after blunt trauma. *Ann. Surg.*, **223**, 395–405.
15. Plank, L.D., Connolly, A.B., and Hill, G.L. (1998). Sequential changes in the metabolic response in severely septic patients during the first 23 days after the onset of peritonitis. *Ann. Surg.*, **228**, 146–58.
16. Gibney, E., Jennings, G., Jebb, S.A., Murgatroyd, P.R., and Elia, M. (1997). Measurement of total energy expenditure in patients with lung cancer and validation of the bicarbonate-urea method against whole-body indirect calorimetry. *Proc. Nutr. Soc.*, **56**, 226A.
17. Aulick, L.H., and Wilmore, D.W. (1979). Increased peripheral amino acid release following burn injury. *Surgery*, **85**, 560–5.
18. Wilmore, D.W., Goodwin, C.W., Aulick, L.H., Powanda, M.C., Mason, A.D., and Pruitt, B.A. (1980). Effect of injury and infection on visceral metabolism and circulation. *Ann. Surg.*, **192**, 491–504.

19. Grande, F., Anderson, J.F., and Keys, A. (1958). Changes in basal metabolic rate in man in semistarvation and refeeding. *J. Appl. Physiol.*, **12**, 230–8.

20. Leibel, R.L., Rosenbaum, M., and Hirsch, J. (1995). Changes in energy expenditure resulting from altered body weight. *N. Engl. J. Med.*, **332**, 621–8.

21. Fleck, A., Colley, M., Myers, M.A. (1985). Liver export proteins and trauma. *Brit. Med. Bull.*, **41**, 265–73.

22. Baumann H., and Gauldie, J. (1994). The acute phase response Imm. Today, *15*, 74–80.

23. Castell, J.V., Gómez–Lechón. M.J., David, M., Fabra, R., Trullengue, R., Heinrich, P.C. (1990) acute–phase response of human hepatocytes: regulation of acute–phase protein synthesis by interleukin 6, *Hepatology*, **12**, 1179–86.

24. Fearon, K.C.H., Falconer, J.S., Slater, C., McMillan, D.C., Ross, J.A., and Preston, T. (1998). Albumin synthesis rates are not decreased in hypoalbuminemic cachectic cancer patients with an ongoing acute-phase protein response. *Ann. Surg.*, **227**, 249–54.

25. Barber, M.D., Fearon, K.C.H., McMillan, D.C., Slater, C., Ross, J.A., and Preston, T. (2000). Liver export protein synthetic rates are increased by oral meal feeding in weight-losing cancer patients. *Am. J. Physiol.*, **279**, E707–E714.

26. Reeds, P.J., Fjeld, C.R., Jahoor, F. (1994). Do the differences between the amino acid composition of acute–phase and muscle proteins have a bearing on nitrogen losses in traumatic states? *J. Nutrition*, **124**, 906–10.

27. Sessler, D.I. (1997). Mild operative hypothermia. *N. Engl. J. Med.*, **336**, 1730–7.

28. Windsor, J.A., and Hill, G.L. (1988). Weight loss with physiologic impairment. A basic indicator of surgical risk. *Ann. Surg.*, **207**, 290–6.

29. Windsor, J.A., and Hill, G.L. (1988). Risk factors for postoperative pneumonia. The importance of protein depletion. *Ann. Surg.*, **208**, 209–14.

30. Hardy, J.R. (2000). Medical management of bowel obstruction. *Br. J. Surg.*, **87**, 1281–3.

31. Scottish Intercollegiate Guidelines Network (1995). *Prophylaxis of venous thromboembolism.* SIGN, Edinburgh.

32. Nygren, J.O., Soop, M., Thorell, A., Efendic, S., Nair, K.S., and Ljungqvist, O. (1998). Preoperative oral carbohydrate administration reduces postoperative insulin resistance. *Clin. Nutr.*, **17**, 65–71.

33. Soop, M., Nygren, J.O., Myrenfors, P., Thorell, A., and Ljungqvist, O. (2001). Preoperative oral carbohydrate treatment attenuates immediate postoperative insulin resistance. *Am. J. Physiol.*, **280**, E576–E583.

34. Lobo, D.N., Bostock, K.A., Neal, K.R., Perkins, A.C., Rowlands, B.J., and Allison, S.P. (2001). Effect of salt and water on gastrointestinal function and outcome after abdominal surgery: a prospective randomised controlled study. *Clin. Nutr.*, **20** (3), 35.

35. Carli, F., and Halliday, D. (1997). Continuous epidural blockade arrests the postoperative decrease in muscle protein fractional synthetic rates in surgical patients. *Anaesthesiology*, **86**, 1033–40.

36. Kehlet, H. (2000). Manipulation of the metabolic response in clinical practice. *World J. Surg.*, **24**, 690–705.

37. Rodgers, A., Walker, N., Schug, S., McKee, A., Kehlet, H., van Zundert, A., *et al.* (2000). Reduction in postoperative mortality and morbidity with epidural or spinal anaesthesia: results from an overview of randomised trials. *B.M.J.* **321**, 1493–7.

38. Basse, L., Hjort Jakobsen, D., Billesbolle, P., Werner, M., and Kehlet, H. (2000). A clinical pathway to accelerate recovery after colonic resection. *Ann. Surg.*, **232**, 50–7.

39. Joris, J., Cigarini, I., Legrand, M., Jacquet, N., De Groote, D., Franchimont, P., *et al.* (1992). Metabolic and respiratory changes after cholecystectomy performed via laparotomy or laparoscopy. *Br. J. Anaesth.*, **69**, 341–5.

40. Maruszynski, M., and Pojda, Z. (1995). Interleukin-6 (IL-6) levels in the monitoring of surgical trauma. *Surg. Endosc.*, **9**, 882–5.

41. Harmon, G.D., Senagore, A.J., Kilbride, M.J., and Warzynski, M.J. (1994). Interleukin-6 response to laparoscopic and open colectomy. *Dis. Colon Rectum*, **37**, 754–9.

42. Vittimberga, F.J., Foley, D.P., Meyers, W.C., and Callery, M.P. Laparoscopic surgery and the systemic immune response. *Ann. Surg.*, **227**, 326–34.

43. Chambrier, C., Shassard, D., Bienvenu, J., Saudin, F., Paturel, D., Garrique, C., *et al.* (1996). Cytokine and hormonal changes after cholecystectomy: effect of ibuprofen pretreatment. *Ann. Surg.*, **224**, 178–82.

44. Abraham, E.A., Wunderink, R., Silverman, H., Perl, T., Nasraway, S., Levy, H., *et al.* (1995). Efficacy and safety of monoclonal antibody to human tumor necrosis factor-α (in patients with sepsis syndrome): a randomised, controlled, double-blind, multicenter trial. *J.A.M.A.*, **273**, 934–41.

45. Cohen, J. and Carlet, J. (1996). INTERSEPT: An international, multicenter, placebo-controlled trial of monoclonal antibody to human tumor necrosis factor-α in patients with sepsis. *Crit. Care Med.*, **24**, 1431–40.

46. Opal, S.M., Fisher, C.J., Dhainaut, J-F.A., Vincent, J-L., Brase, R., Lowry, S.F., *et al.* (1997). Confirmatory interleukin-1 receptor antagonist trial in severe sepsis: a phase III, randomised, double-blind, placebo-controlled, multi-center trial. *Crit. Care Med.*, **25**, 1115–24.

47. Taketa, S., Ogawa, W.R., Nakanishi, K., Kim, C., Miyashita, M., Sasajima, K., *et al.* (1997). The effect of preoperative high-dose methylprednisolone in attenuating the metabolic response after oesophageal resection. *Eur. J. Surg.*, **163**, 511.

48. Jiang, Z-M., He, G-Z., Zhang, S-Y., Wang, X-R., Yang, N.F., Zhu, Y., *et al.* (1989). Low-dose growth hormone and hypocaloric nutrition attenuate the protein-catabolic response after major operation. *Ann. Surg.*, **210**, 513–24.

49. Vara-Thorbeck, R., Guerrero, J.A., Ruiz-Requena, M.E., Capitán, J., Rodriguez, M., Rosell, J., *et al.* (1992). Effects of growth hormone in patients receiving total parenteral nutrition following major gastrointestinal surgery. *Hepatogastroenterology*, **39**, 270–2.

50. Wong, W., Soo, K., Nambiar, R., Tan, Y.S., Yo, S.L., and Tan, I.K. (1995). The effect of recombinant growth hormone on nitrogen balance in malnourished patients after major abdominal surgery. *Aust N.Z.J. Surg.*, **65**, 109–13.

51. Connolly, A.B., and Vernon, D.R. (2000). Manipulations of the metabolic response for management of patients with severe surgical illness: review. *World J. Surg.*, **24**, 696–704.

52. Takala, J., Ruokonen, E., Webster, N.R., Nielsen, M.S., Zandstra, D.F., Vendelinckx, G., *et al.* (1999). Increased mortality associated with growth hormone treatment in critically ill adults. *N. Engl. J. Med.*, **341**, 785–92.

53. Ruokonen, E., and Takala, J. (2000). Dangers of growth hormone therapy in critically ill patients. *Ann. Med.*, **32**, 317–22.

54. Nygren, J.O., Thorell, A., Soop, M., Efendic, S., Brismar, K., Karpe, F., *et al.* (1998). Perioperative insulin and glucose infusion maintains normal insulin sensitivity after surgery. *Am. J. Physiol.*, **275**, E140–E148.

55. Woolfson, A.M.J., Heatley, R.V., and Allison, S.P. (1979). Insulin to inhibit protein catabolism after surgery. *N. Engl. J. Med.*, **300**, 14–17.

56. Sakurai, Y., Aarsland, A., Herndon, D.N., Chinkes, D.L., Pierre, E., Nguyen, T.T., *et al.* Stimulation of muscle protein synthesis by long-term insulin infusion in severely burned patients. *Ann. Surg.*, **222**, 283–97.

57. van den Berge, G., Wouters, P., Weekers, F., Verwaest, C., Bruyninckx, F., Schetz, M., *et al.* (2001). Intensive insulin therapy in critically ill patients. *N. Engl. J. Med.*, **345**, 1359–67.

58. Harper, C.M., and Lyles, Y.M. (1988). Physiology and complications of bed rest. *J. Am. Geriatr. Soc.*, **36**, 1047–54.

59. Wilmore, D.W., and Kehlet, H. (2001). Management of patients in fast track surgery. *B.M.J.*, **322**, 473–6.

60. Nixon, D.W., Lawson, D.H., Kutner, M., Ansley, J., Schwarz, M., Heymsfield, S., *et al.* (1981). Hyperalimentation of the cancer patient with protein-calorie undernutrition. *Cancer Res.*, **41**, 2038–45.

61. Shaw, J.H.F., and Wolfe, R.R. (1989). An integrated analysis of glucose, fat, and protein metabolism in severely traumatised patients: studies in the basal state and the response to intravenous nutrition. *Ann. Surg.*, **207**, 63072.

62. Barber, M.D., and Fearon, K.C.H. (1998). Should cancer patients with incurable disease receive parenteral or enteral nutritional support? *Eur. J. Cancer*, **34**, 279–82.

63. Heys, S.D., Walker, L.G., Smith, I., and Eremin, O. (1999). Enteral nutritional supplementation with key nutrients in patients with critical illness and cancer. A meta-analysis of randomised controlled clinical trials. *Ann. Surg.*, **229**, 467–77.

64. Beale, R.J., Bryg, D.J., and Bihari, D.J. (1999). Immunonutrition in the critically ill: a systematic review of clinical outcome. *Crit. Care Med.*, **27**, 2799–805.

65. Barber, M.D., Ross, J.A., Voss, A.C., Tisdale, M.J., and Fearon, K.C.H. (1999). The effect of an oral nutritional supplement enriched with fish oil on weight loss in patients with pancreatic cancer. *Br. J. Cancer*, **81**, 80–6.

Chapter 5

Psychological response to surgery

Laurie Stevens

Introduction

Medical practitioners deal on a daily basis with the psychological needs and responses of their patients. Practitioners of surgical palliative care, like other medical practitioners, must have a keen eye, intuitive sense, know the right questions to ask of the patient, and the good sense to learn from their own past experiences with an individual patient and with their patients in general.

There is currently little guidance on psychiatric and psychological issues specifically for patients undergoing surgical palliation in the context of interdisciplinary care and when disease is not identified as the enemy. At best we can project what this guidance would be based on our knowledge of surgery and psychiatry as it is, only viewed from the perspective that suffering, not disease, is the opponent.

The aim of this chapter is to provide palliative care practitioners with the tools by which they can determine how best to assess and handle their patient's capacity to tolerate the necessary surgical procedure to treat their symptoms, and what to expect in the postoperative period as the patient continues to face life-limiting illness.

The focus of this chapter will include discussion of preoperative and postoperative psychological issues and how they can contribute to difficulties in caring for patients, the effect of body image issues on the terminally ill patient, and the emotional problems that face both patients and health care-givers during this period of life.

In order to understand how psychological processes may affect patients' reactions to surgery, the foundation must be laid for the understanding of the psyche – how it is formed and how it works, the development of body image, how personality structure may affect patients' experience of surgery and alteration of their body image, and, of course, patients' feelings about having a life-threatening illness and its impact on their lives and the lives of those around them.

The surgeon's difficult role

The surgeon may take on, even when providing palliative care, more of the role of the mutilator than the role more favoured by the surgeon, that of the saviour.[1] Perceived threats to a person's life and body integrity and the surgeon's inability to guarantee a good outcome can produce profound feelings of anger towards the surgeon. The patient may also become depressed and/or anxious about the potential negative outcome and the surgeon's inability to do more than offer palliation – pain relief, relief of obstruction, debulking of a tumour, etc.

Even though patients may have coped well psychologically during their illness and treatment up until now, they may not be able to cope as adaptively with the recognition that the illness is terminal in nature. Anger, sadness, and guilty feelings may be prominent. The patients may be second-guessing their own treatment decisions as well as the advice given to them by their consultants, wondering if different choices had been offered and/or made, whether they would not be facing an imminent death.

One of the most difficult things that a surgeon or other care-givers must do is to tolerate their emotional experience of the patient without having to transform that experience immediately into action. Therefore, the surgeon must be able to tolerate anger, frustration, feelings of helplessness, hopelessness and despair, and fantasies of rescue and magical cures. The patients will desperately want the surgeon to provide magical remedies and solutions and rescue them from their inevitable death. Much as we may want to offer these to the patient, we must resist offering false hope and unrealistic expectations. The danger of magical thinking when selecting a given surgical procedure for palliation of symptoms is by no means limited to the patient. A surgeon can demonstrate the same maladaptive response when proposing a fix for a problem that far exceeds the biological capacities of the patient.

Patients will utilize all the defenses necessary for them to cope with their morbidity and mortality and we do them no favours but trying to strip these away. For example, the defense mechanism of denial is extremely helpful to most patients in coping with illness in general. Unless the patient is not participating in their treatment to their detriment, or is having magical expectations of a 'cure', we need do nothing in response to seeing a patient use denial as a coping strategy.

Patients with advanced illness inevitably have practical, legal, emotional, and spiritual concerns in addition to physical problems. A physician's guidance in these matters can be quite helpful as long as he recognizes his limitations. This includes but is not limited to the preparation of living wills, cooperation in insurance matters, and referrals to hospice or long-term care facilities. Although experienced palliative care practitioners recognize the importance of acknowledging their own vulnerabilities when addressing their patients' emotional needs, this can not be assumed of all practitioners, including surgeons, participating in the care of these patients. The two great fears shared by all patients with advancing disease are fear of loss of control (pain, autonomy, etc.) and fear of becoming a burden to others. These fears may be shared by care-takers as well. For example, obsession with control can motivate a surgeon to pursue aggressively an unwise or unwarranted operative procedure as much as it can motivate its acceptance by a patient with the same obsession. Fears of dependency upon others is often very anxiety-provoking for patients, especially when they have always been independent and self-sufficient. The surgeon may be equally afraid of the patient's dependency upon them for needs that may go far beyond the operating table. A great deal of psychological adjustment may need to take place in order to allow oneself to accept dependency, whether it's the patient accepting assistance in bodily hygiene or the surgeon accepting the guidance of other members of the interdisciplinary team. Dependency may be physical, psychological, or financial. A certain amount of regression is necessary for patients to allow themselves to be cared for when they are ill. However, the threat or fear of unending dependency is a wholly different matter which may bring about profound despair, anger, and a sense of helplessness.

The practitioner may not be able to offer much relief from these fears. However, we can try to help the patient to find ways to continue to function in an independent and autonomous fashion, even if physically or otherwise dependent. For example, the surgeon can suggest to the patient certain tasks, such as medical diary-keeping or colostomy appliance care, allowing them a feeling of participation in their own care and reinforcing their sense of autonomy.

Many practitioners struggle within themselves about how much emotion they will allow themselves to feel and/or to express. This can be particularly difficult for surgeons for whom 'coolness under fire' is a much lauded virtue. All physicians and surgeons have been trained to present a professional demeanor with our patients, which is ordinarily comforting to many patients. However, patients who are dying may experience this demeanor as cold and unfeeling. I have found that patients appreciate honesty and the expression of emotions, allowing them to feel a closer bond to you. You can offer compassion even when telling bad news and allow the patient to start the mourning process with you. After all, all of us do have feelings when our patients are dying and die, despite our attempts to block them out or cut them off.

Transference, counter-reaction and counter-transference

Surgeons are invested with very strong emotions from the patient by virtue of the fact that they are entrusting them with their body and their life. Patients may develop special feelings for their surgeons which are similar to those associated with figures of authority from their past.[2] This may account for the idealization of the surgeon as the 'miracle worker' or 'saviour' as well as for some of the unwarranted angry feelings toward the surgeon. This is a phenomenon known as 'transference'.

The nature of the doctor – patient relationship is extremely important to the success of the treatment of the terminally ill patient. Much as most physicians feel uncomfortable with the fact that patients develop feelings about them, it is important to recognize the phenomena of transference, counter-reaction, and counter-transference.

Transference can be described as the recreation in the doctor – patient relationship of a conflicted relationship with a childhood figure. The transference may be of a paternal or a maternal nature but not necessarily – grandparental, aunt/uncle, and sibling transferences can also occur. When transference is present, the patient will react to the doctor as if they are the transferential figure; in other words, feelings about that figure become 'transferred' onto the doctor. If the transference is positive, generally it need not be addressed. However, if the transference is negative, it does need evaluation.

An example of negative transference would be the patient treating the doctor as if they are sadistic, uncaring, cold, and heartless when the physician is trying his best to be empathic, warm, and caring. The patient is acting in an overly exaggerated fashion out of proportion to the real relationship. Oftentimes, the transference is not totally a distortion of the real relationship between the doctor and patient. The patient may have picked up on an aspect of the doctor's personality or behaviour that has served as the foundation for developing transferential feelings.

Counter-reaction is the doctor's emotional reaction to a patient's expression of feelings. For example, when the patient becomes angry with the doctor, the doctor may wish to withdraw or feel anger in response. The physician has to try to figure out how to respond better to the patient's feelings and responses, without personalizing them. This is easier said than done as physicians, like their patients, are only human and are prey to their own feelings and those of others towards them. Counter-reaction needs to be differentiated from *counter-transference* as it usually is a common or 'normal' response to the patient's emotions or behaviours.

On the other hand, counter-transference is the doctor's reaction to the patient not based on the real circumstances, but rather on issues or conflicted relationships in their own lives; if you will, a 'neurotic' response to a patient's transference. When these feelings occur, they may be quite intense for both the patient and the doctor. Recognizing these feelings and their origins is an important tool to have to improve your relationship with your patient and to avoid pitfalls in the treatment relationship, including the selection of specific treatments.

One example of counter-transference in the palliative care practitioner is the practitioner who has many fears, anxieties, and unsettled feelings about their own mortality and fears of illness or death. If the practitioners have not resolved such anxieties and fears, they may unwittingly interfere with their reaction to a patient's illness or impending death and maybe even their clinical judgement. Patients might be offered false hope and unrealistic expectations because the practitioner cannot let go and allow the patient to die in a dignified way, understanding the course of their illness and the inevitability of their death.

One of the most common reasons for consultation with a liaison psychiatrist in the treatment of the medically ill patient is difficulties in transference, counter-transference, acting out behaviour, and 'splitting' that patients induce between care-givers. 'Splitting' is a defense mechanism in which patients separates their 'good' feelings and objects from their 'bad'. A common example of splitting in medically ill patients is the phenomenon of alternating between overly idealizing staff members who meet their needs and devaluing those whom they feel are trying to frustrate their gratification. What may happen is that the patient complains about one staff member to another and creates a 'split' between staff members. The split then has to be healed by staff members by discussing the problem outside of the patient's presence, and endeavouring to present a unified front to the patient to prevent further splitting.

Speaking the unspeakable

Patients may be reluctant to ask certain questions of their doctor as they feel embarrassed, think their fears or worries are crazy, feel critical of their treatment, or fear their deaths. From 50 to 80% of terminally ill patients experience troubling thoughts or worries about death.[3] Physicians should not be afraid to use the 'D' word (Death). Weisman[4] offers the following points for helping the patient to have an 'appropriate death'. These points include:

- reducing internal conflicts, such as fears about loss of control, as much as possible
- helping the patient to sustain their personal sense of identity as much as possible
- continuing critical relationships and, if possible, resolving conflicted relationships (reconciliation with alienated people in their lives)
- setting realistic and meaningful goals, such as attending a family event like a graduation, in order to provide a sense of continuity of their life into the future.

Patients may sometimes feel that asking questions might be construed by the surgeon as their questioning the surgeon's decisions and competence. A good strategy may be to suggest to the patients that they may have ideas which they think are strange or fears that they worry you may think are silly. By doing this, you give them permission to voice these feelings without fear of humiliation or ridicule and often they feel much relieved and reassured.

Personality and character formation

Much has been written about how personality or character develops in human beings. We all have personality traits which characterize who we are and how we interact with the world. These traits govern how we perceive and relate to our environment and ourselves. These traits are consistent and stable despite outside stimuli and influences.

The ego is the chief executive of the mind, in charge of balancing the internal and external influences that confront it. These influences include memories, drives, anxieties, perceptions, and external needs. To function smoothly, the ego has to have a set of automatic operations which deal with these influences. These operations are called defence mechanisms.

Defence mechanisms

We use defence mechanisms to cope with the stresses of our internal and external worlds. These mechanisms are not under our conscious control and develop in response to our early life experiences. Our repertoire of defences contribute to our character formation and enable us to forget painful experiences, to minimize or deny anxiety-provoking situations, and to evade unwanted impulses (sexual and aggressive). For our purposes of understanding the surgical patient and their response to surgery, the defence mechanisms of regression, denial, projection, repression, distortion, somatization, intellectualization, sublimation, and rationalization will be discussed.[5] These defences are operational not only in the context of impending surgery but also in the context of the underlying illness.

Regression is a return to a previous stage of functioning or development in order to avoid anxiety or conflict. We see regression in both healthy and unhealthy adaptations to illness. Patients have to undergo some degree of regression in order to allow themselves to be cared for when ill and to be in a dependent position. However, regression may get to a pathological level when the patient acts in an infantile and helpless manner, and is unable to participate as a partner in their medical care.

Denial is being consciously unaware of a painful aspect of reality. Through denial, patients invalidate unpleasant or unwanted bits of information and act as though they do not exist. Denial, like regression, can be adaptive or maladaptive in the medical setting. For example, a certain degree of denial can function to allow a patient to cope with an overwhelming feeling of helplessness or hopelessness in response to a diagnosis of terminal cancer. Denial becomes maladaptive when it interferes with a patient's ability to participate in their medical care. Denial need not be confronted when a patient is accepting appropriate medical treatment and participating in their care. Denial can reach psychotic proportions in very psychiatrically ill individuals.

Projection is when one attributes one's unacknowledged feelings to others. Projection may be displayed by falsely attributing or misinterpreting attitudes, feelings, or intentions of others (e.g. 'I'm not angry at her; she's angry at me').

Repression involves keeping unwanted memories, thoughts, or feelings from conscious awareness. The patient who 'forgets' unpleasant news that the physician tells them is likely to be repressing the disturbing thoughts or feelings.

Distortion occurs when patients grossly reshape external reality to suit their inner needs, including magical beliefs and delusional thinking.

Somatization is when patients convert their psychic conflicts and conflicted feelings into bodily symptoms. The most common presentation of somatization is hypochondriasis.

Intellectualization is when the patient controls anxieties and impulses by excessive thinking about them rather than experiencing them. These thoughts are devoid of affect or feeling.

Sublimation is the transformation of drives, feelings, and memories into healthy and creative outcomes.

Rationalization is when the patient justifies their attitudes, beliefs, or behaviour that might be unacceptable by inventing a convincing fallacy.

The patient is not the only one who demonstrates these defences to the reality of progressive, incurable illness – surgical consultants threatened by the uncertainties of incurable illness in their patients can exhibit the same defence mechanisms observable in patients. For example, during a one-year follow-up visit by a patient upon whom the surgeon has performed a mastectomy for poorly differentiated carcinoma, the surgeon finds a hard ipsilateral axillary mass and observes it over several months, convinced it is 'scar tissue' (denial). Another example is the surgeon who insists on a major debulking procedure for a pelvic lesion in a severely malnourished patient with widely metastatic disease, despite the patient's reluctance, with the belief that the procedure will 'give the chemotherapy a better chance' (denial, distortion, and 'magical thinking'). The surgeon who becomes angry with the patient, blaming the patient for not getting better from the surgeon's interventions and treatments, may be projecting their own anger and helplessness to prevent the progression of the patient's disease. The 'somatizing' surgeon will diligently search only for physical causes for distress (more investigations, even operations!) in a patient when anxiety prevails as the basis for the distress. Another example of this is the beeline made by the surgeon for the terminally ill patient's obviously well-functioning drainage tube when the room is roaring with silence.

Psychological reactions to surgery

The preoperative period

Preoperatively, the patient needs careful assessment. The issues of greatest importance are the patients' understanding of their illness and the proposed surgical procedure, the patients' expectations of the surgical outcome, and the providing of informed consent.

Preoperative concerns include the threat to the sense of invulnerability, fears of entrusting one's life to a stranger, separation from their family and home, fears of loss of control, fears of death, and fears of bodily damage or mutilation.[6] After describing the procedure and the team's expectations of the outcome, the surgeon needs to assess whether the patient understands the proposed procedure. The surgeon should ask questions to assess the patient's comprehension. They should also assess whether the patients have realistic or unrealistic expectations of the surgery, and whether they are looking for 'magic' which the surgeon cannot provide. The surgery, if elective, should not be performed until the patient appears to understand that it is palliation that will be provided, not magic.

If the patient is unable to understand the procedure and its sequelae due to psychological problems (like denial of psychotic proportions, magical thinking, severe depression or anxiety interfering with cognitive processing) or organic problems (like dementia or delirium), family members will have to receive the same information and be included in the decision-making process. If you feel that patients are not competent to make a decision for themselves, it is necessary for psychiatric consultation to be obtained to document the patient's mental status.

The surgeon should take the necessary time to sit with the patient and answer all questions and concerns. It is usually helpful to specifically ask patients if they have any particular fears or concerns as many of these can be adequately addressed in the preoperative period, allowing postoperative adjustment to be smoother. If the surgeon expects any possible changes which could affect the patient's body image or functioning, like a colostomy, substantial loss of tissue or amputation, or changes in sexual functioning, it is imperative to prepare the patient in advance for these possible outcomes. This preparation may include preoperative referral to therapists skilled in the management of these problems.

Sexual issues may be particularly difficult for the surgeon and/or the patient to discuss. Surgeons may erroneously make the assumption that when faced with life and death issues or advancing age, sexual dysfunction is or should not be of concern to the patient. Surgeons may need to address their own discomfort with talking about sex in order to make the patient feel comfortable and to give the patient permission to voice these worries. Patients should be reassured that sexual functioning is like all other life functions and should be given similar priority.

Preoperative evaluation of your patient is invaluable to help the patient cope with the aftermath of the procedure and to anticipate specific postoperative problems. This is definitely time well spent both for you and your patient. Being able to anticipate potential problems will make your care of the patient much easier in the postoperative period.

The postoperative period

Just because surgeons have judged the patient preoperatively to be a suitable candidate for surgery does not imply that they should cease to look for signs of psychological disturbance in the patient in the postoperative period. The various psychological reactions include adjustment disorders, depression, anxiety and/or panic symptoms, delirium, psychosis, and somatoform disorders. In addition, the physician has to be alert to psychiatric symptoms that result from medication side-effects.

Much of the psychological response will also be related to the outcome of the surgery. For example, if the surgeon gives 'good news' postoperatively, as in 'we were able to get all of the cancer out', the patient will feel a sense of relief and hopefulness, though the ambiguous meaning of this message can pose serious barriers to communication and trust in the event of recurrence. If they receive 'bad news' postoperatively, the patient may feel hopelessness, despair, and grief.

Depending on the procedure performed, the patient may experience feelings of loss and even start the mourning process. Mourning may begin for the loss of a body part, for loss of specific functioning, and even in anticipation of death. Multiple models for bereavement have been described. Some of these models include the stages of death and dying, beginning with denial and moving on to anger, depression or despair, bargaining, and acceptance. These stages need not occur in any particular order and the surgeon needs to be cognizant of their presence in order to plan the patient's best future treatment, and to gauge how to talk to the patient about the illness and whether to provide additional psychological support to the patient.

Robert Buckman(7) has devised a conceptual framework which does not presuppose a definable sequence of emotional responses to dying. Patients are not preprogrammed by stage or type of illness but instead have idiosyncratic reactions characteristic of the individual's adjustment to previous challenges to their integrity. Their reactions are characteristic of them, not of the diagnosis or proximity of death.

In Buckman's model the process of dying is divided into three stages. The initial stage of facing the threat involves a mixture of emotional reactions as they face the probability of dying. The middle or chronic stage of being ill includes resolution of the elements of the initial response which are resolvable. The final stage is acceptance. Buckman accurately points out that few patients die without ever acknowledging that they are dying (Table 5.1).[7]

Symptomatic and supportive therapies are important. Both pharmacological and non-pharmacological interventions to assist in symptom reduction are recommended. Oftentimes, family members also need supportive treatment as with the impending death of the patient, their own feelings of helplessness and hopelessness may emerge. These emerging feelings in family members may interfere with their ability to be supportive and communicative with the patient.

Table 5.1 The three-stage model of the dying process[7]

Initial stage ('facing the threat')	Chronic stage ('being ill')	Final stage ('acceptance')
A mixture of reactions which are characteristic of the individual and which may include any, or all, of: Fear Anxiety Shock Disbelief Anger Denial Guilt Humour Hope/despair Bargaining	1. Resolution of those elements of the initial response which are resolvable 2. Diminution of intensity of all emotions ('monochrome state') 3. Depression is very common	1. Defined by the patient's acceptance of death 2. Not an essential state provided that the patient is not distressed, is communicating normally, and is making decisions normally

Discussion of body image

Knowledge of body image is quite important in understanding patients' experience of changes in their body parts or appearance as a result of surgery. The obviousness of a physical defect has no direct relationship to the degree of the person's response to a handicap.[8] Some patients cope well with a major scar while others decompensate psychologically when faced with a minor scar. Castelnuevo-Tedesco remarked, 'When an individual acquires a defect in contrast to someone who is born with one, he always feels a sense of loss; loss of hope, loss of his future, loss of normality and the rich experiences that go with it.'[9] However, when a defect is perinatal or congenital, the individual grows up permanently maintaining lower expectations about what he will expect in life, and the sense of loss is hardly present as a psychological issue.* It is important to note that the experience of body image changes may be culturally driven: the psychological impact of changed body image may be amplified or diminished by the person's cultural values.

Body image is comprised of patients' subjective experience of their body as seen through the mind's eye; in other words, the mind – body relationship. Schindler, in 1935, described body image as a tri-dimensional schema of the body involving interpersonal, environmental, and temporal factors.[10] An individual measures their abilities based on their own image of their physical and mental abilities and their success in the world. As a result, people will have differing levels of confidence and/or feelings of inadequacy or anxiety. An outside observer cannot know how people feels about their body based on an objective evaluation of their appearance. Therefore, the physician cannot know how patients will react to their surgery in advance. However, the physician can develop the sensitivity to try to understand the impact of the surgery on the patient and help them adapt to the psychological and physical changes that will or may have already taken place.

Head and neck cancer (see Chapter 10, p. 135)

A discussion of head and neck cancer treatment provides an illustrative example of how cancer surgery that affects both the patient's body integrity as well as his functioning can be quite devastating and complicated for the patient, the family, and the treating team. Similar lessons have been learned elsewhere in surgery, burn care being the most obvious example.

Head and neck cancer precipitates a loss of function and loss of form of the face and oral cavity that can be devastating to both the patient and the family. Facial expression, controlled by the facial muscles, speech, and the ability to eat and drink in a socially acceptable fashion with one's friends and family are of vital importance.[11] Any disfigurement of the face may lead to social, interpersonal, and occupational handicaps. Such is the road for the head and neck cancer patient, disfigured by cancer excision and reconstructive surgery.

In the preoperative period, the patient must be prepared for the likely disfigurement and dramatic change in his face. In the early postoperative period, the patient experiences a great deal of anxiety. This results from difficulty with communication and speech, especially if there is a tracheostomy or nasogastric tube in place, and the need for frequent lengthy dressing periods for wound and flap care.[12] Many patients have severe reactive depression during this time. They may need a great deal of emotional support and reassurance from staff and family. They often feel fearful, abandoned, and intensely alone because of their inability to speak or difficulty with communication. Even if the patients cannot speak, it is important for the staff to communicate with them by talking with them and allowing them to write about their needs and their feelings. This can be a frustrating exercise for all involved and can be quite time-consuming. However, the patient's emotional well-being is dependent on that communication so the surgeon should be prepared during the daily hospital visit to spend the necessary time to facilitate communication.

Pain management may be necessary. A compassionate approach to pain should be maintained. It is important to reassure the patients that you will try to alleviate their pain and discomfort. Using the combination of analgesic agents and/or antidepressant medication is often effective. An overuse of alcohol may be a factor in this patient population. The palliative care team should be on the alert for signs of alcohol withdrawal.

Later in the postoperative period the patients next has to grapple with the change in their appearance and their body image. They are becoming simultaneously aware of the difficulties with swallowing and speech, including possible dribbling. As the patient prepares for discharge, there may be a natural withdrawal of interest and support from the staff. The patients and their families will benefit from good discharge planning, including the initiation of important treatment services such as speech, physical, and occupational therapy, wound care instruction, and psychological support.

Because of the distortions in speech, eating, and drinking, patients may withdraw from their usual lifestyle and important people in their lives. They may become easily frustrated and depressed. Much of the recovery is related to the degree and nature of emotional support available to the patient and their family, and the ability for all to compensate for communication difficulties.

The degree of functional impairment, of course, is related to the nature and extent of excision and reconstruction. After discharge, the family and patient has to spend a lot of time and energy with food preparation and feeding. This may lead to resentment and frustration on both sides. If eating out in restaurants was a usual or pleasurable preoperative activity for the patient and their family, this could be a big loss as they may be uncomfortable eating in such a public setting.

Families tend to experience a great deal of stress while going through the surgical procedure and hospitalization as well as in the post-discharge recovery phase. Some may find the patient difficult to look at because of the disfigurement which tends to lead them to isolate themselves from the patient. The patient will be aware of this withdrawal and may become quite depressed in response. Simultaneously, the patient is trying to cope with the changes in his appearance and functionality.

On top of all of these functional changes is the coming to terms with the cancer diagnosis, the potential need for adjuvant cancer treatment, possibly more surgery, and the frequently guarded prognosis.

Marital relationships may be strained, especially if there is role reversal. For example, if the husband is the patient and normally the dominant partner of the couple, the primary wage earner, and decision maker, surgery and the underlying disease may place him in a very dependent, passive position and create anger and anxiety about the change in the marital relationship. Also, many patients suffer from an odour that accompanies alterations in the oro-nasal anatomy and physiology. This may make the patient feel unattractive and undesirable or may cause the partner to withdraw sexual interest.

For the medical staff, issues arise related to the often disfigured face, speech impairment and drooling, and malodorous smell of the patient. Such reactions may lead treating staff to feel repugnance or pity for the patient.[13] They may avoid looking at the disfigured patient. Health care providers must cope with their own negative affects and attitudes and put them aside in order to help the patients adjust to the dramatic changes in their appearance. Staff can use their own powerful negative reactions to help them understand and be sympathetic to how difficult the patient's psychosocial recovery may be. It is helpful to encourage the patients to discuss their fears and the potential reactions of others, familiar and strangers alike, to their changed physical appearance and function.

All of the above described experiences can set the stage for chronic depression, social with-drawal, loss of self-esteem, anxiety, and feelings of loss and grief. Family relationships may be disrupted, leading to further distress in the patient. Patients may not be able to return to their previous occupation and this may be devastating, especially if their career was an important factor in their self-esteem. When out in public, strangers may stare at their disfigured face, fostering hurt and humiliation in the patient. Many of these negative experiences can be unwit-tingly reinforced by the values and language of the prevailing medical culture: 'He failed chemotherapy', 'She was disqualified from the clinical trial', 'His operation was only palliative', and 'There is no more we can do'.

It is often helpful for the surgeon to suggest a supportive group therapy experience for both the patient and care-givers, to prepare for the physical and emotional changes caused by head and neck cancer surgery. These groups give them a venue to vent their frustrations, anxieties, feelings of loss, and fears with others who have had similar experiences. Critical care experience in surgery has suggested that this type of support may be of value for professionals involved in the care of patients with complex and traumatic illness.

Patients' feelings of profound aloneness and the physician's role

At the end of life, many patients feel quite alone. Family members and friends may feel that they do not know how to comfort the patient or guilty that the patient is dying, so they may visit less often or be uncommunicative when they do visit.

Many physicians may develop cold and detached styles of communication[14] in order to protect themselves from their own feelings of helplessness and hopelessness. Staff members may also feel hopeless to help the patient so they spend less time with the patient or attend them less often. While this may offer some emotional protection for the physician, it creates much anxiety for the patient who experiences this emotional withdrawal as an abandonment.

Even when you have nothing left to offer the patient in terms of medical interventions or treatments, you have the ability to listen, your patience, and the comfort of your interest and presence to offer the patient. Many physicians and surgeons do not realize how powerful the connection is that the patient feels to them and their amazing ability to provide comfort and support, even in the absence of offering disease-directed treatment or cure.

To be a surgeon who can sweep in and save the day by cutting out a malignant growth and effecting a 'cure' is a wonderful thing to be able to offer a patient. However, to be able to provide comfort and solace to a terminally ill patient at the end of his life is the greatest gift a surgical palliative care team can give their patient. This is the true art of medicine.

References

1. Turns, D. (2001). Psychosocial issues: pelvic exenterative surgery. *J. Surg. Oncol.*, **76**, 224–36.
2. Small, S.M. (1976). Psychological and psychiatric problems in aged and high-risk surgical patients. In: *The aged and high-risk surgical patient: medical, surgical and anesthetic management* (ed. J.H. Siegel and P.D. Chodorr), pp. 307–28. Grune and Stratton, Orlando, FL.
3. Cherny, N.I., Coyle, N., and Foley, K.M. (1994). Suffering in the advance cancer patient: a definition and taxonomy. *J. Pall. Care*, **10**, 57–70.
4. Weisman, A.D. (1972). *On death and denying: a psychiatric study of terminality.* Behavioral Publications, New York.
5. Valliant, G.E. and Perry, J.C. (1985). Personality disorders. In: *Comprehensive textbook of psychiatry/IV* (ed. H.I. Kaplan and J.S. Sadock), P. 959. Williams and Wilkins, Baltimore, MD.
6. Strain, J.J. and Grossman, S. (1975). *Psychological care of the medically ill.* Appleton-Century-Crofts, New York.
7. Buckman, R. (1998). Communication in palliative care: a practical guide. In: *The oxford textbook of palliative medicine* (2nd edn) (ed. D. Doyle, G. Hanks, and N. MacDonald). Oxford University Press, Oxford.
8. Castelnuevo-Tedesco, P. (1978). Ego vicissitudes in response to replacement or loss of body parts. Certain analogies to events during psychoanalytic treatment. *Psychoanal. Q.*, **4**, 381–97.
9. Castelnuevo-Tedesco, P. (1997). The psychological consequences of physical illness or defect and the relationship to the concept of deficit. *Psychoanal. Study Child.*, **52**, 76–88.
10. McGrath, M.H. and Mukerji, S. (2000). Plastic surgery and the teenage patient. *J. Pediatr. Adolesc. Gynecol.*, **13**, 105–18.
11. Dropkin, M.J. (1998). Disfigurement and dysfunction with head and neck cancer. *ORL Head Neck Nurs.*, **16**, 28–9.
12. De Boer, M.F., McCormick, L.K., Pruyn, J.F., Ryckman, R.M., and van den Borne, B.W. (1999). Physical and psychosocial correlates of head and neck surgery: a review of the literature. *Otolarygol. Head Neck Surg.*, **120**, 427–36.
13. Petrucci, R.J. and Harwick, R.D. (1984). Role of the psychologist on a radical head and neck surgical team. *Prof. Psychol. Res. Pract.*, **15**, 538–43.
14. Roter, D. and Fallowfield, L. (1998). Principles of training medical staff in psychosocial and communication skills in Holland, In: *Psycho-oncology*, pp. 1074–82. Oxford University Press, New York.

Chapter 6

Spirituality and surgery

Peter Ravenscroft and Elizabeth Ravenscroft

> Healing is understood by religion not only as the natural process of tissue regeneration sometimes assisted by medical means, but also as whatever process results in the experience of greater wholeness of the human spirit.
>
> Kenneth Boyd[1]

Boyd (2000) writes: '. . . we tend to assume that a modern scientific or "objective" picture of the world, in which we ourselves figure as a natural phenomena, is the "true" view of the "real" world. But there is a serious problem about taking this objective scientific picture as the 'true' view of the 'real' world . . . The physicist Schrödinger put it as follows. "The only way scientists can "master the infinitely intricate problem of nature" is to simplify it by removing part of the problem from the picture . . . If science were able to exclude the religious or transcendent dimension from reality (rather than just from the scientific picture of reality), it would be at the cost of excluding the first-person human dimension also." But the idea that science can do this, Schrödinger adds, springs not 'from people knowing too much–but from people believing that they know a great deal more than they do"'.[1] It is a real challenge to integrate spirituality and religion into our view of health and take advantage of some of the benefits in health that may ensue for our patients.

Spirituality and health may seem to have only a tenuous relationship, but in a recent review by Koenig *et al.* (2001) there have been 1200 studies of religion and health and at least two-thirds of them have shown significant associations between religious activity and better physical and mental health or a lower use of health services.[2] Psychologists have been interested in this field as well.[3] Sloan suggests caution in interpreting the studies and believes that evidence for an association between religion, spirituality, and health is weak and inconsistent principally due to methodology.[4,5] This is an area that is evolving rapidly.

Spirituality, religion, and psycho-spiritual distress

One of the problems with research in this area has been to get clear definitions of this construct as it has been for other components of quality of life (QOL). Many investigators have made a distinction between religion and spirituality.

Spirituality is the quest for answers to the ultimate questions of the meaning of life, in contrast to religion, which is a system of beliefs, practices, and symbols designed to bring the believer close to God.[6] Spirituality is more fundamental than religiosity, being a 'subjective experience that exists both within and outside of traditional religious systems'.[7] Brady *et al.* also noted that other features that have been included in definitions of spirituality include 'the way people understand and live their lives in view of their ultimate meaning and value',[8] and is thought to include 'a present state of peace and harmony'[9] and 'dealing with one's adequacy to

Table 6.1 Some relative contrasts of religion with spirituality[6]

Spirituality	Religion
More focused on individual growth	More focused on establishing community
Less objective and measurable	More objective and measurable
Less formal in worship	More formal in worship
More emotion-based, focused on inner experience	More behaviour-based, focused liturgy
Less authoritarian	More authoritarian
More universalizing, discouraging separateness from others	More particularizing, distinguishing one group from another
Less orthodox and systematic in doctrine	More orthodox and systematic in doctrine

see the divinity in the *status quo* of life and then to rely on that transcendence to love above the present troublesome circumstances'.[10] 'These considerations remove this domain from the limiting arena of a particular religious belief system and make it a more widely applicable concept, an important consideration in a QOL construct.'[7]

Spiritual distress is defined as the disruption of the principle of life which pervades a person's entire being and integrates and transcends one's biological and psychosocial nature.[11] Many health professionals, especially in palliative care, refer to these issues as psycho-spiritual issues, highlighting that often psychological and spiritual concerns occur together in those with terminal illnesses. Palliative care has seen spirituality as an important element from its inception and incorporates spirituality into its continuum of care.

Much of the research has been done on religion because its manifestations are more easily measured than those of spirituality. Religion can act as a basis and conduit for the expression of spirituality. The difference between religion and spirituality cannot be absolute but forms a continuum. An individual may have adopted a religion, spirituality, or a combination of both. Table 6.1 illustrates some of the relative attributes of spirituality and religion.

The history of spirituality in the clinical setting

Religion and health have been closely associated from their beginnings. In various cultures this is still so. Our tradition in the West began with the Greeks. Hippocrates, as a particular example, introduced careful observation of patients, both of their disease and their response to treatment, and gradually the benefits of this were seen and there was less emphasis on healing rituals and religion.

Tensions were heightened during the Renaissance when Galileo challenged the Christian view of cosmology with a theory based on scientific observation. Gradually, medicine became more scientific and great benefits were seen to result. Freud equated religion with a 'universal neurosis' and he predicted its ultimate demise.[2] Other psychiatrists followed this line of thought, suggesting that religion was not only irrelevant but harmful. Much of this discussion was based on personal experience and opinion and not on scientific studies. There have been doctors throughout these times who have practised good science and good medicine and have not seen a conflict with their religious life. Some of them, Jung included, have expressed positive views of the relationship of religion and health, but these too have been based on experience and opinion.

In the last century, two factors have greatly impacted on our view of life and death.[12] One has been the deaths as a result of dropping an atomic bomb on Hiroshima and Nagasaki and the Holocaust. The other has been the invention and application of technology that allows life to be maintained long after 'natural' death might have occurred. On one hand, there is a devastation of human life and on the other there is a prolongation of life that has an unacceptable quality to some people. These experiences have caused tensions in our concepts of life and death and have highlighted the spiritual values of life and health.

Medical schools have been bastions of science and have either seen spirituality and religion as irrelevant or have been hostile to any connection between the two. This attitude has been led by the world view of the academics themselves, rather than the suffering people they served, but research of the last two decades has suggested that this attitude is open to question.[13]

A number of surveys have illustrated this discrepancy between the attitudes of clinicians and those of the community. These have been reviewed in an article by Astrow *et al.* (2001). The authors showed that where as 95% of patients in the United States indicate that they believe in God, only 64% of American doctors have the same belief. Figures for psychiatrists and psychologists are lower (about 40%). These types of data suggest there may be a discrepancy between the expectations of patients and the response of doctors. In fact, a study in two states in the US showed that 77% of patients wanted their doctors to consider their spiritual concerns and 48% wanted their doctors to pray with them, but few actually had any spiritual discussion with their doctor.[14] Data like these do not seem to be available for other countries.

Patients and doctors who depend on science alone may understand disease mechanisms and treatment, but what of the larger questions that come with suffering? Is there any meaning in this suffering? Why am I ill? What happens to me when I die? These questions may be very troubling to patients, even if doctors do not share those concerns.

Why has interest in spirituality come to the fore now? There has been a great increase in the technical progress of medicine, but at the same time recognition that it has limits. Patients have found spirituality and religion of assistance in coping with illness and this has been reinforced by the increasing attention that these factors have received in the lay and scientific press. Medical schools have begun to incorporate religion and spirituality into their curricula. Estimates are that some 40 medical schools in the USA have courses on spirituality and religion already and within a few years most if not all will have introduced them.[15] The situation in other countries is not clear from the medical literature.

The measurement of religion and spirituality

There is a strong case for including an assessment of the dimensions of spirituality in QOL questionnaires. This question was addressed by Brady *et al.*[7] They studied a large (n = 1610) and ethically diverse sample in oncology using the Assessment of Chronic Illness Therapy – Spiritual Well-Being (FACIT-Sp). They found that spiritual well-being was correlated with QOL, after controlling for core QOL domains as well as other possible confounding variables. Also they found that spiritual well-being was related to the ability to enjoy life even in the midst of symptoms, making this domain a potentially important clinical target.

There is agreement that QOL is a subjective, multidimensional construct, but there remains controversy over which dimensions should be measured when QOL is measured.[7] As Brady notes, almost 20 years ago, Engel (1980) proposed the 'bio-psycho-social' model. More recently, Hiatt (1986) proposed the 'bio-psycho-social-spiritual' model. Methodology for spirituality has been the subject of ongoing debate. The question is whether the psychological, cultural, and social

Table 6.2 A table of some psychometric tests available for spirituality and religiosity. Modified after Mytko and Knight[16]

Measure	No. of items	Dimensions measured	Reference
Brief RCOPE	14	Positive and negative coping	Pargament et al. (1998)[17]
FACIT-SpWB	12	Meaning/peace, faith	Fitchett et al. (1996)[18]
I/E	12	Extrinsic religiosity	Feagin (1964)[19]
INSPIRIT	7	Spiritual experiences	Kass et al. (1991)[20]
MQOL	6	Existential concerns	Cohen et al. (1995, 1996, 1997)[21–24]
ROS	20	Intrinsic religiosity	Allport and Ross (1967)[25]
SBI-15	15	Belief practices, social support	Holland et al. (1998)[26]
SIBS	26	External/ritual, internal/fluid, existential/meditation, humility/personal application	Hatch et al. (1998)[27]
SCSORF	10	Measure of strength of religious faith	Sherman et al. (2001)[28]
SWBS	20	Existential well-being, religious well being	Paloutzian and Ellison (1982)[29]

Brief RCOPE, Brief version of Religious Coping Scale. **FACIT-SpWB**, Functional Assessment of Chronic Illness Therapy–Spiritual Well-Being Subscale. **I/E**, Intrinsic–Extrinsic Religiosity Scale. **INSPIRIT**, Index of Core Spiritual Beliefs. **MQOL**, Existential Well-Being, McGill Quality of Life Questionnaire–Existential Well-Being Subscale. **ROS**, Religious Orientation Scale. **SBI-15**, Systems Belief Inventory. **SIBS**, Spiritual Involvement and Belief Scale. **SCSORF**, Santa Clara Strength of Religious Faith Questionnaire. **SWBS**, Spiritual Well-Being Scale.

constructs of QOL have captured the impact of spirituality and religion or if spirituality and religion are separate factors. Brady et al. (1999) have made a strong case for including spirituality in QOL measures because spirituality was an important predictor of QOL even when the domains of Physical Well-Being, Emotional Well-Being, and Social/Family Well-Being were controlled.[7] Reviews have addressed these issues and Table 6.2 summarizes some of these instruments.[2,16,5]

The spiritual journey in dying

Threatened with the prospect of dying, almost all patients begin to turn from considerations of achievement, status, money, sexuality, and sport that often occupy their thoughts to spiritual issues such as intimacy and transcendence.[30] Intimacy may be expressed in closeness to family and friends, but also to God and or nature. Transcendence is the search for those things that have a meaning greater than life itself. Transcendence may express itself in terms of religious beliefs that give special value to the person that assures them of special status now or in the afterlife. In terms of spirituality, people may find, for example, an affinity with nature, where there exists a feeling of peace and permanence. Spirituality does not necessarily imply a belief in the afterlife.

This spiritual journey of dying may be difficult for both the patient, their families, and the clinicians caring for them. In the experience of palliative care, the suffering associated with dying is more often due to psycho-spiritual distress than to other symptoms. People often verbalize these problems in statements such as, 'I am a burden on my family and carers'; 'I have lost my dignity'; 'My life lacks meaning', or 'I have been a bad person'. Psycho-spiritual distress is often one of the reasons for calls for euthanasia. Pain or other symptoms alone are infrequent causes of calls from patients for euthanasia, in fact pain alone accounts for 5% of requests in one study.[31]

Dependency is another problem that looms large when a patient needs to be cared for by others. We are all dependent on someone for something whether as a newborn baby, as an adult, or as someone who is terminally ill. The common problem is that we may pretend that we are not dependent. Our Western society promotes a myth of independence as part of the goals of life.

Some see death in terms of tragedy and procrastination.[30] Death is tragic because it comes often unexpectedly and ruins human hopes and dreams. Death is faced with procrastination because if a person takes the position that there is no more life than can be accounted for by biology, increasingly desperate attempts are made to put it off, to delay it, to deny it. Death in reality is part of life; it is the cost of living.

Personal dignity may not only be intrinsic (held as a value of ourselves), but also may be extrinsic (given to us by others). Babies have dignity even though their parents have to change their nappies. The elderly should have dignity given to them because of their past roles in the family, their wisdom, and experience. Eastern cultures are an example to Western cultures in this. In the West, we have chosen to regard youthfulness, good looks, and money as desirable. Personal dignity may be eroded by either real or non-specific feelings of guilt or shame.

Patients may request the right to die. Such a request may indicate that the patient wants to engage in dialogue that might reveal what the request means, including whether the request arises from a clinically significant depression or inadequately treated pain. Muskin (1998) suggests that it might mean, 'Does anyone care enough to talk to me about this request, to want me to be alive, to be willing to share my suffering?' He also suggests a response from a clinician, 'I want to try to do everything I can to work with you and provide you with the best care I can offer. If you die, you will be greatly missed; how can we understand together why you want to die right now?'[32] Other problems that occur in patients who request to die include lack of control, a split in the experience of self, rage and revenge, and a feeling as though they are one of the 'living dead'. These problems will often require psychiatric help as well as spiritual assistance.

The culmination of these types of psycho-spiritual stress is that, if left unresolved, they may lead to hopelessness and depression and even calls for termination of life.[33,34] Hopelessness and lack of meaning may be defined as negative expectancies about oneself and the future. In a study of hopelessness and the risk of dying, Everson et al. (1996) found that hopelessness is a strong predictor of adverse health outcomes, independent of depression and other factors.[35] Dealing with these issues is an important aspect of managing a patient with a life-threatening disease and will be dealt with later in this chapter.

Distinction must be made between the experience of sadness, an emotion that does not require treatment in itself, and that of depression, a treatable medical illness.[32] Making a diagnosis of depression in patients with advanced or terminal disease is very difficult because of the confusion of the somatic symptoms of the physical disease with those of depression. It is necessary to have a high index of suspicion for depression and to use the services of a psychiatrist to confirm it. One good screening test is to ask the patient, 'Are you depressed?' Chochinov et al. (1997) have shown the reliability of this question in suggesting the diagnosis of depression in terminally ill patients.[36]

The impact of spirituality and religion on health

One of the important features of a religious personality is what Allport has called 'extrinsic' and 'intrinsic' religiosity.[37] The extrinsically religious person values religion as a means to an end. Their aim is to gain health, security, status, and power through religion. They may not be aware of their own ulterior motives. What they have to gain is more important to them than their religion's teachings and they are not deeply engaged in the essence of religion, the love for God, and each other. Many of the excesses done in the name of religion are likely to have been performed by those with extrinsic religious personalities.

An intrinsic religious orientation implies that religion is part of a deeply held faith. These people are God-orientated, rather than self-orientated, and maintain a devotional life, praying and reading the scriptures. Their characteristics are humility and gentleness and they often do the unglamorous duties in the religious community, like caring for the chronically ill.

Patients (n = 248) in an ethnically diverse cancer population in the USA indicated that their spiritual and existential needs were: 'overcoming my fears (51%); finding hope (42%); finding meaning in life (40%); finding spiritual resources (39%); or someone to talk to about: finding peace of mind (43%); the meaning of life (28%); and dying and death (25%).'[38] This study emphasizes a number of spiritual and religious needs that frequently occur in cancer patients.

Negative aspects of spirituality and religion

Religion and spirituality can be carried to extremes and can adversely affect both physical and mental health.[39] Religion has been used to justify anger, hatred, aggression, and prejudice as we have seen from the examples of history. It can be used to ostracize others and can be restrictive and confining. If religious beliefs encourage unquestioning obedience to a single religious leader or exclude followers from the benefits of traditional medical care, they are likely to be negative factors in health.[6] In studies comparing extrinsic and intrinsic personality traits, investigators have shown extrinsic personalities are more likely to show evidence of racial prejudice, depression, and grief and distress than those with intrinsic personalities.[6]

Some religious groups directly connect sinfulness and illness. They imply that if a person confesses their sin, they will be cured. If sufferers do not get better from the illness, they may be considered to have inadequate faith or unconfessed sins. These ideas may lead to unnecessary guilt and depression.

Positive aspects of spirituality and religion

There are a number of ways in which religion and spirituality may impact positively on health. These are dealt with in detail by Matthews.[6] He postulates a number of factors, including the 'relaxation response', which can be part of the benefits of mediation and prayer. This is particularly evident in Eastern religions, but is also part of the Western religious tradition. This may buffer stress and enhance immune response. Temperance for alcohol and good nutrition is practised by many religions. An appreciation of religious art and music and a sense of adoration that can lift a person above everyday existence can be a benefit of religion. Confession and the opportunity to start anew are offered in most religions and can contrast to guilt and regret. Developing social networks, as in a church community, is an important factor in mental health and can provide a great deal of loving care to those in need.[37] There can be a sense of unity in a group with shared beliefs and comfort in taking part in familiar activities. These factors enhance patient well-being through stress and coping strategies and social support. Sloan et al. (1999)[5] have raised questions on the methodology of the studies that have been quoted to support an association of religion with health and these questions have been replied to by Koenig *et al.* (1999).[40]

Dealing with spirituality and religion in the clinical context

Taking an open-minded and balanced approach to spirituality and religion without sacrificing scientific integrity seems to be the appropriate way to handle these issues. Surgeons should be concerned with all the factors that affect a patient's health. It is also important that surgeons understand their own spirituality and religious beliefs, biases from their own life experiences and values, so that they remain patient-centred and non-judgemental.

Thoughtful surgeons will prepare for difficult questions (such as 'Why me?') and will put themselves in the place of their patients. They will avoid 'distancing' (acting as if they are pre-occupied with other duties or answering the medical part of the question but not the psycho-spiritual part). They will also avoid casting the answers in incomprehensible medical jargon that is quickly picked up by the patient as avoidance behaviour and may have a major adverse impact on the doctor–patient relationship.

Doctors too are vulnerable. Miles has described the 'emotionally disorientating' nature of the doctor–patient relationship, for the doctor, in caring for a dying patient or their family.[41] Sanderson and Ridsdale (1999) have shown that general practitioners react to the death of patients by feeling guilty and blaming themselves because they have made a mistake. They had the expectation of not making a mistake, something possibly inherited from their medical school education.[42]

In a survey of 267 surgeons assessing perceived level of competence, almost one-third of the sample reported being 'not or not at all competent' in encouraging patients to express anxieties about their condition. Nearly 60% reported a lack of competence in providing bereavement counselling.[43] In a study of surgeons, nurses, and bereaved families, Tinsley *et al.* (1994) found that the majority of surgeons and nurses found it emotionally difficult to support the bereaved family and this was associated with a low frequency of contact with the bereaved families after the patient's death.[44] How surgeons themselves deal with patients in the terminal phase of their disease does not seem to be well studied.

The timing of a spiritual discussion is important. If done too early, some patients feel embarrassed to talk about spirituality or religion. The doctor–patient relationship needs to be one of trust before people will talk about the deepest things that trouble them. It is often better to leave spiritual and religious issues until after physical and psychological issues have been attended to. Discussing such issues as the diagnosis of cancer or terminal illness, severe pain or other symptoms, or grief may allow the opening to introduce the subject of spirituality or religion.

The spiritual assessment

One of the things that can be done during the patient interview is to incorporate a spiritual history into the general clinical history. This will give the surgeon clues that might indicate that there are spiritual problems that are causing stress. It is the surgeon's choice whether they deal with the spiritual issue themselves or refer to a pastoral care person in a palliative care team. The pastoral care person may be able to deal with the issue or refer them to the patient's spiritual advisor.

Anandarajah and Hight (2001) have outlined two ways the spiritual assessment can be done. The first is the informal spiritual assessment.[13] As the patient's story unfolds in the history, there are often clues that suggest spiritual issues. Their symbolic and metaphorical language may suggest themes such hopelessness, fear of the unknown, and isolation. The use of open-ended questions to explore these themes with the patient is recommended. Many patients want their doctors to understand the spiritual issues that concern them even if there may be not a great deal that can be done for them at the time.[45]

The second is a formal spiritual assessment developed for use in the routine medical encounter. These questions do not come from a formally validated questionnaire, but a set of questions that can lead to an open-ended discussion of spiritual and religious issues. This may lead on to dealing with any problems that ensue. These questions do not immediately focus on spirituality and religion and therefore lead to a much broader conversation about concerns that might have an impact on these factors. These are known as the 'HOPE questions' (Box 6.1).[13]

Box 6.1 The HOPE questions for a formal spiritual assessment in a medical interview[13]

H: Sources of **h**ope, meaning, comfort, strength, peace, love, and connection

We have been discussing your support systems. I was wondering, what is there in your life that gives you internal support?

What are your sources of hope, strength, comfort, and peace?

What do you hold onto in difficult times?

What sustains you and keeps you going?

For some people, their religious or spiritual beliefs act as a source of comfort and strength in dealing with life's ups and downs; is this true for you?

If the answer is 'Yes', go on to O and P questions.

If the answer is 'No', consider asking: Was it ever? If the answer is 'Yes', ask: What changed?

O: **O**rganized religion

Do you consider yourself part of an organized religion?

How important is this to you?

What aspects of your religion are helpful and not so helpful to you?

Are you part of a religious or spiritual community? Does it help you? How?

P: **P**ersonal spirituality and practices

Do you have spiritual beliefs that are independent of organized religion? What are they?

Do you believe in God? What kind of relationship do you have with God?

What aspects of your spirituality or spiritual practices do you find most helpful to you personally (e.g. prayer, meditation, reading, scripture, attending religious services, listening to music, hiking, communing with nature)?

E: **E**ffects on medical care and end-of-life decisions

Has being sick (or your current situation) affected your ability to do the things that usually help you spiritually? (Or affected your relationship with God?)

As a doctor, is there anything that I can do to help you access the resources that usually help you?

> **Box 6.1 The HOPE questions for a formal spiritual assessment in a medical interview[13]** *(continued)*
>
> Are you worried about any conflicts between your beliefs and your medical situation/care/decisions?
>
> Would it be helpful for you to speak to a clinical chaplain/community spiritual leader?
>
> Are there any specific practices or restrictions I should know about in providing your medical care (e.g. dietary restrictions, use of blood products)?
>
> *If the patient is dying:* How do your beliefs affect the kind of medical care you would like me to provide over the next few days/weeks/months?

Another screening tool suggested by Post *et al.* (2000)[46] is to include the following questions while taking the history:

1 Do you consider yourself spiritual or religious?
2 How important are these beliefs to you and do they influence how you care for yourself?
3 Do you belong to a spiritual community?
4 How might health providers best address any needs in this area?

It is recommended that surgeons and other medical staff should include a screening tool like one of these into the clinical history and deal with any problems raised either personally or by referral to a pastoral care person or a chaplain.

Being aware of the studies that relate to spirituality, religion, and health that appear in the medical literature

There is a considerable body of evidence relating faith to health. It is summarized in two recent books. Koenig *et al.* (2001)[2] have written an extensive summary of the field and Matthews (1998)[6] has written one for the general reader. Other articles have pointed out that there are methodological difficulties with some of the studies and that the verdict is far from clear at the moment.[4,5]

There are some points of agreement.[40] Religious and spiritual beliefs and activities give many people comfort in the face of illness and death. There is no ethical objection to discussing medical issues between the doctor and his patient in the context of a shared faith tradition. There is ongoing discussion on how doctors should use the published information on the relationship of faith to health where the patient does not have a shared faith with the doctor.

How spirituality relates to clinical practice

Religion, spirituality and clinical outcomes

In this section, some of the evidence for the relationship of spirituality and religion to some surgically relevant conditions is given. The evidence for other conditions can be found elsewhere.[2]

Breast cancer A qualitative study of 33 women aged 65 years who had breast cancer diagnosed within six months in Los Angeles was done by Feher *et al.* (1999). He found that religious and spiritual faith provided emotional support necessary to deal with their breast cancer in 91%, social support in 70%, and meaning in their everyday life in 64%.[47]

Cotton et al. (1999) examined spiritual well-being, quality of life, and psychological adjustment in 142 women with breast cancer.[48] They found a positive correlation with spiritual well-being and quality of life, and between spiritual well-being and specific adjustment styles (e.g. fighting spirit). In regression analyses, controlling for demographic variables and adjustment styles, spiritual well-being contributed very little additional variance in quality of life. The authors concluded that spiritual well-being is correlated with both quality of life and psychological adjustment, but the relationships are more complex than previously considered. Their conclusion was: 'All resources, including spiritual resources, that encourage healing, adjustment, and a better quality of life for patients should be addressed in the clinical arena.'

Gynaecological cancer Roberts et al. (1997) studied a cohort of women with gynaecological cancer at various stages in their disease. For these women fear was the most dominant experience. The fears specified were pain (63%), dying (56%), losing control (48%), or becoming totally dependent (46%). Religion had a serious place in life for 76%, 46% became more religious since their cancer diagnosis while one became less religious. Almost all women (93%) felt that religious commitment helped sustain their hopes, 41% felt their religious life supported their sense of worth.[49]

Melanoma Holland et al. (1999) investigated the role of spiritual and religious beliefs in 117 ambulatory patients coping with malignant melanoma.[50] They used a battery of tests, including the Systems of Belief Inventory (SBI-54). No correlation was found between the SBI-54 scores and the levels of distress. There was a correlation between greater reliance on spiritual and religious beliefs and the use of an active coping style ($r = 0.46$, $p < 0.0001$). The authors suggested that the study showed that the use of religious and spiritual beliefs is associated with an active rather than a passive coping style. They also said that such beliefs provide a helpful active-cognitive framework for many individuals from which to face the existential crises of life-threatening illness.

Colorectal cancer Fernsler et al. (1999) studied 121 patients from 35 states in the USA and six other countries who had colorectal cancer. They used a number of instruments, including the Spiritual Well-Being Scale (SWBS). In correlating the Demands of Illness Inventory (DOII) with the SWBS, the authors reported that subjects who reported higher levels of spiritual well-being indicated lower DOI scores. They concluded: 'The results of this study argue against a mind–body dichotomy and support an integral relationship between spiritual well-being and DOI.'[51]

These examples suggest that supporting patients in their need to have spirituality and religion actively considered by the surgical service will lead to better outcomes for the patient.

Ethical issues

Sloan et al. (1999) have suggested that doctors should not depart from their area of established expertise to promote a non-medical agenda.[5] Koenig (1999) has replied that if religious or spiritual involvement is connected with health behaviours, medical compliance, and coping with illness, then this makes it part of the medical agenda.[40] If the primary task of a doctor is 'to cure sometimes, to relieve often, to comfort always', then if patients use religious or spiritual beliefs as their main way of coping with illness it seems reasonable that 'comforting always' would include support and recognition of what the patient finds comforting.

It might be argued that religion is one of the areas of private behaviour that doctors should not delve into. However, there are many such private behaviours that are commonly regarded as within the province of medicine. For example, smoking, diet, exercise, substance use, and sexual activity are private behaviours that have been linked to health and are considered routine matters for discussion.

Sloan *et al.* (1999) have argued that if religion were suggested as a means of better health, those who had poor health might consider that they were to blame for not having sufficient faith or would feel guilty of moral failure.[5] It might be similarly argued that if we told people to quit smoking, patients might blame themselves in years to come for the chronic lung disease or the lung cancer that they developed through smoking. This type of situation applies to most medical advice that we give and could apply to stressors and cancer, eating and obesity, and AIDS. It seems reasonable then to support patients who enquire about the issues of religion and health, by giving the evidence relating to faith and health or referring them to someone who can do so.

Praying with patients

Prayer may be one expression of spirituality or religion. It is not confined to one religion, but the style and content of prayer may vary from one religion to another and it may vary within religions. It is important that the health professional understands what forms of prayer the patient prefers before they consider praying with a patient. The aim of prayer is to connect the person to their God, to self, and to the health professional.[52] In doing so it may deepen the level of intimacy and help the patient to feel that they have a relationship to God, especially in the areas of forgiveness, strength, and reconciliation. On the other hand, prayer can be imposed on the sick person and therefore may interfere with, rather than promote, the healing relationship. One should not feel compelled to pray on each visit. Above all, prayer should not be used as a subtle form of manipulation by praying for things that the person leading in prayer or the family wishes the person to do.[52]

George Bowman[53] has made a number of suggestions about praying: 'People are better served when prayers are specific. Such questions as "What would you like us to remember?" or "So that our prayer is meaningful to you, would you like us to remember anything in particular?" helps to open doors of communication and to give indications for future support.' The absence of a request for prayer should not be taken as an indication that prayer should not be offered, nor should prayer be automatically offered on every visit to a sick or dying patient.

There are particular moments where prayer may be appropriate:

- with the dying or grieving, particularly if a meaningful religious experience has been shared
- after crisis point or in the process of a life review
- when it seems patients have a new insight into themselves, their relationships, or their illness
- after a confession
- at a time when patients have dealt with their death and find an inner peacefulness and contentment and thanksgiving is appropriate.

Often a prayer after death helps to enable the family to understand that they have joined in community with the fellow sufferers, their own family, and their religious congregation and helps them express deep emotions and feelings.[53]

Bowman offers some pointers for effective prayer:[53]

- Pray in a conversational tone and avoid preaching.
- Prayers should be brief because attention spans are often brief.

- Prayers should be concrete and to the point and not include irrelevant material, trite clichés, or overly sentimental assurances.
- Support, trust, and assurance are important in prayers for the dying and bereaved.
- Prayers are better thought out than given extemporaneously.
- The content should be in the realms of reality for the patient; expressing hopes for cure when they seem unlikely may have a negative effect on faith.
- Prayer for bereaved persons should include:
  - the deep experiences suffered by those who are left behind
  - help and strength for memorial ceremonies
  - thanks for the contribution of the person who has died
  - the use of familiar scripture passages may give comfort.

In summary, polite prayers that leave raw emotions untouched and unexplored are ineffective. A health professional who is sensitive to the wide range of possible feelings experienced by sufferers will be able to help them deal with these feelings.

Public prayer for patients

In the *Journal of Clinical Ethics*, Gross (1995) explores the question 'Is it appropriate to pray in the operating room?'[54] He recalls some anecdotes that indicate that to pray either aloud or with the medical team may impinge on confidence in the team, authority of the surgeon, or lead to disharmony in the surgical team if there were members of other faiths present. He said that it was his routine to offer silent prayer at the scrub sink and not require any others in the room to share his belief.

Dagi (1995), a neurosurgeon, comments on his view of the limits of religious expression in hospitals.[55] He understands prayer in the operating room as involving issues of autonomy, respect for persons, privacy, and culture, thus making the issue very complex. He sees it as exposing the conflict of the healer as a channel of a higher power or the healer as a practitioner of medicine, relying on knowledge and skill. He writes, 'Although prayer in the generic sense may be construed as a quest for the sacred, prayer in the particular sense generally invokes a particular vision of the sacred, and that vision may not be shared. It may, in fact, be remarkably exclusive.' He suggests some guidelines for public prayer in hospitals that might form the basis of discussion (Box 6.2).

Box 6.2 Guidelines for public prayer in hospitals[55]

1. Religious institutions may make participation in ritual a condition for staff privileges so long as this requirement is made explicit, but non-religious institutions should not.
2. Patients and staff should not be coerced into worship or religious practice, but neither should they be permitted to disrupt expressions of faith of others.
3. In order to promote both the atmosphere for worship and the privacy of worshipers and non-worshipers alike, chapels should be provided by religious institutions wherever they deem it important that people pray.
4. Private prayer may be permitted in the operating room with the express permission of all present, including the patient, but without requiring the participation of anyone present.

> **Box 6.2 Guidelines for public prayer in hospitals[55]** *(continued)*
>
> 5. Prayer may not be initiated under circumstances in which bystanders may not leave.
> 6. No one is permitted to openly pray on behalf of another without explicit permission.
> 7. Prayer may be led by an identified religious leader distinct from the treating medical team whenever possible so as to avoid even an appearance of religious coercion.

Prayer may raise some questions for some patients. The spiritual conflicts associated with praying about cancer are considered in the article by Taylor *et al.* (1999).[56] They found in a qualitative study of 30 patients that the themes raised were unanswered prayer, difficulties with petitionary prayers, conflict about control, questions about the nature of God, questions about meaning and of a powerful God in the presence of evil, bargaining, doubts about the efficacy of prayer, doubts about personal spirituality and worth, and praying the 'right' way.

The management of spirituality and religious issues in a surgical unit

The surgeon and spiritual practice

What of the surgeons' own spirituality? Surgeons, like other health care professionals, confront questions of meaning, value, and relationship in their own personal and professional lives. In order to care for patients, surgeons, particularly those whose work encompasses palliative care, need to take time to understand the meaning and value of their work and not to become cynical, or to see that value in primary economic terms.

The General Medical Council (GMC) in Britain has advised doctors that it is wrong for them to use their professional position 'to express personal beliefs in ways which may cause distress or which exploit patients' vulnerability'. They gave examples of doctors who had told patients that they would not recover unless they 'gave their lives to God' or told a patient after the death of her child that she was 'evil' and that the 'devil had taken her baby'. The GMC also pointed out that 'it would be inappropriate to try to prevent doctors from expressing their personal, religious, political, or other views to patients'.[57]

It has been said that 'to heal a person, one must first be a person'. This implies a holistic concept of the person, integrating the professional side of life with the personal and family life that includes recreation both physical and spiritual. This will enable one to find meaning in the stresses that come with caring for dying patients.[58] For many health professionals who are cynical about organized religion, other forms of spirituality may have appeal. Above all, systems must be put in place to monitor and to allow management for those who find being a professional in these circumstances tough. That is most of us! Others in the team can look out for the signs of not coping, but proactive schemes such as the 'buddy system' (associates at work acting as debriefers), regular independent counselling, or spiritual direction should be encouraged for all team members looking after dying patients, including surgeons.

At the end of life, patients are faced with physical, psychological, social, and spiritual challenges.[59] Coping responses range over a continuum from exceptionally good, through adaptive to dysfunctional. Patients want to be appreciated and managed as whole persons, not as diseases. When physical symptoms and suffering are controlled, it is easier to address psycho-spiritual problems. While this is generally true, there are some patients whose psycho-spiritual problems make other symptoms much worse and in these cases physical symptoms and psycho-spiritual issues should be dealt with simultaneously.

Palliative care is generally requested when the expectation of survival is limited. When the patient gets to that stage it is not uncommon for the services of the surgical team to be withdrawn.[12] Krizek (2001) also points out that in one review of trauma where a person had died, families were spoken to by an intern or a medical student, often in a semi-public place and not by a senior member of the surgical team. He writes, 'Surgeons are at our best when we perform that which we can offer uniquely: the performance of operations. Neither should we ask surgeons to deliver palliative care. When the only possible outcome is death, asking surgeons to stay involved is doomed to failure. Surgeons are technicians for whom spirituality of death and the dying process is terrifying.'

There may be disagreement with Krizek's point of view. There are surgeons who play their role very well. Well-planned procedures such as a colostomy, a debulking procedure, or the pinning of a fractured hip can greatly assist a palliative patient. Some surgeons and other medical practitioners have given up their former practices to become palliative care specialists.[60,61] Palliative care requires a palliative care team – the surgeon cannot do it all himself. As Krizek summarizes, 'These complex issues require considerable involvement and reflective deliberation with the patient and the family. It requires a sense of spirituality, involvement with pastoral care, and acceptance of the hopelessness of life-prolonging measures. I do not believe that this is within the scope of the usual surgeon's experience or emotional dispositions. That is not to say that surgeons cannot become disposed and sensitive specialists involved in palliative care, but I am sceptical that they can accomplish this while at the same time conducting a busy surgical practice. Surgical palliative care may become a specialty unto itself, but it is not, in my opinion, now part of the usual surgeon's expertise.'

Some surgeons have been accused of being technicians who have an 'aloof and uncaring demeanour'.[12] Krizek continues, 'Does this mean that we don't care? Of course it does not. And yet the overwhelming experience of the dangers of death on a daily basis demands that we . . . must separate the personal from the professional. We live for hope.' He suggests doctors should acknowledge and respect the spiritual lives of patients. This may take the form of understanding the problems from the patient's point of view, including their religious perspectives.

What should be done for patients? Koenig (2000) has suggested that doctors should not prescribe religious beliefs or activities for health reasons.[62] They should not impose their religious beliefs on patients. Nor should they initiate prayer without knowledge of the patient's religious background or the likely appreciation of such activity by the patient. They should not provide in-depth religious counselling to patients; that is best done by trained clergy.

Encouraging religious practice in the unit

If religious expression is to be encouraged, the surgeon and the clinical team should have done an adequate assessment and have some understanding of the problems they are dealing with. 'They go in where angels fear to tread' is an apt description of clinicians who wade in to a spiritual problem without understanding the matter clearly.

The question of disclosure becomes an issue for any medical or nursing staff who wishes to assist a patient spiritually. The key questions are 'Whose needs are being met by self-disclosure?' and 'Will this self-disclosure assist the doctor–patient relationship?' Avoiding proselytizing or putting inappropriate pressure on vulnerable patients is essential.

Astrow *et al.* (2001) write: 'It is always improper either to proselytize at the bedside or to threaten to make medical services contingent upon any religious belief, expression, or practice. Because it is apparent that religious practice is associated with good health outcomes, some have advocated, mistakenly in our view, that physicians ought actively to encourage religious practice on the part of their patients, much as they now encourage low-fat diets and regular exercise. In the light of the imbalance of power in the doctor–patient relationship, even well-intentioned religious advocacy threatens patient autonomy and should be seen as off limits. It is legitimate though to ask patients who appear to be struggling with spiritual issues whether they have any underlying spiritual concerns regarding their illness and further if they belong to any community of meaning and support. The support of that community or a chaplain might then be helpful.'[14]

Fostering of hope and meaning

Spirituality is important in maintaining hope.[49] Hope and meaning are the two key factors in dealing with major challenges in life.[63] Suffering, particularly in chronic illness, seems to attack hope and meaning directly and may destroy it, leading to hopelessness. Clinicians might consider how they might foster hope as one of their main aims in supporting a patient with a life-threatening illness.

Richardson (2000) quotes Farran *et al.* (1995) as giving a four-dimensional model of hope:[64,65]

1   Hope as an experiential process. The very process of suffering seems to give rise to hope in some patients. Victor Frankl's observations of meaning and hope in the concentration camps of Eastern Europe is one example.[63]

2   Hope as a spiritual or transcendent process. Prayer, meditation, and guided imagery may be used to lift the person out of a hopeless situation.

3   Hope as a rational thought process. This dimension is powerful and practical. Cognitive-behaviour therapists work on this aspect, enabling patients to get some measure of control, not necessarily of their illness, but of their response to it.

4   Hope as a relational process. Relationships with family, friends, and care-givers are important in maintaining hope.

Post-White *et al.* (1996) summarize what gives hope to patients with cancer in five themes: finding meaning, having affirming relationships, using inner resources, living in the present, and anticipating survival.[66] These constructs give some idea of how a clinician may approach hope and meaning to find ways to assist those facing terminal illness.

The saying 'Where there is life, there is hope' is a truth we all recognize. On the other hand, for patients with cancer and other chronic diseases it may be more appropriate to say 'Where there is hope, there is life.'[65] One is a biological, the other is a psycho-spiritual, view of life. There is good reason not only to foster hope for a good outcome from surgery, but also to foster realistic hope for a patient with terminal disease.

Realistic hope does not talk of unrealistic goals nor of predicting long prognoses that bear no relationship to reality. We are talking about exploring life with patients, through their stories, through family and friends, helping them understand that though they have lost much, there are still things to be gained through living in the present and not longing for life the way it used to be.

Part of finding meaning and hope is dealing with guilt and shame. These feelings may come as a result of disfigurement of the disease or surgery making the patient feel shameful. They may experience real or imagined remorse relating to failed relationships. Another aspect is a feeling of being let down by God, to whom they may have been very faithful during their lives. Others may find that they are no longer able to take part in the rituals of their faith and as a result feel abandoned and guilty. Often these matters are not easy to untangle, but it is important for the surgeon to be sensitive to what the patient is saying and ask a pastoral care person or chaplain to see the patient, if these topics arise.

Speck (1999) points out that similar situations, without the religious overtones, may occur in people whose belief system is not a religious one.[67] These people may benefit from a consultation with a pastoral care person, or a spiritual advisor of their choice. This will enable an assessment of the impact of the illness on their coping mechanisms and offer them support.

The surgeon may help by supporting and being with the patient through the illness. Surgeons will realise that there are many calls on their time and will hopefully call in others to help. The pastoral care person will be able to provide spiritual help or arrange with others for this to be given. Counselling may be of value if there are psychological issues to be coped with. There is also great benefit in having an occupational therapist or a volunteer help the patient to write a life story or letters to their children about significant events, to be read after their death. There may be great benefit in having a music therapist or a friend play the music that a patient loves or that reminds them of events in the past that have given their life meaning. The palliative care team can provide many of these services if they are consulted.

With respect to counselling, there are different types of hope that may be recognized. Some patients have 'intrinsic hope'. These people gain hope from finding meaning in their life, from their relationships, their faith, and living in the present. Others may derive 'extrinsic hope' from such things as the attitude of others to them, their body image, and in anticipating survival. Extrinsic hope fades when friends and their surgeon no longer are interested in them as persons. The surgeon may tell the patient 'There is nothing more that can be done for you' and discharge them. This may precipitate hopelessness. If the patient can be reoriented from the extrinsic elements to the intrinsic elements of hope, hope again may be rekindled and meaning can be found even for the most difficult cases.

The potential for conflict in addressing spirituality

Spirituality and religion deal with issues that are central to the person. It would not be surprising to find conflicts, either overt or covert, that arise when clinical staff are dealing with some of these concerns. One obvious one might be the need for blood transfusions in patients whose beliefs preclude them, or people who believe in alternative or complementary therapies. More difficult is the staff member, family member, or carer who feels the need to bring people to faith before they die. Staff members may notice that another staff member is 'getting too close' to a patient and interpret this behaviour as the person giving spiritual support. Such instances can bring great pressures on the patient as they are a 'captive audience'. These issues need to be dealt with individually or in staff meetings and not left unaddressed until they become a crisis.

The place of pastoral care workers and chaplains in the surgical unit

Regardless of the patient's ethnic, religious, or cultural background, the pastoral care persons and chaplains can address existential and spiritual issues. They can understand the problems from the perspective of having a common human experience as well as having a reverence for the patient's background.[68] Surgeons and other doctors may be open to acknowledging and supporting patients in their spiritual concerns, but most lack the skills to address spiritual concerns of patients in depth.

The pastoral care persons and chaplains should usually have completed pastoral care education or equivalent and should be seen as a genuine health care professional. Often the pastoral care person is employed by the palliative care service and they are fully integrated into the palliative care team. This means that spiritual concerns will be seen in the total context of the patient's illness. Sometimes referral can be made to the patient's own religious advisor or a representative of their religion.

Referrals to pastoral care staff or chaplains can be critical to good health care for many patients and can be as appropriate as referrals to other health professionals.[69] Studies, not only in church-affiliated hospitals but over broad samples of patients and hospitals in the USA, have shown that the services of hospital chaplains are appreciated by a high proportion of both staff and patients.[70–72]

Some surgeons and other health care professionals may consider they have the skills to address the spiritual concerns of patients themselves. Merely being a believing person does not qualify a clinician to give spiritual advice, especially to patients who do not share the clinician's particular faith. One should bear in mind that at least part of the separation of the roles of priest and doctor has a salutary effect. There are topics patients may wish to address with their clergy that they do not wish to address with their physicians, and vice versa.[14]

Unfortunately, the pastoral care person or chaplain may be marginalized in health care. In a study of 200 adult deaths at the New York Cornell Medical Center, Fins *et al.* (2000) found that religion and spirituality were infrequently mentioned but often reflected staff frustration with the unrealistic expectations of the family.[73] Only two pastoral care interventions were cited in the records reviewed. These researcher's noted that at the time of the study, pastoral care workers in their centre were not permitted to make notations in the medical record. This, they said, reflected the stature of pastoral care, perpetuated their marginalization, and led to fragmentation of the psychosocial and spiritual dimensions of end-of-life care.

Because many surgeons and other clinicians do not enquire about spirituality in the clinical history, referrals are frequently not made for patients who could benefit from the skills of the pastoral care services.[74] The lack of such referrals has been considered as a form of clinical negligance.[46] For those who wish to see a statement of the functions and activities of pastoral care persons and chaplains, a consensus document has recently been published.[75]

Conclusion

Spirituality is a rapidly developing field and is beginning to have an impact on surgery and other medical specialities. Because of a sense that something is missing from medicine today, spirituality has become a major interest of post-modern society. Even in a pluralist society, it is possible for health care professionals to address the spiritual concerns of patients in a respectful manner without needing to sacrifice any of the obvious gains of scientific medicine.[14] Patients are asking for it to be done, and there is a good deal of scientific evidence to support it. Surgeons ought to work closely with pastoral care, chaplains, or clergy, treating them where possible as members of the health care team. That will enable the spiritual concerns of meaning, value, and relationship that arise naturally in a setting of palliative surgery to be answered appropriately, thereby assisting the patient to cope better with their forthcoming death.

References

1. Boyd, K.H. (2000). Disease, illness, sickness, health, healing and wholeness: exploring some elusive concepts. *J. Med. Ethics: Medical Humanities*, **26**, 9–17.

2. Koenig, H.G., McCullough, M.E., and Larson, D.B. (2001). *Handbook of religion and health*, pp. 1–712. Oxford University Press, New York.

3. Kloos, B., and Moore, T. (2000). Introduction to special issue on spirituality, religion and community psychology. *J. Commun. Psychol.*, **28**, 115–18.

4. Sloan, R.P., Bagiella, E. (2000). Spirituality and medical practice: a look at the evidence. *Am. Fam. Phys.*, **63**, 33–4.

5. Sloan, R.P., Bagiella, E., and Powell, T. (1999). Religion, spirituality and medicine. *Lancet*, **353**, 664–7.

6. Matthews, D.A. (1998). *The faith factor*, pp. 32–59. Viking Penguin, New York.

7. Brady, M., Peterman, A., Fitchett, G., Mo, M., and Cella, D. (1999). A case for including spirituality in quality of life measurement in oncology. *Psycho-Oncology*, **8**, 417–28.

8. Muldoon, M., and King, N. (1995). Spirituality, health care and bioethics. *J. Relig. Health*, **34**, 329–49.

9. Hungelmann, J., Kenkel-Ross, E., Klassen, L., and Stollenwerk, R.M. (1985). Spiritual well-being in older adults: harmonious interconnectedness. *J. Relig. Health*, **24**, 147–53.

10. Brewer, E.D.C. (1999). *Life stages and spiritual well-being*. Washington University Press, Washington, DC.

11. Kim, M.J., McFarland, G.K., and McLane, A.M. (1987). *Pocket guide to nursing diagnoses*. (2nd edn), p. 55. Moseby, C.V., St Louis.

12. Krizek, T.J. (2000). Spiritual dimensions of surgical palliative care. *Surg. Oncol. Clin. North Am.*, **10**, 39–55.

13. Anandarajah, G., and Hight, E. (2001). Spirituality and medical practice: using the HOPE questions as a practical tool for spiritual assessment. *Am. Fam. Phys.*, **63**, 81–9.

14. Astrow, A.B., Puchalski, C.M., and Sulmasy, D.P. (2001). Religion, spirituality, and health care: social, ethical, and practical considerations. *J.A.M.A.*, **110**, 283–7.

15. Ziegler, J. (1998). Spirituality returns to the fold in medical practice. *J. Natl. Cancer Inst.*, **90**, 1255–7.

16. Mytko, J., and Knight, S. (1999). Body, mind and spirit: towards the integration of religiosity and spirituality in cancer quality of life research. *Psycho-Oncology*, **8**, 439–50.

17. Pargament, K.I., Smith, B.W., Koenig, H.G., and Perez, L.M. (1998). Patterns of positive and negative religious coping with major life stressors. *J. Scient. Study Relig.*, **37**, 710–24.

18. Fitchett, G., Peterman, A.H., and Cella, D. (1996). *Spiritual beliefs and quality of life in cancer and HIV patients*. Society for the Scientific Study of Religion, Nashville, TN. 9th November.

19. Feagin, J.R. (1964). Predjudice and religious types: a focused study of Southern Fundamentalists. *J. Scient. Study Relig.*, **4**, 3–13.

20. Kass, J.D., Friedman, R., Leserman, J., Zuttermeister, P.J., and Benson, H. (1991). Health outcomes and a new index of spiritual experience (INSPIRIT). *J. Scient. Study Relig.*, **30**, 203–11.

21. Cohen, S.R., Hassan, S.A., Lapointe, B.J., and Mount, B.M. (1996). Quality of life in HIV disease as measured by the McGill quality of life questionnaire. *Aids*, **10**, 1421–7.

22. Cohen, S.R., Mount, B.M., Bruera, E., Provost, M., Rowe, J., and Tong, K. (1997). Validity of the McGill Quality of Life Questionnaire in the palliative care setting: a multi-centre Canadian study demonstrating the importance of the existential domain. *Pall. Med.*, **11**, 3–20.

23. Cohen, S.R., Mount, B.M., Strobel, M.G., and Bui, F. (1995). The McGill Quality of Life Questionnaire: a measure of quality of life appropriate for people with advanced disease. A preliminary study of validity and acceptability. *Pall. Med.*, **9**, 207–19.

24. Cohen, S.R., Mount, B.M., Tomas, J.J., and Mount, L.F. (1996). Existential well-being is an important determinant of quality of life. Evidence from the McGill Quality of Life Questionnaire. *Cancer*, **77**, 576–86.

25. Allport, G.W., and Ross, J.M. (1967). Personal religious orientation and prejudice. *J. Pers. Soc. Psychol.*, **5**, 432–43.

26. Holland, J.C., Kash, K.M., Passik, S., Gronert, M.K., Sison, A., Lederberg, M., *et al.* (1998). A brief spiritual beliefs inventory for use in quality of life research in life-threatening illness. *Psycho-Oncology*, **7**, 460–9.

27. Hatch, R.L., Burg, M.A., Naberhaus, D.S., and Hellmich, L.K. (1998). The Spiritual Involvement and Beliefs Scale. Development and testing of a new instrument. *J. Fam. Pract.*, **46**, 476–86.

28. Sherman, A.C., Simonton, S., Adams, D.C., Latif, U., Plante, T.G., Burns, S.K., *et al.* (2001). Measuring religious faith in cancer patients: reliability and construct validity of the Santa Clara Strength of Religious Faith Questionnaire. *Psycho-Oncology*, **10**, 436–43.

29. Paloutzian, R., and Ellison, C.G. (1982). *Loneliness, spiritual well-being and quality of life*, pp. 224–37. John Wiley and Sons, New York.

30. Peterson, E.H. (1997). *Subversive spirituality*, p. 10. Erdmanns and Regent College Publishing, Vancouver.

31. Van der Maas, P.J., Van Delden, J.J., Pijnenborg, L., and Looman, C.W. (1991). Euthanasia and other medical decisions concerning the end of life. *Lancet*, **338**, 669–74.

32. Muskin, P.R. (1998). The request to die: role for a psychodynamic perspective on physician-assisted suicide. *J.A.M.A.*, **279**, 323–8.

33. Barnes, L.L., Plotnikoff, G.A., Fox, K., and Pendleton, S. (2000). Spirituality, religion, and pediatrics: intersecting worlds of healing. *Pediatrics*, **106**, 899–908.

34. Brietbart, W., Rosenfeld, B., Pessin, H., Kain, M., Funesti-Esch, J., Galietta, M., *et al.* (2000). Depression, hopelessnes, and desire for hastened death in terminally ill patients with cancer. *J.A.M.A.*, **284**, 2907–11.

35. Everson, S.A., Goldberg, D.E., Kaplan, G.A., Cohen, R.D., Pukkala, E., Tuomilehto, J., *et al.* (1996). Hopelessness and risk to mortality and incidence of myocardial infarction and cancer. *Psychosom. Med.*, **58**, 113–21.

36. Chochinov, H.M., Wilson, K.G., Ennus, M., and Lander, S. (1997). 'Are you depressed?' Screening for depression in the terminally ill. *Am. J. Psychiat.*, **154**, 674–6.

37. Argyle, M. (2000). *Psychology and religion: an introduction*, pp. 30–1. Routledge, London.

38. Moadel, A., Morgan, C., Fatone, A., Grennan, J., Carter, J., Laruffa, G., *et al.* (1999). Seeking meaning and hope: self-reported spiritual and existential needs among an ethnically diverse cancer patient population. *Psycho-Oncology*, **8**, 378–85.

39. Koenig, H.G., Larson, D.B., and Larson, S.S. (2001). Religion and coping with serious medical illness. *Ann Pharmacother.*, **35**, 352–9.

40. Koenig, H.G., Idler, E., and Stanislav, K. (1999). Religion, spirituality, and medicine: a rebuttal to skeptics. *Int. J. Psychiat. Med.*, **29**, 123–31.

41. Miles, S.H. (1994). Physicians and their patients' suicides. *J.A.M.A.*, **272**, 410.

42. Saunderson, E.M., and Ridsdale, L. (1999). General practitioners' beliefs and attitudes about how to respond to death and bereavement: qualitative study. *B.M.J.*, **319**, 293–6.

43. Girgis, A., Sanson-Fisher, R.W., and McCarthy, W. (1997). Communicating with patients: surgeons' perceptions of their skills and need for training. *Aust. N.Z.J. Surg.*, **67**, 775–80.

44. Tinsley, E.S., Baldwin, A.S., Steeves, R.H., Himel, H.N., and Edlich, R.F. (1994). Surgeons', nurses', and bereaved families' attitudes toward dying in the burns centre. *Burns*, **20**, 79–82.

45. Maugans, T.A., and Wedland, W.C. (1991). Religion and family medicine: a survey of physicians and patients. *J. Fam. Pract.*, **32**, 210–13.

46. Post, S.G., Puchalski, C.M., and Larson, D.B. (2000). Physicians and patient spirituality: professional boundaries, competency, and ethics. *Ann. Intern. Med.*, **132**, 578–83.

47. Feher, S., and Maly, R.C. (1999). Coping with breast cancer in later life: the role of religious faith. *Psycho-Oncology*, **8**, 408–16.

48. Cotton, S.P., Levine, E.G., Fitzpatrick, C.M., Dold, K.H., and Targ, E. (1999). Exploring the relationships among spiritual well-being, quality of life, and psychological adjustment in women with breast cancer. *Psycho-Oncology*, **8**, 429–38.

49. Roberts, J.A., Brown, D., Elkins, T., and Larson, D.B. (1997). Factors influencing views of patients with gynecologic cancer about end-of-life decisions. *Am. J. Obstet. Gynecol.*, **176**, 166–72.

50. Holland, J.C., Passik, S., Kash, K.M., Russak, S.M., Gronert, M.K., Sison, A., *et al.* (1999). The role of religious and spiritual beliefs in coping with malignant melanoma. *Psycho-Oncology*, **8**, 14–26.

51. Fernsler, J., Klemm, P., and Miller, M.A. (1999). Spiritual well-being and demands of illness in people with colorectal cancer. *Cancer Nurs.*, **22**, 134–40.

52. Evanson, B., Goodell, E., Handzo, G., and Shulman, S. (1993). Prayer and pastoral care. *Care-giver J.*, **10**, 40–4.

53. Bowman, G.W. (1998). *Dying, grieving, faith, and family*, pp. 110–13. Haworth Pastoral Press, Binghanton, NY.

54. Gross, H.P. (1995). Is it appropriate to pray in the operating room? *J. Clin. Ethics*, **6**, 273–4.

55. Dagi, T.F. (1995). Prayer, piety and professional propriety: limits on religious expression in hospitals. *J. Clin. Ethics*, **6**, 274–9.

56. Taylor, E.J., Outlaw, F.H., Bernardo, T.R., and Roy, A. (1999). Spiritual conflicts associated with praying about cancer. *Psycho-Oncology*, **8**, 386–94.

57. Medicopolitical Digest (1993). Doctors must not proselytise, GMC says. *B.M.J.*, **307**, 1286.

58. Kash, K., and Holland, J. (1990). *Reducing stress in medical oncology house officers: a preliminary report of a prospective intervention study*, pp. 83–195. Indiana University Press, Bloomington, Ind.

59. Block, S.D. (2001). Psychological considerations, growth and transcendence at the end of life. *J.A.M.A.*, **285**, 2898–905.

60. Allbrook, D.B. (2000). A metamorphosis: doctor to chaplain. *Med. J. Aust.*, **21**, 390–1.

61. Faris, I.B. (2000). Perspectives from a surgeon turned hospital chaplain. *Med. J. Aust.*, **172**, 389–90.

62. Koenig, H.G. (2000). Should doctors prescribe religion?. Interview by Anita J Slomski. *Med. Econ.*, **77**, 144–6, 151, 155.

63. Frankl, V. (1985). *Man's search for meaning*, p. 88. Washington Square Press, New York.

64. Farran, C.J., Herth, K.A., and Popovich, J.M. (1995). *Hope and hopelessness: critical clinical concepts*. Sage Publications, Thousand Oaks, CA.

65. Richardson, R.L. (2000). Where there is hope, there is life: toward a biology of hope. *J. Pastoral Care*, **54**, 75–83.

66. Post-White, J., Ceronsky, C., Kreitzer, M., Nickelson, K., Drew, D., Mackey, K., *et al.* (1996). Hope, spirituality, sense of coherence, and quality of life in patients with cancer. *Oncol. Nurs. Forum*, **23**, 1571–9.

67. Speck, P. (1999). *Spiritual issues in palliative care* (2nd edn), pp. 805–14. Oxford University Press, Oxford.

68. Handzo, G. (1996). Chaplaincy: a continuum of caring. *Oncology*, **10**, 45–7.

69. Thiel, M.M., and Robinson, M.R. (1997). Physicians' collaboration with chaplains: difficulties and benefits. *J. Clin. Ethics*, **8**, 94–103.

70. Carey, G.A. (1973). Chaplaincy: component of total patient care? *Hospitals, J.A.H.A.*, **47**, 166–72.

71. Gibbons, J.L., Thomas, J., Vandecreek, L., and Jessen, A.K. (1991). The value of hospital chaplains: patient perspectives. *J. Pastoral Care*, **45**, 117–25.

72. Parkum, K.H. (1985). The impact of chaplaincy services in selected hospitals in the eastern United States. *J. Pastoral Care*, **34**, 262–9.

73. Fins, J.J., Schwager Guest, A.B., and Acres, C.A. (2000). Gaining insight into the care of hospitalized dying patients: an interpretative narrative analysis. *J. Pain Sympt. Manage.*, **20**, 399–407.

74. Larson, D.B., Hohmann, A.A., Kessler, L.G., Meador, K.G., Boyd, K.H., and McSherry, E. (1988). The couch and the cloth: the need for linkage. *Hosp. Commun. Psychiat.*, **39**, 1064–9.

75. A White Paper (2001). Professional chaplaincy: its role and importance in health care. *J. Pastoral Care*, **55**, 81–97.

Chapter 7

Interdisciplinary care

Anne Mosenthal, David Price, and
Patricia Murphy

The concept of surgical palliative care might be considered an oxymoron: the focus of surgery is typically curative, based on procedures and technological interventions, while palliative care is devoted to relief of suffering and symptoms when cure is no longer possible. These two fields of medical care seem dichotomous, in part because their delivery, in practice, has usually been mutually exclusive. Each is immersed in a subculture of medicine that answers to different authorities; that values different patient outcomes, different practice styles, and collegial relationships. The notions of a 'surgical service' and a 'palliative care service' are somewhat artificial constructs, based on historical developments in medicine, not on the needs of a particular patient. The traditional medical framework necessitates delivery of surgical care on a service with a curative, technological imperative. Once prognosis suggests that cure is no longer possible, care may then be abruptly handed over to a palliative care team and surgical care ceases. There is little integration or continuity between the two, and care is necessarily fragmented and not in the best interests of the patient or the family. In reality, this care need not and should not be mutually exclusive; clearly there is common ground as some components of palliative care may require the expertise or skills of a surgeon, while surgical care has always encompassed palliation and pain relief as one of its goals.

To find the common ground between 'surgery' and 'palliative care' in this new field of surgical palliative care is not simple. There are many barriers to the integration of the two. The 'cultures' of surgical and palliative care can be contradictory, with conflicting values and desired outcomes. The professionals of each discipline, while all holding expertise, may find little common language or opportunity for interaction. To surgeons, focus on comfort rather than cure may be tantamount to 'giving up', while to the palliative care professional, surgery may only involve painful procedures for the sake of 'doing something' when time is short at the end of life. Lastly, in many illnesses prognosis is uncertain and when to make the *transition* from cure to comfort is unclear. If comfort and cure remain mutually exclusive because of cultural conflict within medicine, many patients will suffer needlessly because palliative care is offered too late.

Given these cultural conflicts and barriers, surgical palliative care must by definition be an interdisciplinary endeavour. The interdisciplinary team provides the best way to accomplish truly integrated care that will overcome many of these barriers. Surgeons, surgical nurses, and palliative care physicians and nurses as members of such a team can improve communication, cross over cultural barriers between disciplines, and deliver care in a patient-oriented fashion. The interdisciplinary team facilitates the integration of palliative care into the surgical setting, or surgical care into the palliative care setting; it allows curative and palliative care to be delivered *in parallel*, not in an either/or fashion, so that the transition from cure to comfort is less problematic. This care, which may be complex, requires multiple levels of expertise, coordination, and most importantly may have multiple and changing goals. For these reasons, as well as its ethically sound basis, interdisciplinary care is the best way to provide surgical palliative care. In this chapter we will describe the ethical and clinical basis for the interdisciplinary team in surgical palliative care and describe two models for its delivery.

Interdisciplinary care: ethical and clinical foundation

After thousands of years, the core concept of the Hippocratic oath still forms the central commitment of modern health professionals: *the patient's interests are paramount*. Good care, appropriate, properly conceived and executed care begins with the patient and ends with the patient. That is to say, the patient's welfare defines the focus or purpose at the outset and is the reference point for evaluation at the end. Accordingly, the primary ethical consideration that promotes teams and teamwork should be the commitment to patient welfare. Some call this the principle of beneficence, the first and most defining obligation of the health care professional.

Ethically, it follows that the best reason for surgeon, physician, nurse, or social worker to be committed to interdisciplinary palliative care teamwork is that such teamwork is good for patients. Other reasons for a palliative care team might include that it helps surgeons, physicians, and other members of the team; that it is respectful of other professionals and care-givers; that it boosts patient satisfaction ratings; that it is 'politically correct'; and that it may help the hospital's bottom line. Equally important, the shared responsibility between team members when dealing with something as meaningful as death and dying provides intangible rewards for all involved: the patient, the family, and the team members themselves. 'Somehow, no matter what we humans are going through, nothing gives us more comfort than the presence of someone with whom to share our journey.'[1] This mixed bag of values notwithstanding, we assert that an interdisciplinary palliative care team should be considered, organized, and evaluated relative to the most fundamental of all clinical values: the good of the patient.

Good surgical palliative care from the patient's point of view begins with a definition of their goals of care and then the means to attain these goals through the care provided by professionals, regardless of their discipline. Because these goals may be fluid and changeable, defining them and delivering the appropriate end-of-life care to meet them requires an interdisciplinary approach. Singer *et al.* identify five domains of quality of life for the patient at the end of life: adequate pain and symptom management, avoidance of inappropriate prolongation of dying, sense of control, relief of burdens, and strengthening of relationships with loved ones.[2] The complex, varied nature of these domains requires an interdisciplinary team to ensure their realization. For surgical patients near death, optimally addressing these goals requires the coordinated knowledge and skills of both palliative care practitioners and surgical professionals. These skills may include wound care and debridement, palliative surgical procedures, insertion of feeding tubes or other life support *alongside* communication of bad news, pain and symptom management, end-of-life decision making, spiritual care, and bereavement support. While the surgeon's skills in the first group may be considerable, they may not be versed in decision making about *when* to use them, and how to use them to alleviate suffering as well as disease. Here the interdisciplinary team is essential to facilitate decision making and modify goals of care, and weigh the benefits and burdens of various therapies, perhaps while surgical care is ongoing. The traditional hierarchical 'surgical team' must be replaced by an alternative to include professionals who value comfort as their goal while working alongside surgical professionals. The 'medical model' (let alone the surgical model) is quite inadequate as a representation of what is entailed in palliative care. Only a bio-psycho-social-spiritual model can suggest its breadth and complexity and only an appropriate kind of teamwork can implement its promise.

While interdisciplinary care seems ethically and intuitively sound, evidence supports its ability to improve patient outcomes in a variety of settings. Several studies on the use of a 'comprehensive care team' in the intensive care unit for dying patients demonstrated improved processes and efficiency.[3,4] Improvement of outcomes by use of team-driven protocols in specific diseases or practices has been shown in many disciplines in medicine.[5] As end-of-life care has many domains, its quality improvement requires both process and structure changes, sometimes at a system level. This in turn requires an interdisciplinary team with members from system leadership (administrators, medical directors) and day-to-day leadership (nurses, social workers) as well as those with specific technical expertise (physicians, pharmacists, clergy).[6] Evidence-based outcome improvement by an interdisciplinary team approach specifically in surgical palliative care has yet to be demonstrated.

Definition of the interdisciplinary team

Any team by definition is comprised of individuals with differing competencies from various disciplines. However, a multidisciplinary team must be distinguished from the interdisciplinary one as subtle but important differences can affect patient care and team interaction. A 'multi-disciplinary' team is entirely defined and directed by one of the disciplines. Each member is first a representative of his or her discipline with specific skills and secondly, a team member. An operating room team is among the clearest examples imaginable, while the dichotomous relationship of curative surgical team versus the palliative care team is another. Here, surgical patients may become hospice patients. Once a patient is identified as dying, or curative care is deemed unlikely, a palliative care expert comes onto the surgical service as an invited consultant to evaluate a patient. If the consultant decides that the patient is suitable, the patient is discharged from the surgical service to the palliative care service. This transaction, while in theory, multidisciplinary, takes place at or near the cell walls of both the surgical service and palliative service. Other than the patient, little was exchanged and nothing like integration was even contemplated, let alone attempted. This is in effect palliative care *after* surgery, not inter-disciplinary care (Figure 7.1). This sort of arrangement tends to support the fears and clichés of patients and physicians that palliative care is only done 'when there is nothing left to do' and is 'giving up hope'.

By contrast, the 'interdisciplinary' team has essential functions that require collaboration and parallel delivery of care. All members of the team care for the patient over time, so there is no abrupt transition from cure to comfort. Leadership may be shared or fluid depending on patient needs and key decisions emerge precisely from the relatively unscripted interplay of complementary perspectives; the teams' accomplishments are products rather than sums, and the whole is greater than the mere sum of the parts. Even deeper than the level of specific knowledge and skill, a surgical palliative care team embraces complementary perspectives or ways of thinking and perceiving. Communication and coordination between team members in the setting of changing goals are essential to optimal functioning of the team. For example, the

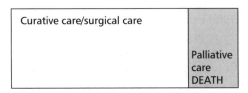

Fig. 7.1 Dichotomous care: surgical versus palliative.

complementary nature of nursing and surgery is not to be found in the differing technical expertise of each profession nor the different relationship to patients and families. It is rather that medicine and nursing have different ways of understanding and responding to the same phenomena. In a *multidisciplinary* team these differences are deliberately and appropriately minimized. In *interdisciplinary* palliative care, the patient is best served when the complementary disciplinary perspectives are recognized, mutually involved, and explored.

These complementary perspectives are essential to address all of the palliative care domains. For example, while a physician or surgeon can address pain and symptom management, inform the patient about prognosis and natural history of the disease process, and guide decision making about therapy, communication of these issues may be facilitated by a palliative care nurse, clergy, or social worker. Decisions regarding therapies must be guided by their relative benefits and burdens, again an understanding relayed by a physician, or nurse, or spiritual counsellor or a combination of all three. A palliative care nurse or nurse practitioner may better provide assessment of symptoms and pain in an ongoing fashion, hour to hour for symptom relief as well as understand patient-oriented experience of the illness. Bereavement counsellors and clergy may be best equipped to facilitate relationships with loved ones and to guide exploration of meaning at the end of life; importantly they inform the other team members of the patient's experience and sense of meaning which may guide other therapies. Social workers and hospice workers may be most qualified to address practical aspects of care, such as financial and care-giving burdens that can lead to inordinate suffering on the part of the family and patient.

While the discipline of palliative care has long been committed to the interdisciplinary team, the notion of *surgical palliative care* adds a new dimension to the team; that is the surgeon or other surgical specialists. The culture of surgery may preclude any comfort on the part of surgeons with their role as a member of the interdisciplinary team, or even with the process of palliative care itself. The surgeon is usually the leader of the surgical team, which is a primarily multidisciplinary entity. Literature describing the culture of surgery alludes to value in action, fixing, and optimism[7] with a modern focus on cure and technology. Death can be seen as a failure in this context.[8] Success is measured in procedural outcomes rather than patient-oriented outcomes. For example, a focus on morbidity and mortality as negative outcomes precludes any value in a 'good death' or the relief of suffering. However, several traditions in surgery can be traced which paradoxically suggest that palliative care by surgeons fits into the larger history of surgical care.[9] Many surgical procedures originated as palliative procedures; relief of suffering through surgical means has a long thread through surgical history. In addition, there is a long tradition of surgical thought which encompasses procedures only in the context of the whole patient. Centuries ago, John Hunter wrote: 'Before undertaking surgery, the surgeon should consider the whole man, his life, history, habits, constitutional idiosyncrasies, the previous ailments, interaction of his mind, emotional and body.'[10] Similarly, in modern times, the surgeon can and should consider surgical procedures and therapy as part of a larger context in palliative care. The question should be asked how does such a procedure or surgery facilitate the particular patient's sense of well-being and alleviate suffering when compared to the burdens it might cause? The surgeon is unique in understanding the benefits and risks of any procedure or therapy as well as the likelihood of different potential outcomes with respect to physical well-being and pain and symptom management. But they may need input from other members of the team to understand the psychosocial benefits and risks of a procedure for the particular patient as well as someone to facilitate communication with the patient.

The interdisciplinary team can create challenges for care that do not occur in the typical medical model due to relative ambiguity of roles. All members of the team must take responsibility and initiative in the comprehensive care of the patient. There is no consistent team leader; without an established hierarchy conflicts must be resolved in other manners. Similarly, decision making must be by consensus and patient oriented. In some instances, the decision maker may be one member of the team by virtue of his or her relationship with the patient, while at other times someone else may take on this role.

While the goal of palliative care is understood, measuring success or accomplishment of the team is more difficult. Its benefits may be intangible or unmeasurable by standard quantitative means. Some team members may gather meaning from one individual's circumstance while others may be relatively untouched. The typical goals of care, such as cure or discharge from the hospital, are not relevant in palliative care. Some may see a particular case as a peaceful death while other team members may not. The quality of bereavement process may be unknown because no feedback is available. Some members of the team may adapt well to this ambiguity while others may not.

Models of interdisciplinary care

Interdisciplinary care can be modelled in many fashions. The critical factor for delivery of surgical palliative care is that the multiple disciplines can be easily integrated with each other and into existing structures of care. The following are two cases which illustrate two approaches to interdisciplinary care. The first demonstrates a model which facilitates integration of palliative care into the surgical service structure while the second describes integration of surgical care into the palliative care setting.

Jack was in the surgical intensive care for several weeks for what intially appeared not to be a terminal condition. He had a history of untreated chronic obstructive pulmonary disease when he was injured in a motor vehicle crash. Although his chest injuries were not life threatening, after several weeks of therapy he remained ventilator-dependent with a tracheostomy. After his initial critical illness resolved, he was more alert. He began to refuse medical care. He pulled out his feeding tube, intravenous lines, and thwarted the nurses' attempts to care for him. He was clearly not delirious or encephalopathic; attempts to talk with him were difficult due to his tracheostomy. He appeared angry and depressed and the nurses and doctors were frustrated.

Both psychiatry and ethics consultations were done as medically a permanent feeding tube seemed indicated, but the patient refused any tube or nutrition. The palliative care counsellor began to see him and his family. After several family meetings she learned that Jack's wife had died after a long illness from laryngeal cancer; Jack had cared for her in her last days when she had suffered immensely with a tracheostomy, unable to speak. Clearly, Jack was most afraid of suffering from suffocation in a similar manner. His family revealed that he had vowed never to be on a ventilator, that his independence was most important, and that to him being unable to talk meant he was closer and closer to death. The advanced practice nurse in palliative care began to work with Jack for help with pain and symptom management, despite the fact that it was not certain that he was dying. A percutaneous gastrostomy tube was placed so that he could receive nutrition comfortably and aggressive nutritional support might allow him to be weaned from the ventilator. The gastrostomy eventually became a secondary issue as alleviation of Jack's spiritual and emotional suffering became paramount concerns. Medications were adjusted and added to treat his depression and anxiety. More importantly, the palliative/ bereavement counsellor saw him daily for conversation, spiritual support, as well as massage. One day Jack's face lit up when she visited him, held his hand, and conversed for quite a while. 'It is so nice to see you today. How are you?' she said. It was the first time anyone had seen him smile.

There were multiple meetings with the team, the patient, and the family. Eventually, as hope for ventilator weaning dimmed, a do-not-resuscitate order was placed and ventilator support was withdrawn in keeping with Jack's wishes. Jack was treated for dyspnoea, with his family at his side as well as the surgeon, counsellor and palliative care nurse. He died peacefully after a six-week intensive care unit stay.

Together, the interdisciplinary team successfully provided surgical palliative care to Jack in the intensive care unit. Because of the team, his care at the end of life was improved in several subtle but significant ways. First, the integration of the team into the intensive care unit provided continuity for both the patient and family. As goals shifted or new ones were added, a change in providers was not required. The original physicians and nurses who knew the full range of medical issues continued to care for him; thus when end-of-life decisions became more acute, new relationships did not need to be formed and decisions were made based on Jack's specific circumstances and wishes. Second, team members versed in ethical and spiritual issues were able to provide comfort and meaning, while critical care and surgical procedures continued on. This allowed palliative care to proceed despite an uncertain prognosis, *alongside* aggressive medical care as appropriate. Third, as life support was withdrawn and spiritual and physical comfort became the most important aspect of Jack's care, team members with this expertise became the primary care providers. Jack did not need to transfer to a hospice or palliative care unit for end-of-life care but was able to die peacefully in the intensive care unit, which was by now a familiar environment.

Jack received integrated care from a surgeon intensivist, critical care nurse, advanced practice palliative care nurse, and spiritual and bereavement counsellor. Each member of the team brought individual expertise to the particular situation, but there was considerable overlap as well. A truly interdisciplinary model must integrate the team members' care delivery with *each other* as well as the patient and the family. The team is more than the sum of its part just as the patient or person is more than the sum of his physical parts. The nature and aetiology of Jack's suffering was unique to him and was not solely related to physical pain. The palliative care counsellor was critical in identifying his particular suffering and interpreting it for the rest of the team. This was especially important for end-of-life decision making regarding withholding and withdrawing of procedures and life support. While the surgeon had the technical expertise for such procedures and the most information about prognosis and possible outcomes of a procedure, they relied on the palliative care counsellor or nurse to place it in an ethical and palliative context for this particular patient. Thus the surgeon's ability to relieve suffering by certain procedures or life support was dependent on other team members, but other team members also relied on surgical expertise for appropriate decision making.

This model of interdisciplinary teamwork is particularly suited to the intensive care unit. We developed a surgical palliative care interdisciplinary team within the surgical intensive care unit (Figure 7.2). This core team includes surgeon/intensivist, advanced practice nurse in palliative care/bereavement, palliative care/bereavement counsellor, and critical care nurse. Other team members such as clergy, social workers, advanced pain management, respiratory therapy, and surgical sub-specialists may be called in. The core members of the team evaluate and treat the critically ill or injured patient and family from admission to the surgical intensive care unit. Because there is often uncertainty about prognosis and who in the intensive care unit is actually dying, the team does not wait for care to become clearly palliative before beginning treatment. The team members are around in the surgical intensive care unit as members of the critical care team. This enables surgical critical care to be delivered in parallel with palliative care. The

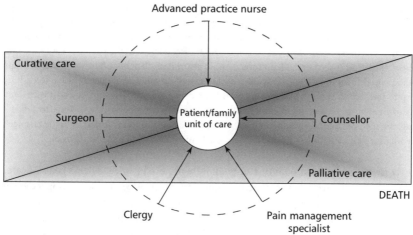

Fig. 7.2 Model of inderdisciplinary care.

advanced practice nurse addresses pain and symptom management, ethical issues around life support, and provides bereavement support for families. The palliative care counsellor focuses on bereavement for families but also provides spiritual and emotional support for patients around their illness and end of life. Together with the surgeon and critical care nurse, they provide therapy in the context of shifting goals of care. Importantly, the counsellor and advanced practice nurse also provide support for the physician and nursing staff. The whole team then can address changing goals of care and end-of-life decisions as they arise as well as relief of suffering without transfer of care to another service.

The above model and case demonstrate the value of the interdisciplinary team as *part* of a surgical service. Here palliative care is successfully integrated into surgical care for patients who are not clearly at the end of life. However, surgical palliative care may be required for patients who are already terminally ill. Consultation for surgical services may be required to improve palliation of suffering, but this necessitates a different type of interdisciplinary approach.

Sylvia was admitted to the surgical intensive care unit after a major debridement of her infected hemipelvectomy wound. She had been diagnosed with sarcoma of the thigh several months before and now had recurrent tumour at the surgery site as well as new lung meta-stases. Initially she was in septic shock and respiratory failure but this improved after hydration, dopamine, and antibiotics. The hope of the orthopaedic oncologist and medical oncologist was that she would heal her wound so that she could undergo chemotherapy for the lung metastases. After some improvement, Sylvia was extubated, oxygenating well, but had a limited mobility due to severe dyspnoea. Her wound was debilitating, requiring multiple dressing changes and debridements.

The palliative care nurse and counsellor collaborated with the critical care and surgical teams for pain management, wound care, relief of dyspnoea, and spiritual support. They learned that Sylvia's only family was her daughter, in Spain, who had just had a baby. Sylvia wanted more than anything to see her only grandchild for the first time. As it became clear that Sylvia would be unlikely to leave the hospital soon, arrangements were made for her daughter and granddaughter to travel to see her. Discussions ensued with the patient, the orthopaedic surgeon, the oncologist, and palliative care nurse and counsellor about advance care planning: Sylvia did not want to be on life-support again but wanted very much to wait for her daughter. Multiple surgical procedures for wound care, while medically indicated, did not seem to meet her goals, and the orthopaedic surgeon agreed to halt them. However, she developed a worsening malignant pleural effusion and progressive dyspnoea and hypoxia, necessitating a chest tube with a return to ventilator support imminent. Sylvia did not want to be on a ventilator again as she wanted the time she had left to be spent with her new grand-daughter. The thoracic surgeon was consulted. After discussion with the palliative care team and the patient, the surgeon recommended thoracoscopic pleurodesis to palliate her symptoms of dyspnoea without need for a long-term chest tube. If successful, it would allow her to leave for a hospice. Despite the risk of surgery and further ventilator dependence, Sylvia agreed and underwent the procedure. She improved significantly and was extubated postoperatively in time to talk to her daughter and hold her new granddaughter. After several days she was transferred to the hospice with ongoing surgical care for her wounds, where her family was able to be at her bedside.

In this case, the procedural skills of a surgeon were required to meet Sylvia's goals of care. Here, the core interdisciplinary team included an oncologist, oncologic nurse, orthopaedic surgeon, wound care nurse, advanced practice nurse in palliative care, and the palliative care counsellor. Shifting goals of care and decision making were facilitated by the palliative care nurse and counsellor, with surgeons providing consultation on the likely benefits and burdens of surgery as well as prognosis. The interdisciplinary nature of care allowed for an important surgical procedure to occur, even though a palliative course of therapy was chosen by the patient. Again, palliative and surgical care were provided in parallel by a team.

This interdisciplinary team was able to overcome the cultural conflicts and barriers that exist between surgical and palliative disciplines. The thoracic surgeon was educated and encouraged by the team to perform palliative thoracoscopy, a major procedure, despite the negative outcome in traditional surgical 'morbidity and mortality' terms. Surgeons and surgical nurses as members of an interdisciplinary team can find value in providing surgical care, despite the unlikely event of a cure, to alleviate suffering. Similarly, the benefits of a surgical procedure became apparent to the palliative care providers as an effective means to treat distressing symptoms. The goal for the interdisciplinary team becomes a good and peaceful death; this overrides individual disciplinary goals. The interdisciplinary team allows for palliative care to be integrated into the surgical setting; it allows curative and palliative care to be delivered in parallel, not an either/or fashion, so that the transition from cure to comfort is smooth. This care has multiple and changing goals and requires multiple levels of expertise and coordination. For these reasons interdisciplinary care is essential to good surgical palliative care.

References

1. Davidson, J.D. (2001). So now what do we do? In: *Care-giving and loss: family needs, professional responses* (ed. K.J. Doka and J.K. Davidson), pp. 299–302. Hospice Foundation of America.
2. Singer, P.A., Martin, D.K., and Kelner, M. (1999). Quality-of-life issues: patients' perspectives. *J.A.M.A.*, **281**, 163–8.
3. Carlson, R.W., Devich, L., and Frank, R.R. (1988). Development of a comprehensive support care team for the hopelessly ill in a university hospital medical service. *J.A.M.A.*, **259**, 378–83.
4. Field, B.E., Devich, L.E., and Carlson, R.W. (1989). Impact of a comprehensive support team on management of hopelessly ill patients with multiple organ failure. *Chest*, **96**, 353–6.
5. Cohen, I.L. (1993). Establishing and justifying specialized teams in intensive care units for nutrition, ventilator management and palliative care. *Crit. Care Clin.*, **9**, 511–20.
6. Lynn, J., Shuster, J.L., and Kabcenell, A. (2000). *Improving care at the end of life*, pp. 11–34. Oxford University Press, Oxford.
7. Katz, P. (1999). *The scalpel's edge: the culture of surgeons*. Allyn and Bacon, Needham Heights, MA.

8. Buchman, T., Cassell, J., Ray, S.E., and Wax, M.L. (2002). Who should manage the dying patient? Rescue, shame, and the surgical ICU dilemma. *J. Am. Coll. Surg.*, **194**, 665–73.

9. Dunn, G.P. (2001). The surgeon and palliative care: an evolving perspective. *Surg. Oncol. Clin.*, **10**, 7–21.

10. Kobler, J. (1960). *The reluctant surgeon: a biography of John Hunter*, p. 165. Doubleday, New York.

Chapter 8

Quality of life issues in palliative surgery

Michael Koller, Christoph Nies, and Wilfried Lorenz

Introduction

Palliative medicine and the topic of quality of life share a common fate in Western medicine: both have no hero status. The hero in medicine and particularly in surgery is the charismatic doctor who understands a clinical problem within seconds, makes the appropriate decision (preferably by means of intuitive judgement),[1] and carries out a complicated operation. All this leads to the healing of the patient. The patient is no longer a patient, the disease is gone, the patient is healed. The desired end-point of survival is established.

Unfortunately, day-to-day medicine is less glamorous and the fact of dying is an indisputable part of the human condition. A life-saving procedure cannot always be the case in a person's history. Technically speaking, survival is not a universal end-point that would allow us to evaluate the efficacy of all medical procedures. Here, considerations such as 'quality of life' come into play as a 'surrogate' parameter. From this seeming discrepancy between survival and quality of life, the QOL issue has the image of the 'weak'. This stereotype corresponds to the belief that QOL is a 'soft' end-point that cannot be measured reliably.

These misconceptions notwithstanding, people cannot avoid the crucial and often uneasy question of what kind of life they would like to live, what kind of death they are afraid of, and what kind of transition from life to death they would prefer.[2] From this description it becomes evident that palliative care and QOL are inextricably interwoven. Quality of life is *the* end-point when it comes to evaluation of the efficacy of palliative/terminal care.

The present chapter is designed to investigate the following arguments:

1 Palliative care and quality of life are conceptually related.

2 Quality of life can be assessed in a satisfactory and methodological way.

3 Quality of life assessment in palliative care poses specific methodological and logistical problems.

4 Quality of life assessment can help to improve patient care.

Concepts of palliative care, outcome, and quality of life

The traditional distinction between active and palliative treatment has been challenged by recent conceptual developments (Figure 8.1). The traditional view proposes that active treatment starts and continues until it becomes clear that there is no chance that it will be effective in prolonging a patient's survival. Then as a second (and last) choice palliative care begins (Table 8.1).

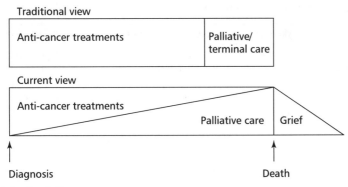

Fig. 8.1 Models of palliative care.

The modern view does not make this strict conceptual distinction between active and palliative treatment. Rather the goal should be both, life-prolonging and comforting at the same time. Literally speaking the term 'palliative' comes from the Latin word 'palliare': to cover with a coat. Thus, both treatment aspects can go side by side, but the relative focus is dependent on the time from start of therapy to death. According to the new concept, palliative care cannot be equated with terminal care. Whereas active treatment satisfies the therapeutic goal of healing, the palliative component tries to ease the symptoms and discomfort that may be associated with the active treatment or the disease. The palliative component also satisfies treatment goals that are not achieved by the active component such as reducing anxiety or depression.

This concept also does justice to recent findings on the relationship between quantity and quality of life. Several studies support the intriguing hypothesis that QOL is a predictor of survival.[3,4] In other words, the better the well-being of a patient at the beginning of the course of therapy, the longer the patient will live. The mechanism of this phenomenon is not understood yet, but the mere empirical facts challenge the strict distinction between quality and quantity of life. Ideally, both go hand in hand and the art of medicine, including palliative care, is to bring both these aspects of human existence into an optimal balance.

Also interesting is the grief section of the model: it reflects the fact that family members and possibly therapists also need time to say goodbye and to cope with the death of a relative, friend, or patient. Bereavement care should be provided for those at risk for complicated grief.[5,6]

Table 8.1 Palliative treatment for various tumours with incurable stages

Tumour	Symptom	Cause of symptoms	Palliative therapy
Oesophageal carcinoma	Dysphagia	Endoluminal tumour growth with stenosis or obstruction	Dilatation of the stenosis, endoscopic laser therapy, implantation of a stent, palliative radiotherapy, or radiochemotherapy
Gastric carcinoma	Upper gastrointestinal bleeding	Bleeding from the tumour	Endoscopic haemostasis, palliative resection of the tumour
	Vomiting	Gastric outlet obstruction	Palliative resection, gastroenterostomy, implantation of a stent

Table 8.1 (continued) Palliative treatment for various tumours with incurable stages

Tumour	Symptom	Cause of symptoms	Palliative therapy
Carcinoma of the head of the pancreas	Jaundice	Obstruction of the common bile duct	Endoscopic implantation of a stent through the papilla of Vater, percutaneous transhepatic implantation of a stent, biliary-enteric anastomosis
	Vomiting	Duodenal obstruction	Gastroenterostomy
	Pain	Infiltration of retroperitoneal nerves	Pain therapy with analgetic drugs, CT-guided alcohol ablation of retroperitoneal nerves, thoracoscopic transection of splanchnic nerves
Carcinoma of the colon	Ileus	Colon obstruction due to tumour growth	Palliative resection, diverting colostomy, intestinal bypass
Carcinoma of the rectum	Lower gastro-intestinal bleeding	Bleeding from the tumour	Endoscopic haemostasis, cryotherapy, palliative resection
	Ileus	Obstruction of the rectum due to tumour growth	Diverting colostomy, cryotherapy, palliative resection

After all, the patient is a social being. Care and dying constitute social processes that affect all participating in this process. As will be discussed later, one of the strengths of the QOL approach is its inclusion of the often neglected social component.

The development of QOL has to be seen in connection with the 'outcome movement'. As A.S. Relman, former editor of the *New England Journal of Medicine*, pointed out, the outcome movement is a response to deficiencies in a health care system that became too costly.[7] The outcome movement tries to bring a crucial rational element into medicine. The idea is to offer and pay only for treatment options that have been proven effective in clinical studies. Now what are the parameters that would indicate good care?

Traditional outcome parameters such as survival, complication rates, recurrence, etc. have long been in use in medicine and medical research.[8] Such outcomes make perfect sense as long as survival is the main therapeutic goal. By definition, however, survival is not the primary goal in palliative care. How can we find out whether the goal of palliation was achieved? The only people who can answer this question are the patients themselves. Therefore, questionnaires have been constructed that allow patients to express their subjective perception and evaluation. The minimum definition that most researchers in this area agree is that QOL measures have to cover well-being and functional capacities in the somatic, psychological, and social domains.

Taking this minimal definition as a starting point, one may ask what determines whether a patient has a good or bad quality of life. Is it the degree of illness, the course of the disease, the treatment, the family, or the type of supportive care? In order to shed some light on this question we carried out a series of studies in cancer patients using the standardized EORTC questionnaire.[9–11] When we had a close look at scores such as global QOL or overall symptom burden, it turned out that 'hard' data such as tumour growth, type of operation, time since operation, age, gender, or physicians' judgements explained a little of the variation. However, psychosocial concepts such as negative affect, experienced social stigma, social desirability, positive thinking, or therapy-related expectations were good correlates of patients' well-being.

This set of findings together with the new conception of active and palliative treatment brings us to suggest that in the palliative situation the following outcome concept would be appropriate (Figure 8.2).[12] Only both sides together portray the full picture of the patient. Which is the true end-point may vary over time; probably it will be more on the left side in the active phase of treatment and more on the right side in the palliative phase, particularly when the palliative phase moves into terminal care.

Quality of life can be measured

Although the concept of QOL has been around in medicine and in medical research for more than 15 years, it still appears vague to many clinicians. Therefore this section is devoted to basic measurement issues.

Research efforts in the past decade have concentrated on developing standardized QOL questionnaires. Several international working groups have been simultaneously active and have independently developed measurement instruments.

Questionnaire development follows a stepwise procedure:[13]

♦ item generation, i.e. developing a list of issues that should be included in the questionnaire; clinicians, nurses, methodologists, and patients should take part in this phase of the project
♦ pruning the list of items according to the relative importance of the issues

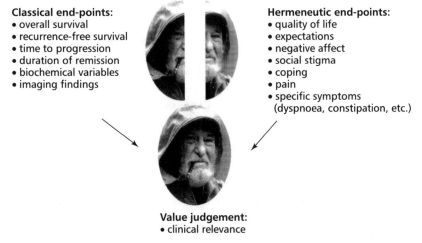

Classical end-points:
• overall survival
• recurrence-free survival
• time to progression
• duration of remission
• biochemical variables
• imaging findings

Hermeneutic end-points:
• quality of life
• expectations
• negative affect
• social stigma
• coping
• pain
• specific symptoms
  (dyspnoea, constipation, etc.)

Value judgement:
• clinical relevance

Fig. 8.2 Three-component outcome model in palliative care.

- pre-testing the questionnaire in small studies, further specification of the questions, and the response scales
- formal validation of the questionnaire in large-scale studies.

In the course of this process, questionnaires are rigorously tested according to their psychometric properties:[14,15]

- reliability: how accurate is the questionnaire (low measurement error, internal consistency); can results be replicated?
- validity: does the questionnaire measure what it is intended to measure?
- sensitivity: is the questionnaire responsive to actual changes in the patient's condition?

These properties can be expressed in statistical terms. Statistical procedures that are commonly used include Cronbachs alpha, group comparisons, before–after tests, multivariate correlational/regression analyses, factor analysis, and structural equation modelling.[14,15] At this point it is sufficient to say that all standardized measures now available have shown satisfactory psychometric results. Details may be found in the original publications and are summarized in several handbooks.[16,17] In the remainder of this section we will focus on the content of the questionnaires.

Given the rigorous psychometric approach, researchers in the field are quite confident about the conception and usefulness of QOL measurements, so that many would agree with a working definition: QOL is what the standardized questionnaire measures. Is it then true that different QOL questionnaires assess the same thing? In order to clarify this point we compared four standardized questionnaires that are widely used in clinical studies.

The European Organization for Research and Treatment of Cancer (headquarters: Brussels, Belgium) initiated a QOL project in 1986 and since then has produced a so-called modular assessment system consisting of a 30-item core questionnaire (the EORTC QOL questionnaire C30) and numerous diagnosis-specific modules (e.g. breast cancer, colorectal cancer, etc.)[18,19]

A very similar approach has been adopted by a research group in Chicago that developed the Functional Assessment of Cancer Treatment (FACT) questionnaire. Versions of this questionnaire are also available for other chronic conditions such as human immunodeficiency virus (HIV) or multiple sclerosis (MS).[20]

The SF-36 has its roots in the medical outcome study (MOS) performed by the RAND cooperation. Given its tireless promotion and the active research environment, it now seems to be the most widely used QOL instrument worldwide.[21]

The PLC (Profile der Lebensqualität chronisch Kranker, profiles of quality of life of the chronically ill) has been developed in Germany and is based on a medico-sociological concept.[22] English and Spanish translations are available and to date international contributions come primarily from Spain.

Despite their different origins, the four questionnaires display – on the surface – striking similarities (Table 8.2). On a technical level all questionnaires make use of Likert scales. This means that each individual question is followed by a numerical response scale with clearly defined intervals (e.g. 1 = not at all, 2 = little, 3 = somewhat, 4 = rather, 5 = very much so) so that responses to questions that capture a common dimension (e.g. somatic distress) can be aggregated.

All questionnaires are self-administered, which means patients are supposed to fill them out themselves. All questionnaires have a moderate length of 30 to 40 items so that they can be completed within 10 to 15 minutes.

Table 8.2 Commonalities among QOL questionnaires

	EORTC	SF-36	PLC	FACT
Technical aspects				
Likert-Scaling	x	x	x	x
Self-assessed	x	x	x	x
Length: approx. 30–40 items	x	x	x	x
Contents				
Somatic symptoms	x	x	(x)	x
Psychological well-being	x	x	x	x
Social aspects	x	x	x	x
Functional capabilities	x	x	x	x
Global QOL	x	x		x

In terms of content, the questionnaires make reference to somatic symptoms, psychological well-being, social aspects, and functional abilities and allow for a score of global QOL (summary score).

However, the questionnaires reveal their individualities when it comes to the details. We start with technical aspects first (Table 8.3). Regarding scaling, the PLC (0 = not at all, 1 = badly, 2 = moderately, 3 = well, 4 = very well) and the FACT (0 = not at all, 1 = a little bit, 2 = somewhat, 3 = quite a bit, 4 = very much) stick uniformly to five response alternatives. The EORTC scales allow for four response alternatives (1 = not at all, 2 = a little, 3 = somewhat, 4 = very much), except the last two items which are accompanied by seven-point scales ranging from 1 (very poor) to 7 (excellent).

Most versatile is the SF-36 that includes several scale formats allowing for either two (yes, no), three (yes, limited a lot; yes, limited a little; no, not limited at all), five (excellent, very good, good, fair, poor), or six (all of the time, most of the time, a good bit of the time, some of the time, a little of the time, none of the time) response options.

The SF-36 is also flexible regarding other aspects. In addition to the patient version of the questionnaire, there is also an observer version, in which health care providers, family members, or others may assess the patient. There exists a four-week time-frame version ('indicate your well-being during the past four weeks') in addition to the standard one-week version. Furthermore, there is also a short form of the questionnaire containing only 12 instead of the usual 36 questions.

The most notable discrepancies appear, however, when it comes to the relative weighting of the content of the questionnaires. The classification in Table 8.3 was done by the authors in a straight-forward way, taking into account the face validity and semantic meaning of the individual items of the questionnaires. A few examples should illustrate the classification rationale: somatic symptoms (nausea/vomiting, difficulty breathing), psychological (tense, worry), social (impairment of social encounters, family life), functional (climbing stairs, ability to relax), global (overall quality of life), positive (feel happy, enjoy meals), negative ('I expect my health will deteriorate'). Sometimes one item could be assigned to more than one category (e.g. psychological and positive; somatic and functional; social and negative). A few items could not be classified (items with a neutral tone, e.g. usage of nutritional supplements).

Table 8.3 Differences between QOL questionnaires

	EORTC	SF-36	PLC	FACT
Technical aspects				
Scaling (response options)	4, 7	2, 3, 5, 6	5	5
Self and other ratings	no	yes	no	no
Short version	no	yes	no	no
Time period (past . . .)	7 days	7 days or 4 weeks	7 days	7 days
Translations (no. of languages)	>20	>20	3	3
Contents				
Somatic symptoms	27%	6%	(0%)*	25%
Psychological well-being	13%	25%	33%	29%
Social aspects	10%	6%	23%	39%
Functional capabilities	23%	50%	53%	32%
Global QOL	7%	6%	0%	100%**
Positive experiences	3%	14%	45%	54%
Negative experiences (complaints, impairments)	97%	72%	25%	43%

Note: Percentages relate to the number of items containing a particular characteristic divided by the number of total questions of the questionnaire (i.e. EORTC, n = 30; SF-36, n = 36; PLC, n = 40; FACT, n = 28).

* additional symptom modules exist

** summary score across the total number of items

As can be seen in Table 8.3, the proportion of physical symptoms is highest in the EORTC and FACT. Psychological as well as social issues are extensively covered by PLC and FACT. The SF-36 and FACT are strong in functional aspects. The EORTC and SF36 include separate questions to indicate overall quality of life/health, whereas FACT allows for the computing of a summary index across the total of all items.

SF36 and particularly the EORTC focus on impairment, thus tap into negative aspects of life, whereas PLC and FACT capture positive aspects of health, well-being, and everyday encounters.

It is also important to note that one should be careful in interpreting the names and labels of subscales or questionnaires. There are marked discrepancies in how different authors use these labels. For instance, what is called 'emotional functioning' in the EORTC questionnaire is commonly referred to as 'negative affect' in the personality literature.[9,23] A new, methodologically sound, and brief measure that is intended to assess 'habitual well-being'[24] comes very close to what is seen as a particular functional aspect (capacity to enjoy) in the PLC. The SF-36 is commonly discussed under the rubric quality of life, but some authors have used the term 'health status assessment'.[25]

Given this lack of conceptual clarity, it is not surprising that studies comparing questionnaires with one another have found disappointingly low correlations.[26] Transformation procedures have been proposed that should lead to higher equivalence of test scores stemming from different questionnaires.[27] The chances are that the future will see a generation of so-called calibration studies in order to reconcile issues. The outcome of such research efforts, however, is uncertain. Quality of life assessment is becoming an industry (including computerized questionnaire versions)[28,29] and – quite understandably – research groups have a vital interest in demonstrating that their own assessment approach looks particularly good!

On a deeper level, the problems mentioned above ought to be seen in connection with Popper's criticism regarding the value of definitions: a human being can be defined as a 'biped without feathers'.[30] This definition is correct, but makes little sense. In the same vein, questionnaires tapping into humans' experiences related to health or illness may be called measures of 'quality of life', 'health-related quality of life', 'subjective well-being' or 'health status'. No label is better than the other and which one to choose is ultimately an arbitrary decision.

A subject matter is preferably described by its components and attributes.[31,32] In respect to the QOL issue this means that we have to be sure about the content of the items, the time frame, whether the patient or someone else fills out the questionnaire, and the exact situation in which the questionnaire data are collected. These considerations have implications for the very obvious question of which questionnaire is the 'best' and which to choose for a particular study. Decision algorithms have been published,[33] but we suggest that the most important part is actually to read the items one by one and to make clear whether the questions asked will answer the research question. When a definitive decision is hard to make, spilot studies, including patients, nurses, and research personnel, will help to decide on the most appropriate measurement device.

Specific measurement problems in the palliative/terminal situation

Measurement issues

There are certain problems in the palliative/terminal situation that are not covered in the standardized QOL questionnaires described. These include spiritual and existential problems, the care situation, family support/social isolation, and specific somatic symptoms. Furthermore, most standardized questionnaires are too long for those palliative patients who have reached their final stages. Timing is an important issue.[34] Taking the time axis in Figure 8.1 as a frame of reference, we would guess that the standard instruments described in the previous section are viable in the first half of the course of the disease and treatment. Later on, more specific instruments will be more appropriate. Such instruments have been developed in recent years and the progress in this field can best be evaluated when comparing the present list[35–40] (Table 8.4) with earlier reviews.[41,42]

The questionnaires vary in length containing between five and 17 items (the TIQ with 36 being an exception). They address typical symptoms and therapy side-effects (pain, fatigue, nausea), and psychological and social issues and worry (family concerns) about the future, the illness, and about dying. As detailed above, a close look at the content of questionnaires, together with a clarification of the research or clinical question to be resolved, will help researchers/clinicians to find the appropriate instrument.

To date, most publications have used the STAS and the MQOL. International translation procedures and validation studies have not been performed yet for a palliative-specific instrument. However, a short form of the EORTC QLQ-C30 for palliative settings and specific scales addressing spiritual and existential dimensions are under development.

A major issue in palliative QOL research is whether the patient or someone else (care provider, family member) should fill in the questionnaire. Studies have been published in which questionnaires were completed either by the patients,[43] by health providers,[43] or in a more sloppy manner either by patients or others (depending on how ill the patients felt).[35] This constitutes

Table 8.4 QOL questionnaires specifically developed for use in palliative care settings

	STAS[43]	MQOL[37]	PEPS[39]	TIQ[35]	ESAS[40]	HRCA-QL[38]	POS[36]
Contents of individual items or dimensions	Patient and family items	Overall QOL	Part I:	Physical symptoms resulting from disease or therapy (24 items)	pain fatigue nausea depression anxiety drowsiness appetite sense of well being shortness of breath (nine visual analogue scales)	mobility health support daily living outlook (modified Spitzer Index)	Pain
	pain control symptom control	Most troublesome symptoms	Patients generate list of problems that are troublesome				Other symptoms
	patient anxiety patient insight family anxiety family insight	Feeling phys. terrible depressed worried sad future	Part II: Global rating of QOL on a scale from 0 to 10	Functional condition (capacity to work, enjoy, look after oneself; 3 items)			Worry about illness or treatment (patient)
	predictability planning spiritual communication between patient and family	Life: meaningful/ -less goals (not) achieved worthwhile/ worthless under control		Psychological conditions (emotion and cognition; 6 items)			Worry about illness or treatment (family)
	Service Items	self-worth burden world (un)pleasant support/no support		Family and social relationships (2 items)			Information giving to patient and family
	Practical aid financial waste wasted time communication			Global judgement (1 item)			Patient ability to show emotion

	professional anxiety advising professionals					Life worth living
						Feeling good about themselves
						Wasted time
						Addressing of practical matters
						Performance status (ECOG)
No. of items	17	17	36	9	5	12
Rating scales	0–4	Numerical scales 0–10	free format; global QOL: 0–10	0 = best; 10 = best	0 = worst, 1, 2 = best	0 = not at all; 4 = yes, overwhelmingly

a problem, since a considerable number of studies have consistently shown that patient responses and proxy ratings are not closely related.[44] However, it appears that the correlation between doctor and patient ratings rise the better the doctor knows the patient.[9]

It is also unclear what is the criterion of 'good overlap'. Whereas some researchers[43] may judge a correlation of rho = 0.66 as high, others might find this 40% of common variance less satisfying. The critical question is: would an even higher correlation make any difference for practical purposes? From a pragmatic standpoint one might argue that proxy measures are good enough and certainly better than having no account of patients' pain and emotional and functional situations. It can also be argued that routine documentation of patients' (assumed) quality of life may enhance care. This argument gains its credence from the well-known Hawthorne effect in clinical studies. Participants in clinical studies are better off than 'ordinary' patients, regardless of whether they are assigned to the treatment or to the control group. In any event, they receive more attention and better care. The value of proxy assessments may be further enhanced when assessors have sufficient background information (patients' preferences for particular treatments [e.g. no machines!], last will). In the present state of uncertainty, randomized studies are called for to clarify whether proxy measures really enhance the quality of care and patient outcome scores (self-assessed quality of life!).

The most common argument to use proxy measures is patients' inability to fill out an entire questionnaire. One solution to the problem is to reduce the assessment to a single item. Indeed, single visual analogue scales (VAS) and other practical check-lists[45] are widely used in pain research. VAS simply ask patients to indicate their degree of pain along a continuum ranging from 'no pain' to 'worst pain'. The indisputable advantage of such devices is their feasibility (easy use) that guarantees high compliance and allows for multiple assessment (before–after comparisons).

Caveats, however, come from conceptual considerations. Pain is often associated with other somatic symptoms,[9,10] and it is socially more acceptable to report pain than other problems.

Saunders coined the phrase 'total pain' in order to highlight the psychological and social aspects or other specific symptoms that are present when patients report their pain.[46]

Qualitative investigations showed that death is not necessarily the major threat to critically ill patients: social isolation and loss of coherence are major concerns and are even rated higher than fear of pain.[47]

Other studies showed that although patients complain about pain they would rather tolerate a moderate amount of it than increase dosage of pain medication.[48] Undoubtedly, there are clinical situations where pain reduction and pain assessment are the major concern. Fortunately, due to refined therapeutic options, pain can be successfully treated in most terminal cases. Therefore, clinicians should consider the above warnings and not ignore other issues.

Another method to overcome assessment problems due to a limiting condition is a qualitative approach. The stunning simplicity of this method is illustrated with a surgical example. In one study of ours we investigated the relative inconvenience of gastric decompression devices (nasogastric tube versus gastrostomy tube).[49] We took several measures that either showed a weak difference between groups (VAS) or no difference (EORTC QOL questionnaire), but the most sensitive measure was a simple question asked shortly after the operation: 'which tube system is most inconvenient for you?' (Patients had various tubes at that time, such as urinary catheters or drains.) In 44% of cases the nasogastric tube was rated most inconvenient, in only 4% the gastrostomy tube. (The validity of this finding was further confirmed since interviewer effects could be ruled out by having the interviews taped and presented to external reviewers.)

It is interesting to note that the beginnings of the palliative care movement followed a strictly empirical approach, underscoring the need to 'listen to patients'.[46,50] Qualitative methods in severely ill patients have also been described by other authors.[51]

A further novel approach would be observing patients systematically and inferring QOL from body movements, muscle tonus, or gestures. Studies are needed that investigate the connection of such external signs with brain activities related to discomfort or well-being. A somewhat related research example comes from a recent animal experiment where sickness behaviour as a proxy of QOL was telemetrically assessed and related to the animals' immune function.[52] Some readers may find this example remote or even unethical in the context of palliative medicine. However, it must be noted that the fundamentals of learning theory have been discovered in animal models (Pavlov's dog). Even the standard theory to explain reactive depression in humans (learned helplessness) has its roots in animal experiments.[53]

Psychological issues

The description of specific QOL assessment issues would be incomplete without reference to two major psychological forces that play a role in the palliative/terminal setting, namely *expectations* and *denial*.

In a study on radiotherapy inpatients, 58% of the patients expected healing from therapy although the majority followed a palliative regimen.[11] Healing expectation was associated with high QOL at therapy onset. However, patients whose healing expectations were not fulfilled had lowest QOL at the end of the therapy. Another important finding was that patients had multiple expectations. When certain symptoms were prevailing (pain, dyspnoea), the desire for symptom relief was higher than healing expectations. In sum, across the entire sample of patients investigated a good portion of optimism was accompanied by a sense of reality. Such findings have implications for the ongoing discussion on how to inform patients. Full information may reduce QOL immediately; lying to patients may have an equally dramatic effect when patients later find out that the healing goal was unrealistic.

When patients neglect indisputable aspects of reality they engage in denial.[54] Denial has been shown to be an important force in cancer patients and may be prominent particularly in emotionally stressful situations, namely time of diagnosis or when the issue of death becomes indisputable.[55] Denial and fear of death can affect symptom reporting. In an experimental study involving students, one group of students was made to think about death and then fill out a somatic symptom list. Compared to others, the death-group had the lowest symptom score.[56] This has implications for the interpretation of QOL test results. Clinicians have often been puzzled by the observation that patients in their final stages report surprisingly good quality of life, a phenomenon called 'well-being paradox' in the literature.[57] Only a sensitive clinician can find out whether the patient's coping efforts are successful or whether the patient masks a problem that constitutes an ongoing plague. Several further recent publications on the issues of expectations[58,59] and denial[60–63] underscore the importance of these topics.

In summary, it appears that the palliative situation poses specific problems for QOL assessment and research. Partially these challenges have been met, particularly in the development of short, easy-to-handle questionnaires. Measurement approaches that go beyond questionnaires would be an additional option that merits more attention in the future. The data gained from such efforts, however, are only interpretable when the psychology behind the expression (denial, expectation) is better understood. Research efforts should be focused on an empirical basis of how to inform patients and how to interpret test results from QOL assessments.

The quality of life concept may enhance care

Whether or not routine QOL assessment has the potential to improve health care is an emerging issue. To date, randomized studies are not available in sufficient quality and quantity to allow an unequivocally positive answer.[64] However, existing data and conceptions allow some optimistic extrapolations.

In a recent study it was shown that the use of pain assessment scales increased the frequency of diagnosing pain among nursing home residents, particularly among elderly or cognitively impaired patients.[65] In another study, marked discrepancy was shown in the quality and quantity of symptoms as reported by patients in standardized QOL questionnaires and as actually reported by physicians in the medical records. This was particularly true for psychological problems and diffuse physical symptoms such as fatigue.[66] In other words, the use of standardized QOL scales has huge informational value.

Before, however, QOL data can be used in a clinical setting, data of individual patients have to be presented in such a way that the physician can make sense out of it. A so-called QOL profile fulfils these requirements.[67,68] Figure 8.3 presents the profile of a patient who had undergone inpatient radiotherapy for lymphoma. The patient filled out the EORTC QOL questionnaire C30 before and after therapy. From the range of possible QOL scores we selected those that were rated as most important by clinicians. Individual questionnaire items were aggregated according to the scoring manual; however, in order to increase understanding, 0 uniformly represented the negative and 100 the positive pole. A computer software program had been prepared in order to generate such profiles automatically from a SPSS file. From practical and theoretical arguments it can be concluded that the a value of 50 is the threshold level of intervention.[32] That means QOL scores <50 merit closer inspection by clinicians and, if possible, therapeutic action.

Although the 82-year-old female patient was undergoing a palliative treatment approach, she expected healing from the radiotherapy.[11] In fact, a glance at the right-hand-side line of the

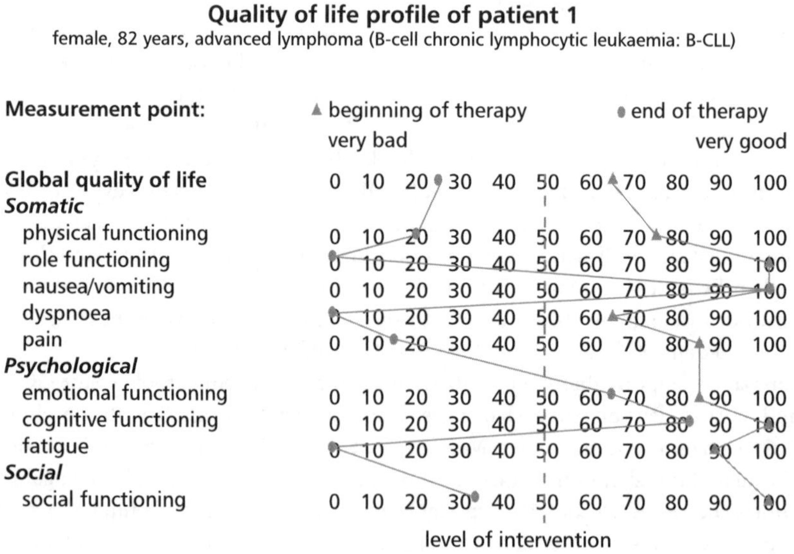

Quality of life profile of patient 1
female, 82 years, advanced lymphoma (B-cell chronic lymphocytic leukaemia: B-CLL)

Measurement point:	▲ beginning of therapy	● end of therapy
	very bad	very good

Global quality of life	0	10	20	30	40	50	60	70	80	90	100
Somatic											
physical functioning	0	10	20	30	40	50	60	70	80	90	100
role functioning	0	10	20	30	40	50	60	70	80	90	100
nausea/vomiting	0	10	20	30	40	50	60	70	80	90	100
dyspnoea	0	10	20	30	40	50	60	70	80	90	100
pain	0	10	20	30	40	50	60	70	80	90	100
Psychological											
emotional functioning	0	10	20	30	40	50	60	70	80	90	100
cognitive functioning	0	10	20	30	40	50	60	70	80	90	100
fatigue	0	10	20	30	40	50	60	70	80	90	100
Social											
social functioning	0	10	20	30	40	50	60	70	80	90	100

level of intervention

Fig. 8.3 Quality of life profile.

diagram indicates that the patient is doing very well. All values are above 50 and she even has optimal QOL scores regarding role, cognitive, and social functioning. At the end of therapy, the patient found that the goal of healing had not been achieved. This insight was accompanied by a dramatic drop in her quality of life. Global QOL declined from 67 before therapy to 25 after therapy. Specific QOL aspects that show very low results include physical, role, and social functioning, as well as the symptoms dyspnoea and fatigue.

The advantage of presenting individual QOL data in this manner is its high clinical practicability. Even a non-expert in QOL methodology gets an impression of a person's subjective situation at a glance and can intuitively appreciate the clinical implications of the findings. Furthermore, a QOL profile like this meets the current standards in the design of medical records[69] and does justice to the notion of cognitive psychology that 'sometimes a picture can say more than a thousand words'.[70]

However, it should be noted that a QOL profile is no substitute for a patient–physician interaction: quite the contrary. The patient–physician interaction remains the cornerstone of medicine, particularly in palliative care. A profile, however, may serve as a welcome supplement, may help direct the conversation in the right direction, and signals to the patient that the mentioning of ostensibly 'non-medical' problems such as psychological or social issues is appropriate.

Quality of life assessment and documentation is one thing. Patients, however, will only profit when the QOL concept is being implemented into the health care system. In the famous SUPPORT study, for instance, the intervention phase enhancing opportunities for more patient–physician communication did not lead to improvement of patient outcomes such as pain or number of days spent in the ICU.[71] Apparently, more forceful strategies of change are called for. In a recent study conducted in an outpatient palliative care unit, it was found that physicians failed to address serious QOL problems (particularly emotional problems and fatigue) in up to 50% of the cases.[72]

The conclusion is that before any changes can be expected, a concept, particularly a colourful one such as quality of life, has to be implemented. Implementation is an idea stemming from quality assurance and health care research and involves its stepwise introduction with the aim of changing the behaviour of health care providers. In a project on improving the regional health care for cancer patients we have followed such an approach. The first step was establishing a quality circle, including representatives of all parties involved in regional cancer patient care (hospitals, practitioners, self-help groups). One of this group's accomplishments was compiling a list of QOL-enhancing therapeutic options available in the region. The physicians in the region were introduced to the concept and assessment of QOL through a variety of methods: outreach visits at the practitioners' through a study physician, regular meetings of the quality circle, and local conferences.[73]

In an assessment phase, a cohort of breast and rectal cancer patients filled out a standardized QOL questionnaire at every follow-up visit in their practitioner's office. During an implementation/evaluation phase, practitioners received QOL profiles of their respective patients and were asked to judge their usefulness.[74] The profile was seen to be understandable in all cases (100%). Physicians indicated that the profile contained useful additional information and led to a more complete diagnosis (55%). Furthermore, the communication between physicians and patients became more problem focused (42%). Interestingly, in 95% of the cases the physicians indicated that the profile overlapped with their intuitive perception of the patient. In the light of studies showing marked differences between doctors' and patients' ratings, this response is likely to be a judgement bias.[3] Furthermore, physicians caring for breast cancer patients were more cooperative in the course of this implementation study (67%) and in attending meetings of the quality circle (82%) than were physicians caring for rectal cancer patients (25% and 35%, respectively).

The results of this first experience were discussed in our quality circle and a barrier analysis was performed.[75] The analysis revealed that the following aspects were barriers to the application of the QOL concept: lack of medical education, lack of transparency about regional therapeutic options, communication barriers between hospitals and practitioners, and lack of financial support.

In summary, this study highlights the fact that attitudinal (physicians, patients) and systemic (health care environment, insurance companies) barriers have to be overcome before the concept of quality of life will have the degree of bearing on patient care that it deserves.

Conclusion

The present chapter started with the proposition that both 'palliative care' and 'quality of life' lack a hero status within current Western medical thinking. This overview makes clear that nevertheless both can be dealt with from a scientific standpoint. This may increase the respect for both topics and attract new generations of enthusiastic physicians and researchers. Eventually, increased scientific efforts will also shape public attitudes toward death, dying, and incurable disease.

It cannot be denied that the importance of palliative care will increase in the future. One reason is the ever-growing proportion of elderly people. The other reason is that in an age of molecular biology with its claims of getting rid of all major diseases and of prolonging life up to 200 years, medical thinking runs the danger of hybris – the issue of palliation helps to keep a sense of proportion. Under the assumption that 'Frankensteinian medicine'[76] will never become a reality, palliation is something that is of interest to everyone. In contrast, the treatment of rare genetic disorders will be of interest only to a few.

Therefore, issues of a good life and of a good death merit more financial support from granting agencies. The current imbalance in funding between molecular research and palliative research has to be overcome.[77]

Palliation research can profit a lot from the QOL movement. The present chapter has introduced the reader to basic conceptual and methodogical issues. It has alerted the reader that simple cookbook solutions do not exist and also do not do justice to the complexities of the field. Although this may sound disappointing to some, we believe this constitutes the strongest argument for adopting a scientific, empirical orientation to palliative care research.

References

1. Abernathy, C.M., and Hamm, R.M. (1995). *Surgical intuition*. Hanley & Belfus, Philadelphia.
2. Loewy, E.H. (2000). Living well and dying not too badly: integrating a whole life into a tolerable death. *Wien. Klin. Wochenschr.*, **112**, 381–5.
3. Coates, A., *et al.* (1992). Prognostic value of quality-of-life scores during chemotherapy for advanced breast cancer. *J. Clin. Oncol.*, **10**, 1833–8.
4. Ringdal, G.I., *et al.* (1996). Prognostic factors and survival in a heterogeneous sample of cancer patients. *Br. J. Cancer*, **73**, 1594–9.
5. Finlay, I. (2001). UK strategies for palliative care. *J. Roy. Soc. Med.*, **94**, 437–41.
6. Stroebe, M. *et al.* (2003). Bereavement research: methodological issues and ethical concerns. *Palliat. Med.*, **17**, 235–40.
7. Relman, A.S. (1988). Assessment and accountability. The third revolution in medical care. *N. Engl. J. Med.*, **319**, 1220–2.

8. Blazeby, J.M. (2001). Measurement of outcome. *Surg. Oncol.,* **10**, 127–33.

9. Koller, M., *et al.* (1996). Symptom reporting in cancer patients: the role of negative affect and experienced social stigma. *Cancer,* **77**, 983–95.

10. Koller, M., *et al.* (1999). Symptom reporting in cancer patients. II: Relations to social desirability, negative affect, and self-reported health behaviors. *Cancer,* **86**, 1609–20.

11. Koller, M., *et al.* (2000). Expectations and quality of life of cancer patients undergoing radiotherapy. *J. Roy. Soc. Med.,* **93**, 621–8.

12. Lorenz, W., and Koller, M. (2002). Empirically-based concepts of outcome and quality of life in medicine. In: *Health and quality of life: philosophical, medical and cultural aspects* (ed. A. Gimmler, C. Lenk, and G. Aumüller) pp. 123–136. LIT-Verlag, Münster.

13. Vickery, C.W., *et al.* (2001). The EORTC Quality of Life Group. Development of an EORTC disease-specific quality of life module for use in patients with gastric cancer. *Eur J Cancer,* **37**, 966–71.

14. Nunnally, J.C. (1978). *Psychometric theory.* McGraw-Hill, New York.

15. Lienert, G.A. and Raatz, U. (1994). *Testaufbau und Testanalyse* (5th edn). Beltz, Weinheim.

16. Bowling, A. (2001). Measuring disease. *A review of disease-specific quality of life measurement scales* (2nd edn). Open University Press, Buckingham.

17. Westhoff, G. Handbuch psychosozialer Messinstrumente. Göttingen: Hogrefe, 1994.

18. Fayers, P., Aaronson, N., Bjordal, K., Groenvold, M., Curran, D., and Bottomley, A. (2001). *EORTC QLQ-C30 scoring manual* (3rd edn). EORTC Study Group on Quality of Life, Brussels.

19. Aaronson, N.K., *et al.* (1993). The European organization for research and treatment of cancer QLQ-C30: a quality-of-life instrument for use in international clinical trials in oncology. *J. Natl. Cancer Inst.,* **85**, 365–76.

20. Cella, D.F., *et al.* (1993). The functional assessment of cancer therapy (FACT) scale: development and validation of the general measure. *J. Clin. Oncol.,* **11**, 570–9.

21. Stewart, A.L., and Ware, J.E. (1992). *Measuring functioning and well-being. The medical outcomes study approach.* Duke University Press, Durham.

22. Siegrist, J., Broer, M., and Junge, A. (1996). *PLC – Profil der Lebensqualität chronisch Kranker.* Beltz Test, Göttingen.

23. Watson, D., and Pennebaker, J.W. (1989). Health complaints, stress, and distress: exploring the central role of negative affectivity. *Psychol. Rev.,* **96**, 234–54.

24. Basler, H.D. (1999). Marburger Fragebogen zum habituellen Wohlbefinden. *Schmerz,* **13**, 385–91.

25. Bullinger, M., and Kirchberger, I. (1998). *SF-36 Fragebogen zum Gesundheitszustand.* Hogrefe, Göttingen.

26. Kemmler, G., *et al.* (1999). Comparison of two quality of life instruments for cancer patients: the functional assessment of cancer therapy-general and the European Organization for Research and Treatment of Cancer Quality of Life Questionnaire-C30. *J. Clin. Oncol.,* **17**, 2932–40.

27. Cella, D. (1998). Quality of life. In: J.C. Holland, *et al.* (Ed.), *Psycho-oncology.* Oxford University Press, New York, pp. 1135–46.

28. Velikova, G., *et al.* (1999). Automated collection of quality-of-life data: a comparison of paper and computer touch-screen questionnaires. *J. Clin. Oncol.,* **17**, 998–1007.

29. Sigle, J., and Porzsolt, F. (1996). Practical aspects of quality-of-life measurement: design and feasibility study of the quality-of-life recorder and the standardized measurement of quality of life in an outpatient clinic. *Cancer Treat. Rev.,* **22** Suppl A, 75–89.

30. Troidl, H., McKneally, M.F., (1998). Toward a difinition of surgical research. In: H. Troidl, *et al. Surgical research. Basic principles and clinical practice.* Springer, New York, pp.3–7.

31. Lorenz, W. (1998). Outcome: definition and methods of evaluation. In: H. Troidl, *et al. Surgical research. Basic principles and clinical practice* (3rd edn) Springer, New York, pp. 513–20.

32. Koller, M., and Lorenz, W. (2002). Quality of life: a deconstruction for clinicians. *J.R.Soc.Med.,* **95**, 481–8.

33. Osoba, D., Aaronson, N.K., and Till, J.E. (1991). A practical guide for selecting quality-of-life measures in clinical trials and practice. In: D. Osoba (Ed.) *Effect of cancer on quality of life.* CRC, Boca Radon, pp. 90–104.

34. Klee, M.C., King, M.T., Machin, D., and Hansen, H.H. (2000). A clinical model for quality of life assessment in cancer patients receiving chemotherapy. *Ann. Oncol.*, **11**, 23–30.

35. Paci, E., *et al.* (2001). Quality of life assessment and outcome of palliative care. *J. Pain Sympt. Manage.*, **21**, 179–88.

36. Hearn, J., and Higginson, I.J. (1999). Palliative Care Core Audit Project Advisory Group. Development and validation of a core outcome measure for palliative care: the palliative care outcome scale. *Qual. Health Care*, **8**, 219–27.

37. Cohen, S.R., *et al.* (1997). Validity of the McGill quality of life questionnaire in the palliative care setting: a multi-centre Canadian study demonstrating the importance of the existential domain. *Pall. Med.*, **11**, 3–20.

38. Higginson, I.J., and McCarthy, M. (1994). A comparison of two measures of quality of life: their sensitivity and validity for patients with advanced cancer. *Pall. Med.*, **8**, 282–90.

39. Rathbone, G.V., *et al.* (1994). A self-evaluated assessment suitable for seriously ill hospice patients. *Palliat. Med.*, **8**, 29–34.

40. Philip, J., *et al.* (1998). Concurrent validity of the modified Edmonton Symptom Assessment System with the Rotterdam Symptom Checklist and the Brief Pain inventory. *Support. Care Cancer*, **6**, 539–41.

41. Ahmedzai, S. (1991). Quality-of-life research in the European palliative care setting. In: D. Osoba (Ed.) *Effect of cancer on quality of life.* CRC Press, Boca Raton, pp. 323–42.

42. Bullinger, M. (1992). Quality of life assessment in palliative care. *J. Pall. Care*, **8**, 34–9.

43. Higginson, I.J., and McCarthy, M. (1993). Validity of the support team assessment schedule: do staff's ratings reflect those made by patients or their families? *Pall. Med.*, **7**, 219–28.

44. Osoba, D. (1994). Lessons learned from measuring health-related quality of life in oncology. *J. Clin. Oncol.*, **12**, 608–16.

45. Duke Pain Initiative (2000). Pain and palliative care reference cards. Duke University Medical Center, editor. Unpublished work.

46. Saunders, C. (2001). The evolution of palliative care. *J. Roy. Soc. Med.*, **94**, 430–2.

47. Lavery, J.V., *et al.* (2001). Origins of the desire for euthanasia and assisted suicide in people with HIV-1 or AIDS: a qualitative study. *Lancet*, **358**, 362–7.

48. Weiss, S.C., Emanuel, L.L., Fairclough, D.L., and Emanuel, E.J. (2001). Understanding the experience of pain in terminally ill patients. *Lancet*, **357**, 1311–15.

49. Hoffmann, S., *et al.* (2001). Nasogastric tube versus gastrostomy tube for gastric decompression in abdominal surgery: a prospective, randomized trial comparing patients' tube-related inconvenience. *Langenbeck's Arch. Surg.*, **386**, 402–9.

50. Saunders, C. (1998). Caring for cancer. *J. Roy. Soc. Med.*, **91**, 439–41.

51. ten Kroode, H.F.J. (1998). Active listening to cancer patients' stories. *Netherlands J. Med.*, **53**, 47–52.

52. Bauhofer, A., *et al.* (2002). Quality of life in animals as a new outcome for surgical research: G-CSF as a quality of life improving factor. *Eur. Surg. Res.*, **34**, 22–9.

53. Seligman, M.E.P. (1975). *Helplessness: on depression, development, and death.* Freeman, San Francisco.

54. Kreitler, S. (1999). Denial in cancer patients. *Cancer Investig.*, **17**, 514–34.

55. Lazarus, R.S. (1993). Coping theory and research: past, present, and future. *Psychosom. Med.*, **55**, 234–47.

56. Matzen, K., *et al.* (1997). Defensive Reaktion im Angesicht des Todes: Das Verleugnen korperlicher Symptome. Abstractbook: 6. Tagung der Fachgruppe Sozialpsychologie Univ. Konstanz.

57. Staudinger, U.M. (2000). Viele Gründe sprechen dagegen, und trotzdem geht es vielen Menschen gut: Das Paradox des subjektiven Wohlbefindens. *Psychol. Rundsch.*, **51**, 185–97.

58. Chow, E., *et al.* (2001). Patients with advanced cancer: a survey of the understanding of their illness and expectations from palliative radiotherapy for symptomatic metastases. *Clin. Oncol.*, **3**, 204–8.

59. Jordhoy, M.S., Fayers, P., Loge, J.H., Ahlner-Elmqvist, M., and Kaasa, S. (2001). Quality of life in palliative cancer care: results from a cluster randomized trial. *J. Clin. Oncol.*, **19**, 3884–94.

60. Goldbeck, R. (1997). Denial in physical illness. *J. Psychosom. Res.*, **43**, 575–93.

61. Ness, D.E. and Ende, J. (1994). Denial in the medical interview. Recognition and management. *J.A.M.A.*, **272**, 1777–81.

62. Moyer, A., and Levine, E.G. (1998). Clarification of the conceptualization and measurement of denial in psychosocial oncology research. *Ann. Behav. Med.*, **20**, 149–60.

63. Miceli, M., and Castelfranchi, C. (1998). Denial and its reasoning. *Br. J. Med. Psychol.*, **71**, 139–52.

64. Sprangers, M.A.G. (2002). Quality-of-life assessment in oncology. Achievements and challenges. *Acta Oncol.*, 41, 229–37.

65. Kamel, K.H., *et al.* (2001). Utilizing pain assessment scales increases the frequency of diagnosing pain among elderly nursing home residents. *J. Pain Sympt. Manage.*, **21**, 450–5.

66. Strömgren, A.S., *et al.* (2001). Does the medical record cover the symptoms experienced by cancer patients receiving palliative care? A comparison of the record and patients' self-rating. *J. Pain Sympt. Manage.*, **21**, 189–96.

67. Koller, M., Kussmann, J., Lorenz, W., and Rothmund, M. (1994). Die Messung von Lebensqualität in der chirurgischen Tumornachsorge: Methoden, Probleme und Einsatzmöglichkeiten. *Chirurg*, **65**, 333–9.

68. Koller, M., and Lorenz, W. (1998). Quality of life research in patients with rectal cancer: traditional approaches versus a problem-solving oriented perspective. *Langenbeck's Arch. Surg.*, **383**, 427–36.

69. Wyatt, J.C., and Wright, P. (1998). Improving medical records. Part 1: Can records be improved? *Lancet*, **280**, 1321–4.

70. Larkin, J.H., and Simon, H.A. (1987). Why a diagram is (sometimes) worth ten thousand words. *Cognit. Sci.*, **11**, 65–99.

71. SUPPORT Principal Investigators (1995). A controlled trial to improve care for seriously ill hospitalized patients: the study to understand prognoses and perferences for outcomes and risks of treatments (SUPPORT). *J.A.M.A.*, **274**, 1591–8.

72. Detmar, S.B., *et al.* (2001). Patient–physician communication during outpatient palliative treatment visits. *J.A.M.A.*, **285**, 1351–7.

73. Gross, P.A., *et al.* (2001). Optimal methods for guideline implementation: conclusions from the Leeds Castle meeting. *Med. Care*, **39** (8, Suppl. II), 85–92.

74. Albert, U.S., *et al.* (2002). Quality of life profile: From measurement to clinical application. *Breast*, **11**, 324–34.

75. Margolis, C.Z., and Cretin, S. (1999). *Implementing clinical practice guidelines*. AHA Press, Chicago.

76. Harris, J. (2000). Essays on science and society: intimations of immortality. *Science*, **288**, 59.

77. Kaasa, S., and De Conno, F. (2001). Palliative care research. *Eur J Cancer*, **37**, S153–S159.

Chapter 9

Anaesthesia and perioperative pain management

Karen H. Simpson and Dudley J. Bush

Anaesthesia differs from many medical interventions because it does not directly benefit the patient, yet it is highly invasive. It is therefore important to identify and minimize the risks specifically associated with anaesthesia. Surgical palliation is not complete without careful perioperative pain control.

Anaesthesia

Risks of anaesthesia and surgery

Patients presenting for palliative surgery will usually have a number of systemic disorders that are known to increase perioperative risk, including nutritional, cardiac, respiratory, hepatic, renal, or haematological dysfunction.

ASA grade

The most widely used assessment of perioperative risk is the classification of the American Society of Anesthesiologists.[1] This uses the presenting surgical problem and underlying medical status of the patient (Table 9.1). Although the ASA grading system is non-specific, it remains useful because it reliably predicts risk and is easy to apply. The annual National Confidential Enquiry into Peri-operative Death (NCEPOD) in the United Kingdom records most deaths occurring within 30 days of surgery, with surgical, anaesthetic, and pathological data.[2] In 1998–99 approximately 20 000 deaths were recorded; 84% occured in patients of ASA grade 3 or higher, while the mortality in ASA grade 1 was only 0.5%. Identification of higher risk patients according to ASA grade may allow corrective strategies or modifications of anaesthetic technique that improve outcome.

Age

Age is a risk factor for perioperative morbidity and mortality, mainly because of increasing co-morbidity and reduction in physiological reserve. The 1998–99 UK NCEPOD data show that 73% of deaths occured in surgical patients older than 70 years.

Urgency of surgery

The urgency of surgery influences perioperative risk. Data from the UK NCEPOD indicate that 67% of deaths occured in patients having surgical procedures performed as an emergency (immediate) or urgent (performed with minimal delay). Mortality attributable to surgery was 1:2860.

Table 9.1 ASA physical status classification system[1]

P1	A normal healthy patient
P2	A patient with mild systemic disease
P3	A patient with severe systemic disease
P4	A patient with severe systemic disease that is a constant threat to life
P5	A moribund patient who is not expected to survive without the operation
P6	A declared brain-dead patient whose organs are being removed for donor purposes

Direct risk of anaesthesia

The risk due to anaesthesia independent of the underlying condition of the patient and surgical factors is very small with current anaesthetic drugs and techniques. Anaesthesia was the single factor responsible for death in only 1:185 056 cases in the UK NCEPOD study. This represents a mixture of adverse drug reactions, equipment problems, and human error. The report concluded that senior, more experienced anaesthetists achieve better results in high-risk groups.

Many patients presenting for palliative surgery will be in the high-risk categories. They will be older, have co-existing conditions, and will often present for urgent surgery. Data reported on 16 220 patients having cancer-related surgery at the University of Texas M.D. Andersen Cancer Center between 1992–93 indicated an overall 2% mortality within 31 days. The 30-day mortality did not increase with age until the eighth decade, but was 11% in ASA class 4 and 44% in ASA class 5 patients.[3] Pedersen[4] has presented prospective data on the factors associated with perioperative morbidity in over 7000 surgical patients (Table 9.2).

Pre-anaesthetic assessment

The purpose of the pre-anaesthetic assessment is no longer to determine absolute 'fitness for anaesthesia'. Using modern drugs and techniques any patient can be anaesthetised, no matter how sick, although to do so may not be in the best interests of the patient. Rather the main objectives of pre-anaesthesia assessment are to:

◆ obtain a relevant medical history, including the condition requiring surgery, pre-existing medical conditions, medication, drug allergies, previous surgical and anaesthetic history, and family history. The medical history will usually be biased towards evaluating the cardiovascular and pulmonary systems

◆ arrange any further investigations that are necessary

◆ suggest interventions and alterations in management that may improve outcome by rendering the patient in better physical condition, termed 'optimisation'

◆ facilitate informed consent

◆ alleviate patient anxiety by discussing the various anaesthesia options.

Routine investigations

Untargeted evaluation of many laboratory, radiographic, and physiological variables contributes little to patient management. In a recent systematic review of routine preoperative investigations, detection of abnormal results were very low, e.g. 4.4% for chest x-ray and less than 2% for full blood count and biochemistry. Patient management was changed on the basis

Table 9.2 Factors associated with increased perioperative complications[4]

Risk factors	Number of anaesthetics	Cardiovascular complication (%)	Pulmonary complication (%)	Mortality in hospital (%)
Male	2634	8.8	6.6	2.2
Female	4587	4.9	3.7	0.7
Age <50 years	3965	2.6	2.3	0.3
Age 50–69 years	2043	8.2	6.7	1.8
Age 70–79 years	886	14.3	8.9	2.9
Age >80 years	293	16.7	10.2	5.8
Myocardial infarct within 1 year	26	38.5	10.4	7.7
Chronic heart failure	199	35.2	15.1	9.1
Hypertension	380	11.8	7.1	1.3
Hypotension systolic BP <90 mmHg	127	16.5	17.3	9.4
Chronic obstructive lung disease	201	12.4	12.4	5
Renal failure	153	14.4	11.8	5.9
Cancer surgery (abdominal)	1257 (242)	7.0 (19.8)	5.5 (19.4)	1.1 (5.0)
Emergency surgery	2454	7.4	6.3	2.8
Procedure >300 minutes	162	20.4	30.0	4.9
Total	**7221**	**6.3**	**4.8**	**1.2**

of unexpected abnormal results less that 1% of the time.[5] In the patient population presenting for palliative surgery, investigations need to be requested and updated according to the patient's history and underlying physical condition, as well as with regard to the planned surgery. Some abnormal investigations, such as hypoalbuminaemia, reliably predict adverse outcome. They are not easily correctable because they reflect the patient's underlying poor condition.[6] Two preoperative investigations merit discussion because they often result in postponed surgery and are responsible for potentially harmful and unjustified intervention.

Haemoglobin

Mild chronic normovolaemic anaemia at or above 8 g/dl is not associated with adverse perioperative outcome. Preoperative transfusion for this degree of anaemia is not associated with improved outcome.[7] Most anaesthetists accept a preoperative haemoglobin of 8 g/dl if intraoperative blood loss is expected to be less than 500 ml, and 10 g/dl if there is severe cardiorespiratory disease or major blood loss at surgery is expected. Ideally, any preoperative transfusion should be performed at least 24 hours before surgery because the metabolite 2,3 DPG in stored erythrocytes needs to be regenerated for the transfused blood to be fully functional for oxygen delivery.

Serum potassium

This must be considerably outside the normal range of 3.5–5.5 mmol/l before there is additional risk from anaesthesia. Chronic hypo or hyperkalaemia is less harmful than acute change. Overzealous potassium replacement is hazardous. It may produce cardiac dysrhythmias and contractility problems as severe as those due to hypokalaemia. Most anaesthetists would accept a range of serum potassium of 2.8–5.8 mmol/l, providing the patient is in otherwise optimal condition. In acute renal failure or acute hypovolaemia from gastrointestinal loss secondary to obstructive vomiting, then corrective measures should be considered before surgery.

Management of co-existing medical disease

Cardiovascular disease

Pre-existing cardiovascular impairment is important in anaesthesia because nearly all anaesthetic drugs and techniques impair cardiovascular function. Exercise tolerance from the patient history is very informative, although specific tests, e.g. echocardiogram, may be needed in selected patients. Identification and specific treatment of residual myocardial ischaemia, e.g. by angioplasty, will improve outcome[8] but may not be possible. Anaesthesia within six months of a significant myocardial infarction is associated with a 1.5–10 times increase in the risk of re-infarction, and a 20–86% increase in excess mortality, compared to a longer interval.[9] A delay of six months after myocardial infarction minimizes risk of re-infarction, but is often impossible in the context of palliative procedures. If surgery is urgent, then aggressive management to maintain cardiovascular parameters within 20% of awake values may reduce perioperative risk. To achieve this control requires invasive haemodynamic monitoring followed by high-dependency postoperative care.

Inadequately treated or refractory congestive heart failure confers great perioperative risk.[10] There is less evidence that aggressive perioperative management can reduce this risk unless the heart failure can be improved, although aggressive management is standard practice. Similarly valvular heart disease, particularly aortic stenosis, confers additional risk, but can often not be easily improved preoperatively.

Untreated hypertension is associated with increased risk of perioperative cardiovascular and cerebrovascular complications. A diastolic blood pressure greater than 110 mmHg precludes all but emergency operations untill investigated and treated. There is evidence that treatment of hypertension, even for a short period of time, particularly β-blockade, reduces intraoperative circulatory lability and significantly improves outcome.[11]

Pulmonary disease

General anaesthesia causes several pulmonary complications. Most anaesthetic agents cause ventilation/perfusion mismatch and decrease functional residual capacity. These effects lead to perioperative hypoxaemia unless the inspired oxygen concentration is increased, especially when recovering from anaesthesia. Barotrauma from prolonged positive pressure mechanical ventilation may permanently worsen pulmonary function in chronic obstructive pulmonary disease (COPD). The duration of any controlled ventilation should be minimized or completely avoided by use of regional anaesthesia.

Risk factors for pulmonary complications in order of importance include upper abdominal surgery, poorly controlled asthma and COPD, smoking, and obesity. Exercise tolerance is the most useful form of assessment, supplemented by additional specific respiratory function tests in a few cases.[12] There is often little that may be done to improve respiratory disease in the time available before palliative surgery. Bronchospasm should be actively treated and smoking avoided perioperatively. Supplementary oxygen is required for several days after major surgery.

Renal disease

Stable, well-managed, chronic renal impairment can be accommodated by the anaesthetist. There are now many anaesthetic agents and techniques not dependent upon renal clearance; chronic anaemia is well tolerated. Patients with acute severe hyperkalaemia or acidosis need dialysis before anaesthesia. Too vigorous dialysis performed immediately preoperatively should be avoided as there will be insufficient time for fluid redistribution and major hypotension may occur at induction of anaesthesia.

Diabetes mellitus

Diabetes is a multi-system disorder causing small- and large-vessel occlusive disease, including ischaemic heart disease, diabetic cardiomyopathy, renal impairment, and autonomic neuropathy. All of these will increase the risk of anaesthesia. Perioperative management of diabetes is primarily directed at avoiding hypoglycaemia that is potentially lethal. The signs are masked by general anaesthesia, and there is no evidence that short-term mild hyperglycaemia is harmful. There are many possible strategies (Table 9.3).

Neurological impairment

Patients already taking large doses of analgesia may require more analgesia than predicted perioperatively. The patient with intracerebral metastases poses special problems for the anaesthetist. If there is raised intracranial pressure then spinal techniques are contraindicated because leak of spinal fluid may alter the pressure dynamics and cause lethal medullary herniation. The residual sedative effects of anaesthesia drugs are greater and more prolonged in such patients. Drugs that are epileptogenic must be avoided.

Table 9.3 Strategies for intraoperative management of diabetes

Controlled non-insulin-dependent diabetes mellitus
Minor procedures
Change from long- to short-acting oral hypoglycaemic drugs 48 hours preoperatively and omit on day of surgery
Check blood glucose preoperatively:
<4 mmol/l commence intravenous 5% dextrose infusion
>10 mmol/l commence intravenous insulin/dextrose/potassium regimen
Major procedures
As for insulin-dependent diabetes mellitus
Insulin-dependent diabetes mellitus: all procedures except minor local anaesthesia
Convert from long- to short-acting insulin 24 hours preoperatively
Ensure meal is taken night before surgery
Omit normal subcutaneous insulin on day of surgery
Commence dextrose and insulin intravenous infusion with regular blood sugar monitoring and continue until oral intake resumed

Patients with small cell lung tumours or other malignancy may have Eaton–Lambert syndrome (a myasthenia-like condition in which reduced amounts of acetylcholine are released at the neuromuscular junction). This makes the effects of muscle relaxants unpredictable and causes autonomic lability.[13]

Sepsis

Infection or other insult, particularly in the immunocompromised patient, may lead to sepsis. This is characterized by a generalized inflammatory response with myocardial depression, hypotension, and metabolic and pulmonary impairment. The condition may progress to multi-organ failure. Anaesthesia requires aggressive monitoring and resuscitation for optimal outcome. There is evidence that anaesthesia may directly precipitate deterioration in clinical condition, requiring admission to a critical care facility.[14] Thorough multidisciplinary discussion and decision making is appropriate before embarking upon palliative procedures in such patients.

Anti-tumour treatments

Chemotherapy Several chemotherapy agents may influence the course of anaesthesia. Alkylating agents, including cyclophosphamide, act as anticholinesterases and may prolong the action of neuromuscular blockade. Doxorubicin may rarely produce myocardial depression leading to congestive cardiac failure and interstitial lung fibrosis; the onset may be delayed for up to one year. Risk factors include doses exceeding 550 mg/m^2, thorax radiotherapy, and concurrent alkylating therapy. This toxicity may occur at any age. It increases the risks of anaesthesia and requires more aggressive monitoring. Mithramycin in doses in excess of $30 \text{ }\mu\text{g/kg/day}$ may cause hepato-renal damage and coagulopathies. Bleomycin produces pulmonary impairment in up to 25% of patients, presenting as a restrictive fibrosis. Rarely this is severe and can be fatal. Exposure to increased concentrations of inspired oxygen, such are used in routine anaesthesia practice, may aggravate this damage. It may be prudent to use the minimum inspired oxygen concentration required in this group.[15]

Radiotherapy Radiotherapy may be used locally as total body radiotherapy or in combination with chemotherapy. Each may have implications for anaesthesia. The patient with head and neck cancer, who has had localised radiotherapy, may have post-radiation fibrosis. This may make direct laryngoscopy and intubation impossible. If general anaesthesia, including muscle relaxation, is used in this situation, it may prove impossible to manually ventilate or intubate the patient, producing potentially life-threatening hypoxaemia. Preoperative assessment of the airway with consideration of awake intubation under local anaesthesia using a flexible fibrescope is mandatory in this group.

Do not resuscitate (DNR) orders and anaesthesia

Some patients presenting for palliative surgery may have pre-existing 'do not resuscitate orders' or other advance directives. This may conflict with the performance of clinical anaesthesia because of the inevitable physiological trespass involved, particularly regarding general anaesthesia and the cardio-respiratory systems. In this situation the American Society of Anesthesiologists[16] has recommended that discussion with the patient, or a suitable surrogate, should precede surgery to clarify the patient's wishes. It is important to pre-empt any conflicts that arise that may compromise the patient's previously expressed autonomy. A range of options may then be formulated and documented. At one extreme is complete suspension of the advance directive perioperatively. More common would be agreement not to undertake certain courses of action, such as instituting cardiopulmonary resuscitation with chest compression, so long as this is compatible with a workable plan for clinical anaesthesia. Lastly the patient may devolve any necessary clinical decisions to the operating team after having expressed a general indication of their desires and goals, e.g. prolonged mechanical ventilation would be avoided, while dysrhythmias or tension pneumothorax would be treated. Management of blood loss in the Jehovah's Witness might be considered a special case of an advance directive, and would be managed in a similar way. This situation is far more common in clinical practice. Most institutions have policies and specific consent documentation to allow such patients to decline blood transfusion.

Anaesthesia techniques

Techniques can be divided into general and regional or local anaesthesia (Table 9.4). There are few absolute indications for either type of anaesthesia. Despite widespread belief that regional techniques are inherently safer, there are only a few procedures where there is undisputed evidence of improved outcome. Orthopaedic procedures have not yet been demonstrated to

Table 9.4 Comparison of general and regional anaesthesia

General anaesthesia

Advantages

Usual choice for major abdominal or thoracic procedures

Suitable for virtually any type or site of surgery

Requires less cooperation in the confused patient

More predictable in sepsis

Disadvantages

Significant cardio-respiratory depression from drugs

Usually requires airway instrumentation and ventilation

Significant postoperative side-effects, e.g. nausea, hypoxaemia

Regional/local anaesthesia

Advantages

Suitable for any peripheral or lower abdominal procedure

Less effect on cardio-respiratory system

May be safer than general anaesthesia alone

May be combined with general anaesthesia

? Reduced phantom pain after amputation

Can be continued for postoperative analgesia

Disadvantages

Unsafe in sepsis and coagulopathy

Unsuitable for very confused patients without sedation

Spinal techniques unsafe if intracranial pressure raised

Spinal techniques unsafe if spinal cord compression impending be safer when performed under any particular type of anaesthesia.[17] In some high-risk cases, the benefits are demonstrable, e.g. epidural analgesia after thoracic surgery[18] or bowel surgery.[19] Regional anaesthesia does reduce the risk of deep vein thrombosis. Modern general and regional anaesthesia is now so safe that it has little effect upon outcome that is primarily dependent upon patient and surgical factors. In practice, the type of anaesthesia is determined according to preoperative assessment and clinical experience, taking account patients' preference. General and regional techniques will often be combined to achieve optimal effect.

Fasting and gastric contents

Induction of general anaesthesia results in a loss of protective laryngeal reflexes and reduction in lower oesophageal sphincter tone. All anaesthetized patients are at risk of life-threatening airway obstruction and pulmonary soiling from regurgitation of gastric contents. Fasting for a period of four hours before anaesthesia reduces this risk. Patients presenting for palliative surgery may remain at extra risk because gastric emptying is severely delayed in the presence of opioids, fear, autonomic neuropathy, and intestinal obstruction.

General anaesthesia

Induction of general anaesthesia is usually achieved using intravenous drugs that produce loss of consciousness within seconds of reaching the brain. Induction agents include thiopentone, etomidate, ketamine, and most commonly, propofol. Etomidate causes the least cardio-respiratory depression in the debilitated patient, but is more nauseating. Propofol is rapidly metabolized which facilitates early recovery. It is the only intravenous agent suitable for maintaining anaesthesia by infusion. Ketamine is unlike any other induction agent. A state of catalepsy-like dissociative anaesthesia is produced, with relative preservation of airway and other reflexes and profound analgesia. There may be unpleasant emergence hallucinations. It has a limited role for short procedures such as radiotherapy in children and painful dressing changes.

Inhalation of volatile anaesthetic agents such as halothane or sevoflurane can also be used as an alternative to intravenous induction of anaesthesia, especially in children; the distress of awake cannulation can be avoided. Volatile anaesthetics are either halogenated hydrocarbons, e.g. halothane, or halogenated ethers, e.g. isoflurane or sevoflurane. All are myocardial depressants and vasodilators. They differ in their speed of onset and recovery, cost, degree of metabolism, and toxicity.

Following induction of anaesthesia, maintenance of the airway and ventilation assume primary importance because protective reflexes and ventilatory drive are compromised. For simple procedures, lasting less than 60 minutes, the patient may continue to breathe spontaneously; the airway is maintained by the anaesthetist using a facemask. The cardio-respiratory depression of more prolonged general anaesthesia is not well tolerated by the spontaneously breathing patient and recovery becomes prolonged. General anaesthesia for longer procedures, or for intra-abdominal surgery, is usually provided by administration of a muscle relaxant and tracheal intubation. This is followed by controlled positive pressure ventilation of the lungs with oxygen-enriched nitrous oxide or air. Opioids are used for intraoperative analgesia. Anaesthesia is maintained with volatile anaesthetics or infusions of intravenous drugs, e.g. propofol.

Polypharmacy is the rule in general anaesthesia. Most modern anaesthesia drugs have been developed for specificity and relative lack of side-effects and interactions. Modern neuromuscular blocking agents are amongst the most specific of any class of drugs. With the exception of suxemethonium, they are largely devoid of unwanted adverse effects and are very safe, even in sick patients with multiple organ impairment. Morphine remains the most common opioid used intraoperatively, although there are several other opioids, e.g. fentanyl, sufentanil, and remifentanil. These share the basic properties of morphine, but have greater potency and faster onset and recovery times, making them more suitable for intraoperative use. The combination of different induction and maintenance agents, opioid, and muscle relaxant is termed balanced anaesthesia. It produces less morbidity and more rapid recovery than larger amounts of single agents. Regional anaesthesia may be combined with general anaesthesia as an extension of the balanced anaesthesia concept.

Regional anaesthesia

Regional anaesthesia involves injection of local anaesthetic and other drugs to block sensory, and sometimes motor, nerve transmission in two or more nerve trunks proximal to the site of surgical stimulation. Spinal anaesthesia is the most common regional technique either as intrathecal or epidural injection. In intrathecal blockade small volumes of local anaesthetic are injected directly into spinal fluid, acting on bare nerve fibres to produce reliable anaesthesia. Direct intrathecal injection can only be safely performed below the termination of the spinal cord in the lower lumbar area, and so is primarily used for abdominal, pelvic, or lower limb surgery. An indwelling catheter is not normally used for anaesthesia practice because of risk of infection and neurological damage. Epidural blockade depends upon larger volumes of local anaesthetic placed in the epidural space outside the dura that then diffuse to block adjacent nerve roots. It may be performed safely at any intervertebral level. A catheter is often introduced to permit repeat injections. It is not quite as predictable as intrathecal blockade. The volume of local anaesthetic used for epidural anaesthesia will cause life-threatening systemic toxicity if inadvertently injected intravenously, and brain stem anaesthesia if injected intrathecally.

The two spinal techniques share many advantages, adverse effects, and complications. Both provide surgical anaesthesia in the lower part of the body, while avoiding the adverse systemic and pulmonary effects of general anaesthetic drugs. Both techniques produce variable blockade of thoraco-lumbar sympathetic outflow that results in vasodilatation, hypotension, and bradycardia; this effect is exaggerated by hypovolaemia. Neither technique is safe in the presence of coagulopathy or full therapeutic anticoagulation because of the neurological risks of epidural haematoma. Heparin prophylaxis for thromboembolism should be given several hours before or after spinal blockade.[20] Both techniques are relatively contraindicated in bacteraemia and sepsis because of the risk of spinal infections.

For any surgery of the upper limb, the brachial plexus can be easily blocked with large volumes of local anaesthetic placed at one of several sites. There are techniques for unilateral blockade of the lower limb but these are rarely performed because of the ease of use of spinal techniques.

Pain management

Incidence and causes of pain in cancer

Patients with cancer may experience acute and/or chronic pain; they often have more than one site of pain. Pain is often multifactorial due to:

- Primary or secondary tumour
- Investigations or procedures, e.g. stents
- Oncology treatments, e.g. surgery or radiation

- General debility, e.g. pressure sores
- Intercurrent problems, e.g. osteoarthritis.

Breakthrough pain (flares of pain that interrupt a tolerable background pain) and pain on movement (incident pain) are common and important. These cause more functional impairment, worse mood, and more anxiety.[21]

Specific issues in cancer pain management

Pain may be nociceptive (mediated by normal pain pathways), e.g. pathological fracture, or neuropathic (generated from within the nervous system), e.g. brachial plexus invasion or mixed. Neuropathic pain can be partially opioid-sensitive or opioid-unresponsive;[22] it may require specialist treatment. Cancer pain in children, those with cognitive impairment, and the elderly can be difficult to assess and manage; these groups have special needs.

Patients with malignant disease may have altered anatomy and physiology due to weight loss or tumour progression. Patients may be unable to swallow or absorb drugs enterally, thus limiting prescribing. Patients with end-stage disease may have cachexia or hepato-renal compromise that alter the pharmacokinetics of analgesic drugs. Patients may present for surgery already taking large doses of opioids and adjuvant analgesics for pre-existing pain; establishing the requirement for postoperative pain relief can be difficult. Coincident use of steroids, chemotherapy, or biological therapies may narrow analgesic options, e.g. NSAIDs may be contraindicated. Coagulopathy or impending spinal cord compression may limit the provision of regional blocks.

Effects of cancer pain on outcomes

Pain adversely affects sleep, mood, and function. However, the influence of postoperative pain on tumour mediators is less well understood. Stress, including surgery, may promote tumour development, metastases, and tumour recurrence. Suppression of natural killer (NK) cells occurs during surgery; this is associated with a higher mortality from many common tumours. Acute pain also suppresses NK cell activity and promotes tumour development in animals. Perioperative analgesia with opioids or intrathecal local anaesthetics and opioids in animals attenuates some of these effects.[23] However, anaesthetic and analgesic drugs may also suppress immune function, e.g. morphine has more profound deleterious effects on immunity than tramadol.[24] Whether these studies can be transferred to clinical situations remains to be seen. However, pain and its relief after surgery may be important immunologically.

Assessment of pain

Good pain management is based on careful assessment. Pain should be seen as the 'fourth vital sign'. The nature of the assessment tools is less important than generating a culture where pain assessment is a regular and routine part of clinical practice. Assessment is difficult in neonates, those in intensive therapy units, preverbal children, confused, cognitively impaired, and some elderly patients. There are specific validated tools for all of these groups, e.g. pictorial scores for children or behavioural scores for the elderly. Most assessment in acute pain requires simple, quick methods, e.g. visual analogue scores. Chronic pain needs more global assessments of the sensory, functional, psychosocial, and spiritual domains of the pain experience.

Education about pain

There are many studies showing that health care professionals are poor at assessing pain.[25] Education of staff in assessment and management of pain and analgesic side-effects is essential. Fear of opioid addiction amongst professionals[26] and patients[27] still exists. Therefore education of patients and their carers is important.

Teams in pain management

Chronic Pain Management and Palliative Care Services have been established for many years. Anaesthesia-based, postoperative pain management services have developed since the late 1980s. These have improved the quality of postsurgical care and patient satisfaction by developing analgesia guidelines in collaboration with other disciplines.[28] The main role of these teams is educational.[29] Quality of care is closely related to the provision of pain management; this relies on cooperation between teams. Mutual education, respect, and communication are essential. This collaboration in hospital practice should blend seamlessly into community care.

Pre-emptive analgesia

Animal studies show that analgesic intervention provided prior to trauma can prevent or reduce subsequent pain. There are discrepancies between this and clinical situations.[30,31] Animals are often healthy and pain free prior to injury that usually occurs peripherally. Clinically, patients have complex disease, pre-existing pain, and surgical stimuli applied to viscera as well as peripherally. Complete blockade of nociceptors throughout surgery is needed if pre-emptive analgesia is to be effective; this is not always possible even with epidural blocks. Analgesia must be evident before surgery and continued without interruption throughout surgery, otherwise its effect is negligible. Pre-existing pain, e.g. limb ischaemia, or postoperative infection or inflammation may impair pre-emptive analgesia.

Local anaesthetic infiltration can only provide pre-emptive analgesia for very superficial surgery; once visceral structures are stimulated, then its effect is small. Pre-emptive analgesia using epidural drugs is insignificant after laparotomy, but significant after limb surgery or mastectomy. The effect of pre-emptive epidural block on development of phantom limb pain is controversial.[32,33] The pre-emptive effect of NSAIDs is usually insignificant. In the absence of presurgical pain, systemic opioids may give significant pre-emptive analgesia in all types of surgery. However, the doses needed may produce significant side-effects. Evidence that the animal model of pre-emptive analgesia can be transferred to the clinical situation is weak. Pre-emptive analgesia can provide high-quality perioperative care, but this must be balanced against risks in each case.

Pain management

Pain management should be based on research evidence whenever possible. Most acute pain can be managed with drugs. There are many systematic reviews of analgesics for acute pain that can be used to develop local and national guidelines.[34] Efficacy can be expressed as number needed to treat (NNT). In acute pain this is the number of patients who need to receive the active drug for one patient to achieve at least 50% relief of pain compared with placebo over a treatment period of four to six hours. Effective drugs have a NNT of about 2; meaning that for every two patients treated one will get 50% relief because of treatment (Table 9.5). The same concept can be applied to adverse effects, as number needed to harm (NNH). However, NNHs do not take

Table 9.5 Single-dose number needed to treat (NNT) compared with placebo for oral analgesics

Drug	Dose (mg)	NNT	Comment
Paracetamol	600–650	5.3	Adverse effects no different from placebo
	1000	4.6	
Dextropropoxyphene	65	7.7	No better than placebo
Paracetamol/ dextropropoxyphene	650 65–100	4.4	Transient dizziness and drowsiness
Codeine	60	16.7	Not effective
Paracetamol/ codeine	600/650 60	3.6	Drowsiness and dizziness, no increased emesis
Dihydrocodeine	30		No better than placebo
Tramadol	50	8.3	Headache, emesis, sedation, and dizziness
	75	5.3	similar to comparators
	100	4.8	
	150	2.9	
Aspirin	600–650	4.4	Higher incidence of drowsiness, gastric
	1000	4.0	irritation, not emesis
	1500	2.4	
Ibuprofen	100	5.6	No difference in adverse effects from placebo
	200	3.3	
	400	2.7	
	600	2.4	
	800	1.6	
Diclofenac	25	2.6	No difference in adverse effects from placebo
	50	2.3	
	100	1.8	
Ketorolac	10	2.6	More adverse effects than placebo
	20	1.8	
Rofecoxib	50	1.9	
Celecoxib	200	2.8	
Morphine	10	2.9	Intramuscular

into account occasional but catastrophic effects, e.g. agranulocytosis; these are captured by case reports. Chronic pain often requires more complex treatments that may involve adjuvant drugs, nerve blocks, or spinal drug delivery. In chronic pain, there are fewer good studies. However, the absence of evidence is not the same as evidence of inefficacy. Systems for risk management and critical incident reporting should be incorporated into all guidelines for pain management. Proposals must match local circumstances and resources; they must be supported by education.

Drug treatments

Simple analgesics and weak opioids (Table 9.5)

Paracetamol is an important analgesic; the NNT for 1000 mg is 4.6. It is not associated with adverse effects.[35] Single-dose dextropropoxyphene is not effective. Paracetamol with dextropropoxyphene has an NNT of 4.4, but adverse effects are commoner than after placebo.[36] Therefore it is logical to use 1000 mg paracetamol alone for mild to moderate pain. A single dose of oral codeine 60 mg is not effective. Paracetamol with codeine is effective even in single dose (NNT 3.1). Drowsiness and dizziness are more common after the combination, but nausea and vomiting are not increased.[37]

Dihydrocodeine is a synthetic opioid commonly used in acute pain. Single-dose 30 mg dihydrocodeine is not effective. There is no data for a 60 mg dihydrocodeine against placebo, however 60 mg dihydrocodeine is less effective than 400 mg ibuprofen. Tramadol is a weak opioid that has activity at 5-hydroxytryptamine and noradrenaline receptors; it shows a clear dose response. Side-effects include headache, emesis, dizziness, and somnolence. These data on single-dose trials may be applied only cautiously to chronic pain. Repeated dosing may improve analgesia and patients may become tolerant to some side-effects.

NSAIDs and coxibs (Table 9.5)

NSAIDs and coxibs are powerful analgesics that block the production of mediators of pain and inflammation by cyclo-oxygenase (cox) inhibition. Cox-1 is found in most tissues; it serves physiological functions such as gastric protection, renal blood flow, and platelet function. Cox-2 is inducible and mediates the synthesis of inflammatory prostaglandins; analgesia is probably mediated by cox-2 inhibition.

NSAIDs inhibit cox-1 and cox-2. They are effective in relieving cancer pain.[38] After single dose, they are as effective as intramuscular morphine, oral weak opioids, or paracetamol/weak opioid combinations. After multiple doses there is no difference in efficacy or side-effects between NSAIDs and weak opioid or paracetamol/weak opioid combinations. There is no evidence for superiority of one NSAID over another after single dosing; this may not be true in chronic use. Aspirin is an important analgesic with a clear dose response. Paracetamol and aspirin are comparable mg for mg. However, even in single dose, aspirin has a higher incidence of drowsiness, nausea, and gastric irritation (one in 40 patients). There is an increased risk of bleeding. These findings have implications for long-term aspirin use. Oral NSAIDs are very effective in moderate to severe postoperative pain. There is no difference in adverse effects in single dose between ibuprofen or diclofenac and placebo; the same is not true in chronic use. Ketorolac is an effective analgesic, but there are more adverse effects after 10 mg oral ketorolac than placebo (NNH 7.3), e.g. drowsiness, dizziness, and emesis. There have been case reports of serious gastrointestinal and postoperative wound haemorphage after ketorolac.

When choosing analgesic drugs, benefits should always be balanced against risks. NSAID use is limited by side-effects that can occur after single dose, but are more common in chronic use. Their efficacy dose response curve is quite flat compared with that for side-effects; this is unlike opioids. Increasing NSAID dose may not improve analgesia, but will cause more side-effects, e.g. gastrointestinal bleeding, renal impairment, exacerbation of asthma, cardiac failure with peripheral oedema, and platelet inhibition. Chronic use of NSAIDs leads to fatalities usually due to gastrointestinal bleeding.[39] Annual NSAID data are: UK – 25 million prescriptions and 2600 deaths; USA – 70 million prescriptions and 16 500 deaths; Canada – 10 million prescriptions and 365 deaths. The risks increase with: age over 50 years, females, previous peptic ulcers or bleeds, and previous heart disease; there is synergism of risk. Some NSAIDs are more risky than others, e.g. ibuprofen (below 2400 mg daily) is much safer than piroxicam or ketorolac. NSAIDs produce a clinically insignificant reduction in creatinine clearance and potassium excretion after surgery. They should not be withheld from those with normal kidneys because of concerns about renal function. However, chronic NSAID use is associated with an increased risk of renal failure, especially in those with previous heart or renal problems or gout. Those taking loop diuretics, or who have had more than a 10% loss of blood volume, are also at increased risk. The renal risk is greatest with NSAIDs with a half-life of more than 12 hours, e.g. naprosyn or piroxicam rather than ibuprofen or diclofenac. The risk reduces after 30 days of stopping NSAID treatment. NSAIDs may precipitate congestive cardiac failure in the elderly; this is more likely in the longer-acting drugs. Postsurgical bleeding may be increased by NSAID use.

Cox-2 inhibitors, e.g. rofecoxib, celecoxib, and paracoxib are as effective as NSAIDs. Rofecoxib has a longer duration of action and can be given as a once-daily dose. The major advantage of coxibs is that they do not produce endoscopic ulcers and are unlikely to cause gastrointestinal bleeding. Cox-2 inhibitors act within the kidney, so they can still cause renal problems and peripheral oedema. Cox-2 inhibitors have no effect on platelet aggregation, and will not substitute for the use of aspirin. Many patients requiring palliative surgery are at high risk for NSAID-induced adverse effects. Cox-2 inhibitors may have advantages for acute and chronic use in such cases.

Strong opioids (Table 9.5)

Many strong opioids have been used for postoperative pain management; all have advantages and disadvantages. Morphine is commonly used for severe or moderate pain. It is the 'gold standard' against which other drugs are tested. The most important principle for safe and effective use of opioids is to titrate the drug to achieve analgesia and treat side-effects early.

In single-dose studies of intramuscular morphine 10 mg, the NNT is 2.9,[40] however chronic dosing is likely to be different. Morphine produces active glucuronides that may accumulate; therefore it should probably be avoided in those with renal impairment. Diamorphine is a pro-drug of morphine. It is very lipid soluble. It has the advantage of powder form so that it can be reconstituted as a very concentrated solution. Pethidine should not be used at all; it has no advantages over other opioids in its action on smooth muscle. It is metabolized to nor-pethidine that can accumulate and causes CNS toxicity. Oxycodone, fentanyl, or hydromorphone may be useful in patients who do not tolerate morphine. These do not have clinically important metabolites and so may be used in patients with renal problems. There may be differences in side-effects, e.g. fentanyl may be less constipating than morphine in long-term use. Methadone can be a useful drug because of its action on other receptors. Enzyme induction or inhibition can alter its metabolism and it has a long half-life. Titration in the postoperative period is difficult. There is evidence that in chronic pain the response to opioids is quite individual. If a patient does not respond to one opioid, then it may be worth switching to another.

Routes of drug delivery

The route of drug administration is important in the perioperative period. Oral administration of ibuprofen, diclofenac, or ketorolac is more effective than 10 mg intramuscular morphine (Table 9.5). Injectable or rectal NSAIDs are popular, but they have similar efficacy and side-effects as oral drugs. In most situations (except renal colic), oral administration is as good as parenteral or rectal use. Topical NSAIDs are effective; they may be used for coincidental musculoskeletal pain. In multiple doses NSAIDs have fewer side-effects than intramuscular morphine. Therefore oral drugs should be used if possible.

Altered consciousness, fasting, and ileus often occur; therefore other routes of drug delivery are needed. Sustained release or transdermal formulations are not applicable immediately after surgery, either because of difficulty in titration or uncertainty about gut function. Regular intramuscular or fixed-rate intravenous opioid administration can be used. However this may not deal with the 10-fold difference in opioid requirement that can occur between patients. The use of patient-controlled analgesia (PCA) allows the patient to match the dose of opioid to activity.[41] Patients must be titrated to comfort, with a loading dose of intravenous opioid, before the commencement of PCA. There are risk management reasons for using a standard opioid in a standard concentration, e.g. 50 mg/50 ml morphine, with which all staff can become familiar. The bolus dose is set at the minimum dose required to produce analgesia, e.g. 1–2 mg morphine or 10–20 μg fentanyl. The lockout interval relates to the time to reach peak effect, e.g. 5–10 minutes. Patients need to maintain the plasma opioid concentration above the minimum effective analgesic concentration (MEAC) and below the minimum toxic concentration (MTC), i.e. within the analgesic window. In some patients or situations this can be difficult and side-effects occur. The use of a background infusion does not improve analgesia or sleep in the perioperative period; it increases adverse effects. In cancer patients taking regular high-dose opioids prior to surgery, the use of a background infusion may be helpful. Not all patients can use PCA, e.g. very young, cognitively impaired, and those with confusion. Great care is needed with the use of PCA in children, problems of toxicity can occur in nurse- or parent-controlled analgesia. There is little evidence that analgesia, patient satisfaction, bowel or ventilatory function, and hospital stay are better with PCA than with an optimal intramuscular regimen.[42] However, staff numbers and education do not always lead to an optimal regimen. Routes such as intranasal, subcutaneous, rectal, and spinal (see below) may have a place in selected patients. Breakthrough and incident pain in otherwise stable patients may be managed by oral transmucosal fentanyl.

Adjuvant analgesics

Patients with complex pain problems, e.g. neuropathic pain, may have resistance to opioids and may benefit from the use of adjuvant analgesics. Antidepressants should probably be used as first-line therapy for neuropathic pain, often at less than half the dose needed to treat depression.[43] The NNT is about 3 in a variety of neuropathic pain conditions. Side-effects, e.g. sedation, dry mouth, arrhythmias, and retention of urine, occur in about 30% of patients; 4% have to stop treatment. Giving a single dose two hours before bed can reduce sedative side-effects. The elderly should start with a low dose, e.g. 10 mg amitriptyline, slowly titrated to effect. Modern antidepressants such as serotonin reuptake inhibitors are less effective, but have a 50% reduction in side-effects.

Anticonvulsants may be effective in some neuropathic pains, but the dose needed is usually in the anticonvulsant dose range.[44] Carbemazepine has an NNT of about 2.5 for trigeminal pain. There are very few trials of other anticonvulsants, e.g. phenytoin and gabapentin; they have NNTs of about 3. There is a high risk for minor adverse effects (NNHs 2–4). Newer drugs such as gabapentin have fewer side-effects, and are probably the first choice if an anticonvulsant is indicated.

Clonidine is an α2 adrenergic agonist with analgesic effects in nociceptive and neuropathic pain. It can be used spinally. It is synergistic with local anaesthetics and opioids. It may produce sedation and hypotension. Ketamine has been used in anaesthesia for many years as a dissociative anaesthetic. It has potent analgesic actions via the N-methyl-D-aspartate (NMDA) receptor channel complex. It produces unpleasant psychomimetic effects. Its oral bioavailability is poor, but it is metabolized to nor-ketamine that is an analgesic. It has been used orally as an infusion or spinally in various doses to manage a variety of chronic pain conditions.[45] The immunological and psychomimetic effects of ketamine have not been fully elucidated in palliative care patients. Ketamine has abuse potential.

Drug side-effects

NSAIDs should be avoided in those with asthma, renal problems, or at high risk from surgical bleeding. All patients with risk factors for gastrointestinal bleeding who are prescribed NSAIDs should receive proton pump inhibitors. This probably includes all patients undergoing palliative surgery, who may be better treated with coxibs. There is no advantage for co-administration of proton pump inhibitors with coxibs. Opioid side-effects must be monitored and treated early. All opioids produce side effects, e.g. ventilatory depression, itching, sedation, emesis, and constipation; they can cause cognitive effects. Severe opioid-induced ventilatory depression is uncommon, especially in those who are not opioid naïve; supplementary oxygen should be used for at least 48 hours after surgery. High-risk patients, e.g. those with pre-existing chest disease or some elderly, require careful monitoring after surgery. Itching can be managed with nalbuphine or ondansetron. Emesis requires regular anti-emetic drugs. Constipation must be pre-empted by bowel care and aperients. Severe cognitive impairment may respond to a change in opioid.

Risk increases with high-technology analgesia methods.[46] The use of such methods must have demonstrable benefits, otherwise it is better to use low technology. It may be necessary to manage high-risk patients in a high-dependency or intensive therapy unit. This depends on local circumstances, but there should be clear local policies on this issue.

Local and regional analgesia

Drugs are effective analgesics in more than 80% of patients with cancer. Others may benefit from interventions such as nerve blocks, spinal drug delivery, or neurosurgery. Local and regional blocks can be useful for patients requiring palliative surgery. A variety of techniques are available that must be considered in the context of the patient's pain problem, the skill of the anaesthetist, and local resources. Patients and their carers need a full explanation of any proposed techniques; consent must be as informed as possible.

Wound infiltration and nerve blocks

Local wound infiltration may be helpful for several hours after inguinal herniorraphy, but there is no evidence of efficacy after other procedures.[47,48] Further trials are needed before firm conclusions can be reached. Plexus and paravertebral blocks can be very useful during surgery, but efficacy in the postoperative period is quite operator-dependent. They are probably best done by enthusiasts rather than as part of general postoperative pain management guidelines.

Spinal analgesia

The use of epidural analgesia is popular after major surgery, however there is little evidence that it alters outcome, except in some high-risk cases. There is no evidence that epidural local anaesthesia contributes to anastomotic breakdown.[49] It is not clear whether the use of epidural opioids contributes, in the same way as systemic opioids, to gastrointestinal paralysis after bowel surgery. The use of spinal local anaesthetic and opioid together is synergistic, with reduced dose requirement and side-effects. There are several studies showing that, with adequate education and staffing, epidural analgesia can be used safely in a ward setting for many patients.[50] Epidural PCA has been used with some success, but can only be introduced if local circumstances are optimal.[51]

Risks of spinal drug delivery include infection or haematoma, cardiac or central nervous system local anaesthetic toxicity, or opioid side-effects such as itch, retention of urine, or ventilatory depression. The use of newer agents such as ropivacaine or levobupivacaine may reduce local anaesthetic side-effects.[52] The risk of serious adverse effects is probably about 0.45 per 10 000 spinals and 0.52 per 10 000 epidurals.[53] The risk of neurological sequelae after epidural is about one in 5000.[54,55] Therefore postoperative spinal analgesia should only be used if the benefits outweigh the risks in each case and if local circumstances permit safe spinal drug delivery. The practical problems around delivery of a safe and effective postoperative epidural service are often considerable.[56]

Neurolytic blocks

Some patients with cancer pain can benefit from neurolytic blocks, but should be warned of potential complications. Coeliac plexus block is effective for relief of pain from intra-abdominal pancreatic and non-pancreatic cancers.[57,58] Fluoroscopic guidance should be used for the percutaneous technique, but there is no advantage in using computerized tomography. It can be performed during open surgery. About 90% of patients have acceptable relief at three months. In 73–92%, at least partial relief is maintained until death. Transient adverse effects include local pain (96%), diarrhoea (44%), and postural hypotension (38%). If diarrhoea is troublesome it can be treated with octreotide. Impotence may result. Neurological complications, such as paraplegia and incontinence, are rare. Neurolytic lumbar sympathectomy can be useful for ischaemic leg pain in those who are unfit for surgery. Bilateral block has also been used to treat tenesmus from perineal tumours. The technique is simple, but must be performed under fluoroscopy. Adverse effects include postural hypotension, lateral thigh pain due to genitofemoral neuritis, impotence, and renal or ureteric trauma. Neurolytic block of the superior hypogastric plexus may be useful in malignant pelvic pain. Intrathecal injection of small amounts of hyperbaric phenol can be used to treat the pain of perineal, gynaecological, or bladder tumours. Risks include motor block and bladder/bowel disturbance. Only those with experience should use these techniques.

Physical methods of analgesia

The physiotherapist may have a lot to offer patients with cancer undergoing palliative surgery. Careful positioning of limbs, manoeuvres to help with spinal pain, and general postural advice are helpful.

Transcutaneous electrical nerve stimulation (TENS)

TENS has limited efficacy in the management of postoperative pain;[59] it should not be used as it may lead to delay in offering more effective methods. There are no good trials of TENS in chronic and cancer pain. If it is used, it is clear that patient and staff education is vital. The patient must be carefully instructed on the optimum use of TENS, e.g. where to put the electrodes and how long to stimulate.

Acupuncture

Although acupuncture has been used for pain control for many centuries, and is popular with patients, there is no good evidence for its efficacy. Acupuncture trials are difficult to design and carry out in chronic pain. It may be justified to offer it as an adjunct in some cases. Acupuncture practitioners need to be adequately trained. The treatment must be integrated into more routine analgesic management. It should not cause delay in administering more conventional and proven treatments.

Neurosurgery

Occasionally patients with difficult cancer pain may benefit from neurosurgical intervention. Techniques such as percutaneous cordotomy may be appropriate. It is vital to involve a neurosurgeon with interest and expertise in pain management.

Recommendations for analgesia

◆ Consider the needs of the individual and co-existing pathology.

◆ Allow the patient as much control as possible.

◆ Assess and record pain regularly and accurately.

◆ Choose evidence-based analgesia when possible.

◆ Use safe and simple techniques.

◆ Multi-modal approaches produce better analgesia and reduce side-effects.

◆ Always consider the benefits and risks in each case.

◆ Use appropriate drugs, routes, and drug delivery techniques.

◆ Monitor and treat adverse effects.

◆ Educate health care professionals, patients, and their carers.

◆ Choose methods that fit local needs, e.g. staff training and availability, equipment.[60]

Analgesia can be enhanced using techniques other than drugs, nerve blocks, and physical methods. The effects of good nursing care, psychological interventions, and spiritual support should never be forgotten in the context of total pain control. This approach requires a team of committed professionals with training in palliative care and pain management. They must work in a complementary way to the patient's team, providing support and education when required. The management of pain in this vulnerable group has to be a team effort. Effective postoperative pain management may improve outcome only if it is integrated with a multi-modal rehabilitation programme.[61]

References

1. American Society of Anesthesiologists, Inc. (1963). New Classification of Physical Status. *Anesthesiology*, **24**, 111–17.

2. Callum, K.G., Gray, A.J.G., Hoile, R.W., *et al.* (2000). *Then and Now – the 2000 Report of the National Confidential Enquiry into Perioperative Deaths.* NCEPOD, London.

3. Rahlfs, T.F., and Jones, R.L. (1998). Risks and outcomes in oncology patients undergoing anesthesia and surgery. *Int. Anesth. Clin.*, **36**, 141–9.

4. Pedersen, T. (1994). Complications and death following anaesthesia. A prospective study with special reference to the influence of patient-, anaesthesia-, and surgery-related risk factors. *Danish Med. Bull.*, **41**, 319–31.

5. Munro, J., Booth, A., and Nicholl, J. (1997). Routine preoperative testing – a systematic review of the evidence. *Hlth Tech. Assess.*, **1** (12).

6. Khuri, S.F., Daley, J., Henderson, W., *et al.* (1997). Risk adjustment of the postoperative mortality rate for the comparative assessment of the quality of care. Results of the National Veterans Affairs Surgical Risk Study. *J. Am. Coll. Surg.*, **185**, 315.

7. Carson, J.L., Duff, A., Berlin, J.A., *et al.* (1998). Perioperative blood transfusion and postoperative mortality. *J.A.M.A.*, **279**, 199–205.

8. Potyk, D., and Raudaskowski, P. (1998). Preoperative cardiac evaluation for elective non-cardiac surgery. *Arch. Fam. Med.*, **7**, 164–73.

9. Shah, K.B., Kleinman, B.S., and Sami, H., *et al.* (1990). Re-evaluation of perioperative myocardial infarction in patients with prior myocardial infarction undergoing non-cardiac operations. *Anesth. Analges.*, **71**, 231–5.

10. Eagle, K.A., Brundage, B.H., Chaitman, B.R., *et al.* (1996). Guidelines for perioperative cardiovascular evaluation for non-cardiac surgery. Report of the American College of Cardiology/American Heart Association Task Force on perioperative cardiovascular evaluation for non-cardiac surgery. *Circulation*, **93**, 1278–91.

11. Wallace, A., Layug, E.L., Tateo, I., *et al.* (1998). Prophylactic atenolol reduces postoperative myocardial ischemia. *Anesthesiology*, **88**, 7–17.

12. Klotz, H.P., Candinas, D., Platz, A., *et al.* (1996). Preoperative risk assessment in elective general surgery. *Br. J. Surg.*, **83**, 1788–91.

13. Small, S., Ali, H.H., Lennon, V.A., *et al.* (1992). Anesthesia for unsuspected Lambert–Eaton syndrome. *Anesthesiology*, **76**, 142–5.

14. Baxter, F. (1997). Septic shock. *Can. J. Anesth.*, **44**, 59–72.

15. LaMantia, K.R., Glick, J.H., and Marshall, B.E. (1984). Supplemental oxygen does not cause respiratory failure in bleomycin-treated surgical patients. *Anesthesiology*, **60**, 65–7.

16. American Society of Anesthesiologists (2001). Ethical guidelines for the anaesthesia care of patients with do-not-resuscitate orders or other directives that limit treatment. http://www.asahq.org/publicationsandservices/standards/09.html.

17. O'Hara, D.A., Duff, A., Berlin, J.A., *et al.* (2000). The effect of anesthetic technique on postoperative outcomes in hip fracture repair. *Anesthesiology*, **92**, 947–57.

18. Ballantyne, J.C., Carr, D.B., de Ferranti, S., *et al.* (1998). The comparative effects of postoperative analgesic therapies on pulmonary outcome: cumulative meta-analysis of randomized controlled trials. *Anesth. Analges.*, **86**, 598–612.

19. Lui, S.S., Carpenter, R.L., Mackey, D.C. *et al.* (1995). Effects of peri-operative analgesic technique on rate of recovery after colon surgery. *Anesthesiology*, **83**, 757–65.

20. Checketts, M.R., and Wildsmith, J.A.W. (1999). Central nerve blockade and thrombo-prophylaxis – is there a problem? *Br. J. Anaesth.*, **82**, 164–7.

21. Portenoy, R.K., Payne, D., and Jacobsen, P. (1999). Breakthrough pain: characteristics and impact in patients with cancer pain. *Pain*, **81**, 129–34.

22. Dellemijn, P. (1999). Are opioids effective in relieving neuropathic pain? *Pain*, **80**, 453–62.

23. Page, G.C., Blakely, W.P., and Ben-Eliyahu, S. (2001). Evidence that post-operative pain is a mediator of the tumor-promoting effects of surgery in rats. *Pain*, **90**, 191–9.

24. Sacerdote, P., Bianchi, M., Gaspani, L., *et al.* (2000). The effects of tramadol and morphine on the immune responses to pain after surgery in cancer patients. *Anesth. Analges.*, **90**, 1411–14.

25. Klopfenstein, C.E., Herrmann, F.R., Mamie, C., Van Gessel, E., and Forster, A. (2000). Pain intensity and pain relief after surgery: a comparison between patients' reported assessments and nurses' and physicians' observations. *Acta Anaesthesiol. Scand.*, **44**, 58–62.

26. O'Brian, S., Dalton, J.A., Konsler, G., and Carlson, J. (1996). The knowledge and attitudes of experienced oncology nurses regarding the management of cancer-related pain. *Oncol. Nurses Forum*, **23**, 515–21.

27. Ward, S.E., Goldberg, N., Miller-McCauley, V., *et al.* (1993). Patient-related barriers to management of cancer pain. *Pain*, **52**, 319–24.

28. Miaskowski, C., Crews, J., Ready, B., Paul, S.M., and Ginsberg, B. (1999). Anesthesia-based pain services improve the quality of postoperative pain management. *Pain*, **80**, 23–9.

29. Gould, T.H., Crosby, D.L., Harmer, M., *et al.* (1992). Policy for controlling pain after surgery: effect of sequential changes in management. *B.M.J.*, **305**, 1187–93.

30. Niv, D., and Devor, M. (1996). Does pre-emptive analgesia work, and why? *Pain Rev.*, **3**, 79–90.

31. Aida, S., and Shimoji, K. (2000). Pre-emptive analgesia: recent findings. *Pain Reviews*, **7**, 105–17.

32. Nikolajsen, L., and Jensen, T.S. (2001). Phantom limb pain. *Br. J. Anaesth.*, **87**, 107–17.

33. Lambert, A.W., Dashfield, A.K., Cosgrove, C., Wilkins, D.C., Walker, A.J., and Ashley, S. (2001). Randomized prospective study comparing preoperative epidural and intraoperative perineural analgesia for the prevention of postoperative stump and phantom limb pain following major amputation. *Reg. Anaesth. Pain Med.*, **26**, 316–21.

34. Smith, L.A., Moore, A.R., McQuay, H.J., and Gavaghan, D. (2001). Using evidence from different sources: an example using paracetamol 1000 mg plus codeine 60 mg. *BMC Med. Res. Method.*, **1**, 1–12.

35. Moore, A., Collins, S., Carol, D., and McQuay, H.J. (1997). Paracetamol with and without codeine in acute pain: a quantitative systematic review. *Pain*, **70**, 193–201.

36. Collins, S.L., Edwards, J.E., Moore, R.A., and McQuay, H.J. (2001). Single-dose dextropropoxyphene, alone and with paracetamol (acetaminophen) for postoperative pain (Cochrane Review). In: *The Cochrane Library*, **3**. Update Software, Oxford.

37. Moore, A., Collins, S., Carol, D., McQuay, H.J., and Edwards, J. (2001). Single-dose paracetamol (acetaminophen), with and without codeine, for postoperative pain (Cochrane Review). In: *The Cochrane Library*, **3**. Update Software, Oxford.

38. Eisenberg, E., Berkley, C.S., Carr, D.B., Mosteller, F., and Chalmers, T.C. (1994). Efficacy and safety of non-steroidal anti-inflammatory drugs for cancer pain: a meta-analysis. *J. Clin. Oncol.*, **12**, 2756–65.

39. Hernandez-Diaz, S., and Garcia Rodriguez, L.A. (2000). Association between non-steroidal anti-inflammatory drugs and upper gastrointestinal tract bleeding and perforation: an overview of epidemiological studies published in the 1990s. *Arch. Intern. Med.*, **160**, 2093–9.

40. McQuay, H.J., Carroll, D., and Moore, R.A. (1997). Injected morphine in postoperative pain: a quantitative systematic review. *J. Pain Sympt. Manage.*, **17**, 164–74.

41. Ballantyne, J.C., Carr, D.B., Chalmers, T.C., Dear, K.B., Angelillo, I.F., and Mosteller, F. (1993). Postoperative patient-controlled analgesia: meta-analyses of initial randomized controlled trials. *J. Clin. Anaesth.*, **5**, 182–93.

42. Macintyre, P.E. (2001). Safety and efficacy of patient controlled analgesia. *Br. J. Anaesth.*, **87**, 36–46.

43. McQuay, H.J., Tramer, M., Nye, B.A., Carroll, D., Wiffen, P., and Moore, A. (1996). A systematic review of antidepressants in neuropathic pain. *Pain*, **68**, 217–27.

44. Wiffin, P., Collins, S., McQuay, H.J., Carroll, D., Jahad, A., and Moore, A. (2000). *Cochrane Database Systematic Review*, **2**, CD001133.

45. Schmid, R.L., Sandler, A.N., and Katz, J. (1999). Use and efficacy of low-dose ketamine in the management of acute postoperative pain: a review of current techniques and outcomes. *Pain*, **82**, 111–25.

46. Bates, D.W., Cullen, D.J., Laird, N., *et al.* (1995). Incidence of adverse drug events and potential adverse drug events. *J.A.M.A.*, **274**, 29–34.

47. Dahl, J.B., Moiniche, S., and Kehlet, H. (1994). Wound infiltration with local anaesthetics for postoperative pain. *Acta Anaesthesiol. Scand.*, **38**, 7–14.

48. Moiniche, S., Mikkelsen, S., Wetterslev, J., and Dahl, J.B. (1998). A qualitative systematic review of incisional local anaesthesia for postoperative pain relief after abdominal operations. *Br. J. Anaesth.*, **81**, 377–83.

49. Holte, K., and Kehlet, H. (2001). Epidural analgesia and the risk of anastomotic leakage. *Reg. Anesth. Pain Manage.*, **26**, 111–17.

50. de Leon-Casasola, O.A., Parker, B., Lema, M.J., and Harrison-Massey, J. (1994). Postoperative epidural bupivacaine – morphine therapy: experience with 4227 surgical cancer patients. *Anesthesiology*, **81**, 368–75.

51. Wigfull, J., and Welchew, E. (2001). Survey of 1057 patients receiving postoperative patient-controlled epidural anaesthesia. *Anaesthesia,* **56,** 47–81.

52. McLeod, G.A., and Burke, D. (2001). Levobupivacaine. *Anaesthesia,* **56,** 331–41.

53. Aromaa, U., Lahdensuu, M., and Cozanitis, D.A. (1997). Severe complications associated with epidural and spinal anaesthesia in Finland 1987–1993: a study based on patient insurance claims. *Acta Anaesthesiol. Scand.,* **41,** 445–52.

54. Kane, R.E. (1981). Neurologic deficits following epidural or spinal anesthesia. *Anesth. Analges.,* **60,** 150–61.

55. Yuen, E.C., Layzer, R.B., Weitz, S.R., and Olney, R.K. (1995). Neurologic complications of lumbar epidural anesthsia and analgesia. *Neurology,* **45,** 1795–801.

56. McLeod, G.A., Davies, H.T.O., Munnoch, N., Bannister, J., and Macrae, W. (2001). Postoperative pain relief using thoracic epidural analgesia: outstanding success and disappointing failures. *Anaesthesia,* **56,** 47–81.

57. Eisenberg, E., Carr, D.B., and Chalmers, T.C. (1995). Neurolytic coeliac plexus block for treatment of cancer pain: a meta-analysis. *Anesth. Analges.,* **80,** 290–5.

58. Mercadante, S., and Nicosia, F. (1998). Celiac block: a reappraisal. *Reg. Anesth. Pain Med.,* **23,** 37–48.

59. Carroll, D., Tramer, M., McQuay, H.J., Nye, B., and Moore, A. (1996). Randomization is important in studies with pain outcomes: systematic review of TENS in acute postoperative pain. *Br. J., Anaesth.,* **77,** 798–803.

60. McQuay, H.J., Moore, A., and Justins, D. (1997). Fortnightly review: treating acute pain in hospital. *B. M. J.,* **314,** 1531–43.

61. Rosenberg, J., and Kehlet, H. (1999). Does effective postoperative pain management influence surgical morbidity? *Eur. Surg. Res.,* **31,** 133–7.

Part II

Chapter 10

Symptom palliation of diseases of the head and neck (including dentistry)

Simon Rogers

Introduction

It has been estimated that there are around 250 000 new cases of mouth and pharynx cancers annually amongst men worldwide and half that number for females. This corresponds to 8% of all cancers in men and 4% all cancers in females.[1] The commonest sites of head and neck cancers in the United Kingdom are larynx, oral cavity, pharynx, thyroid, and salivary gland, with about 2400, 2100, 1200, 1000, and 700 new case per annum, respectively.[2] The management of patients with advanced, incurable, or recurrent head and neck cancer is a relatively common occurrence as unfortunately many patients have advanced disease at presentation[3] and despite radical treatment one-third will have persistent or recurrent disease. The survival of patients with head and neck cancer has improved substantially over recent decades and the five-year survival is between 60% to 70% for all stages combined. For both males and females, the overall increase in relative survival between 1971–75 and 1986–90 has been much less for head and neck sites compared with other tumours such as melanoma of skin, leukaemia, bladder, and colon.[4] Oral cancer has a similar death:registration ratio as breast and invasive carcinoma of the cervix.[5]

Head and neck malignant neoplasms have a diverse pathology[6] (Box 10.1), occuring in a variety of sites and subsites[7] (Table 10.1). The commonest histopathology is squamous cell carcinoma arising from the mucosal surfaces of the upper aerodigestive tract. This malignancy is most often related to smoking and alcohol. Sites are divided into lip, tongue, salivary gland, mouth, oropharynx, nasopharynx, larynx, hypopharynx, pharynx unspecified, and paranasal sinuses. Table 10.1 illustrates the complexity of subsites stratification of the oral cavity and further consideration of tumour node metastasis (TNM) staging is beyond the scope of this chapter. Other locations include thyroid, skull base, craniofacial, and tracheo-oesphagus. It can be appreciated that with such a diverse anatomical distribution there can be a variety of symptoms that require palliation, depending on the structures involved.

Head and neck cancer patients who present with incurable tumours or develop inoperable recurrent disease pose the surgical team with unique problems different from patients with cancer of other areas. The dying process tends to be slow, lingering, and painful; and the anatomic areas involved tend to be visible, and difficult to shield from the patient and carers.[8] It is extremely important to involve the multidisciplinary team in the decision process.

In this chapter surgical palliation of the major symptoms (Box 10.2) will be discussed rather than specific tumours and locations. Medical management for conditions such as hypercalcaemia,[9] pain,[10] or mouth care[11] will not be considered nor will palliative radiotherapy[12,13] or chemotherapy.[14–17] The chapter will focus on the surgical aspects of palliation and will reflect the author's clinical experience in the management of incurable disease.

Box 10.1 Examples of the range of head and neck malignancy

- ◆ Squamous cell carcinoma
- ◆ Variants of squamous cell carcinoma, e.g. verrucous carcinoma
- ◆ Carcinomas of salivary glands, e.g. acinic cell, mucoepidermoid, adenoid cystic
- ◆ Malignant melanoma
- ◆ Cutaneous tumours such as basal cell carcinoma
- ◆ Lymphoma
- ◆ Fibrosarcoma
- ◆ Liposarcomas
- ◆ Osteosarcoma
- ◆ Maligant fibrous histiocytoma
- ◆ Malignant nerve sheath tumours
- ◆ Rhabdomosarcoma
- ◆ Odontogenic tumours
- ◆ Thyroid
- ◆ Metastatic tumours

Table 10.1 Examples of subsites for tongue (ICD 141) and mouth (ICD 143-5)

ICD-9 code	Subsite description
141	**Tongue**
141.1	Dorsal surface
141.2	Tip and lateral border
141.3	Ventral surface
141.4	Anterior two-thirds, part unspecified
141.9	Unspecified
143	**Gum**
143.0	Upper
143.1	Lower
144	**Floor of mouth**
144.0	Anterior
144.1	Lateral
144.9	Unspecified
145	**Other and unspecified parts of mouth**
145.0	Cheek mucosa
145.1	Vestibule

Table 10.1 (continued) Examples of subsites for tongue (ICD 141) and mouth (ICD 143-5)

ICD-9 code	Subsite description
145.2	Hard palate
145.6	Retromolar area
145.9	Unspecified

Before the issue of symptom control by surgery is considered in greater detail there are six strands that interleave in the decision process.

Natural history of head and neck cancer

It is essential to have an appreciation of the natural history of the disease. A familiarity with the natural history of head and neck cancer gives the necessary background when contemplating surgery with curative intent versus palliation. Kowalski and Carvalho (2000)[18] reported the characteristics of 808 untreated head and neck cancer patients followed up until their death. Although some patients survived up to four years, approximately half were dead within four months. Performance status was the most significant predictor of survival but other factors, notably co-morbidity, was important. Jones (1995)[19] reported that of 3482 patients, 539 were unsuitable for radical treatment, and in the untreated group advanced age, poor general condition, and advanced nodal disease adversely affected survival. The majority of patients whose cancer cannot be controlled are confronted with recurrence at the primary site, neck, or overlying skin (Figures 10.1 and 10.2). A detailed account of the patterns of recurrence and

Box 10.2 Common symptoms requiring control

- Airway obstruction
- Communication difficulties
- Conductive deafness
- Dysphagia (obstruction directly by tumour – oral/oropharyngeal obstruction)
- Facial nerve – corneal abrasion
- Fatigue
- Fistula
- Fungating wound
- Haemorrhage
- Mucosal dryness
- Nasal obstruction
- Nausea and vomiting
- Oral thrush
- Pain
- Weight loss and poor oral intake (nutritional)

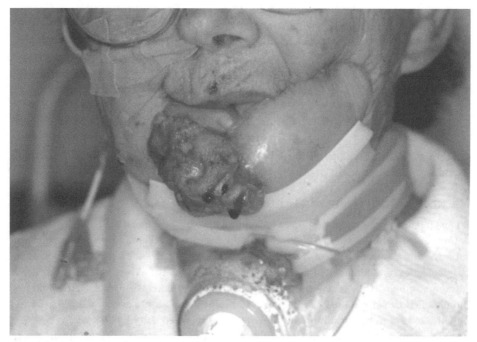

Fig. 10.1 Recurrence involving the oral cavity and skin of the lower lip. This woman developed three new primaries over a 10-year priod. Recurrence occurred following the most recent floor of mouth and alveolus tumour for which resection, fibula free flap reconstruction, and adjuvant radiotherapy were employed. The anticipated functional deficits and relatively small chance of cure were such that the patient declined further intervention.

survival of 200 oral cancer patients treated by radical surgery and neck dissection has been published by Woolgar *et al.* (1999).[3] Thirty per cent of this cohort died of/with their cancer, 18% of local recurrence, 7% of regional disease, 3% of systemic metastases, and 2% with metachronous disease. Recurrence tends to occur within the first year to 18 months and the prognosis is generally poor with survival in terms of months rather than years. Although experience will differ between units, Burns *et al.* (1987)[20] reported a mean survival of 8.4 months following palliative treatment for unresectable head and neck cancer. Skin involvement from mucosal squamous cell carcinoma of the head and neck indicates a poor prognosis[21,22] and resection tends to offers only short-term palliation. Salivary gland disease tends to be much more indolent, particularly in the low-grade tumours, and patients with incurable disease may live months and even years in the presence of metastatic disease.

Morbidity and health-related quality of life

The second issue concerns the effect of treatment in terms of morbidity and health-related quality of life.[20,23] This is a very important concept as intervention can have a substantial detrimental impact on fundamental activities such as breathing, mastication, swallowing, speech, and appearance. Poor function has an unfavourable bearing on self-esteem and psychological well-being. Although there is a body of literature on health-related quality of life (HRQOL) outcomes following primary treatment,[24–26] information on HRQOL in palliation is lacking. Magne and Marcy (2001)[27] reported the HRQOL in patients with unresectable cancer treated by radiotherapy and

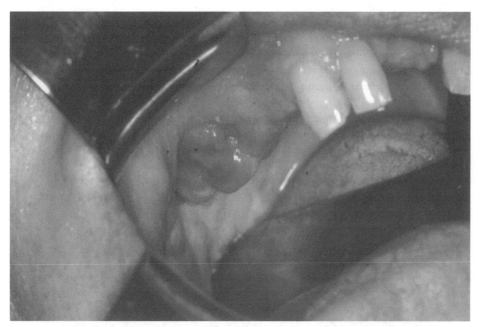

Fig. 10.2 Intraoral recurrence at the margin of a radial free flap. This photograph shows a small discrete recurrence in a previous surgical field (right tuberosity/soft palate). Further resection, reconstruction using local tissues, and adjuvant radiotherapy was 'curative'.

chemotherapy. They demonstrated a regime of increased total radiotherapy equivalent dose which was well tolerated by the patients and accompanied by improved loco-regional control, survival, and long-term quality of life. Clinical experience is such that patients undergoing treatment for recurrence following previous surgery tend to have greater morbidity, poor functional outcome, longer hospital stay, and a poor HRQOL. The situation is made worse if the patient's initial treatment also included adjuvant radiotherapy. It is critical to include the relative subjective benefit of palliative intervention so that the quality of the time remaining for the individual is optimized. The decision process, however, is complex.[28] Only around half of patients[29] die in the hospital setting and it is pertinent to avoid surgery if this is likely to reduce the opportunity for home care. An example is the insertion of a 'temporary tracheostomy' for airway compromise, which then becomes permanent and hinders discharge arrangements.

Surgical rehabilitation

The third consideration is the ability and appropriateness of modern surgical techniques to rehabilitate patients following tumour ablation.[30] Although there have been substantial advances in surgical rehabilitation during the last quarter of the twentieth century, such techniques are seldom appropriate for palliation. A loco-regional approach to salvage therapy is an attractive concept, primarily because distant metastases are uncommon,[31] however radical salvage surgery all too often confers only a short-term benefit because the tumour regrows. One-stage ablation and microvascular reconstruction can have a relatively short hospital stay and therefore makes operating on larger lesions more of an attractive proposition.[28] Because of the associated morbidity, further radical surgery should be considered only if removal of all macroscopic disease is feasible.

Previous cancer treatment

The fourth matter when contemplating palliative surgery is the type and extent of previous treatment. Primary therapy may have been by surgery alone, radiotherapy alone, or combination therapy. Previous therapy will influence the survival versus morbidity benefit of further surgery. There is greater opportunity for worthwhile salvage surgery in cases that have been treated by single modality treatment, had limited initial resections, or present with small-volume recurrent disease (Figure 10.2). If the primary treatment required was radical surgery with free flap reconstruction and adjuvant radiotherapy, major palliative surgery tends not to be indicated for the reasons outlined above (Figure 10.3).

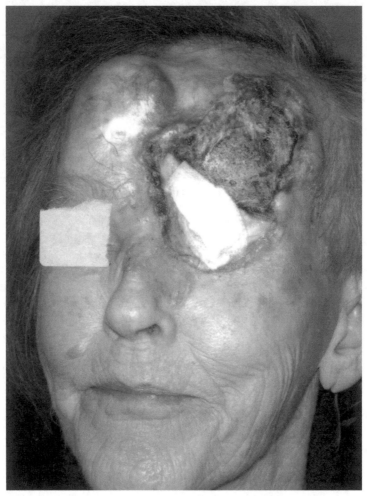

Fig. 10.3 Craniofacial recurrence. This photograph illustrates the indolent nature of some types of head and neck pathology. This woman had undergone major surgery, including left orbital exenteration and radiotherapy over the course of two decades. Surgical palliation was considered for tumour extension involving the right eye with the purpose of preventing complete blindness. Unfortunately, the tumour involved the anterior cranial fossa and its contents and was deemed inoperable for palliation.

Symptoms

The fifth area to be discussed is symptom control. There are a variety of symptoms, some of which are more appropriately managed surgically and others non-surgically (Box 10.2). Patients with head and neck cancer have particular problems because of the impact of the tumour on the airway, the upper gastrointestinal tract, and the major senses.[8,28,32–36] In one study of 150 patients with head and neck cancer (Aird *et al.* 1983),[33] the eight major complaints were pain (50%), dysphagia (38%), airway obstruction (28%), fungating wound (14%), nausea and vomiting (12%), mucosal dryness (10%), conductive deafness (<5%), and bleeding (<1%). A smaller North American study (Shedd *et al.* 1980)[32] reported a higher incidence of pain (85%), feeding problems (62%), and respiratory difficulties (43%). Forbes (1997)[35] reported on 38 patients in the hospice setting and found that pain, weight loss, feeding difficulties, dysphagia, respiratory symptoms, xerostomia, oral thrush, and communication difficulties were the major problems.

Surgical palliative procedures

The final consideration is the variety of surgical procedures for palliation. The concept of surgery for recurrent disease has been reviewed (Ridge 1993, Walton and Ridge 1998),[37,38] but surgery for recurrence does not necessarily equate with surgery for palliation. In the palliation of symptoms surgery has a relatively small part to play compared to supportive care, chemotherapy, and radiotherapy.[8,32,39]

Surgery has a role in palliation for nutritional support and loco-regional control (Box 10.3).

Box 10.3 Options in the surgical armamentaruim

Nutritional support

◆ Percutaneous endoscopic gastrostomy (PEG)
◆ Open jejunostomy and gastrostomy

Loco-regional control

◆ Airway patency (tracheotomy)
◆ Pain control (nerve ablation)
◆ Scleral protection (tarsorrhaphy)
◆ Fistula
◆ Tumour debulking:
　– palliative embolization, image-guided ablation, CO_2 laser
　– photodynamic therapy
　– cryosurgery
◆ Tumour ablation with reconstruction:
　– pedicled myocutaneous flaps
　– microvascular free tissue transfer (latissimus dorsi, scapula, fibula, ilium, jejunum, radial)
◆ Arrest of haemorrhage

Nutritional support

The need for fluid and nutritional support in patients with head and neck cancer is widely appreciated and the palliative situation is no exception. Percutaneous endoscopic gastrostomy (PEG) is an effective method for providing alimentation in patients with upper aerodigestive tract carcinoma,[40] and has all but superseded open jejunostomy and gastrostomy. Percutaneous endoscopic gastrostomy is valuable if the expected survival is more than two months. They are usually inserted under intravenous sedation and the presence of loco-regional recurrence can pose a risk of life-threatening respiratory compromise. On occasion a temporary tracheotomy is advisable. In situations where tumour prevents the passage of the gastroscope, gastric insufflations techniques can facilitate percutaneous insertion without recourse to surgical intervention.

Loco-regional control

Surgery is aimed at maintaining airway patency, pain control, sclera protection, closure of fistula, tumour debulking, tumour ablation, and arrest of haemorrhage.

Airway patency

The decision to perform a tracheostomy for palliation is a difficult one. A tracheostomy may help with breathing difficulties but will limit communication (Figure 10.1). The decision should not be made in the acute situation, rather it should be part of a structured care plan. A tracheostomy does not guarantee airway patency and in the presence of uncontrolled disease in the laryngeal region, problems occur with occlusion of the tracheal lumen by tumour or secretions. This leads to considerable anxiety and distress for the patient, family, and carers (Forbes 1997).[35] Another indication for a tracheostomy is to secure the airway at the time of palliative surgery. Awake fibre-optic intubations can suffice but there must be a readiness in the surgical team to undertake a tracheostomy if the awake intubation proves impossible or hazardous. If a tracheostomy is required it can be performed using local anaesthesia with sedation and personal experience favours a bjork flap.[41,42] A bjork flap gives a window into the trachea and a flap of anterior wall hinged at the inferior aspect, held forward by a suture. This allows for easier replacement of the tracheostomy tube at a later date. Although percutaneous dilatational tracheostomy under ultrasound guidance is successful,[43] an open procedure by an experienced surgeon is favoured because of the difficult airway with distorted anatomy due to previous surgery, radiation, or tumour infiltration.

Pain control

Pain control is an important issue in patients with incurable disease and analgesic preparations are the mainstay of treatment.[10,44] Increasing pain can denote the presence of recurrence.[45] The role of surgery in the palliation of pain in head and neck cancer is limited because of the anatomical configuration of nerves. Nerve block with alcohol or phenol and surgical nerve transection can be applied if pain is limited to a discrete neural distribution. It is relatively easy to block the maxillary (infra-orbital) and mandibular divisions (mental, inferior alveolar) of the trigeminal nerve, glossopharyngeal nerve, and the cervical plexus (C3/4). Trigeminal ganglion ablation, percutaneous radio-frequency rhizotomy, sterotaxic thalamotomy, or leuko-tomy though described are seldom indicated.[46] Pain of dental cause needs to be treated by an experienced, hospital-based practitioner. Dental extractions can invariably be performed using local anaesthesia. Caution is necessary in situations where the jaws have been exposed to previous radiotherapy as extraction sites may fail to heal and osteoradionecrosis might ensue.

Tarsorrhaphy

In the presence of facial nerve weakness affecting the upper branches, there is inability to adequately close the eyelids. Drying out of the sclera leads to corneal ulceration and pain. A lateral tarsorrhaphy can be performed under local anaesthetic and is a well-tolerated procedure. It would be indicated for longer-term palliation in patients with slowly going, inoperable salivary gland tumours, particularly where simple measures such as eye patches have failed.

Fistula

An orocutaneous or pharyngocutaneous fistula represents a considerable problem (Fortunato and Ridge 1995, Ball *et al.* 1999).[46,47] Fistulae are more common after laryngectomy, particularly following large resections in previously irradiated patients and in those who have additional co-morbidity. Once a fistula has developed, the tract should be opened, necrotic tissue debrided, and local wound care instituted. In the palliative situation most fistulae respond sufficiently to conservative measures, though it may be necessary to consider protecting the carotid artery from infection and rupture by the introduction of healthy tissue as described below.

Tumour debulking

The aim of tumour debulking is to reduce the size of an intraluminal mass that is causing obstructive symptoms such as interference with speech, swallowing, or breathing. Alternatively, debulking is worthwhile for dirty, fungating, malodorous, and unsightly neck/cutaneous mass (Figure 10.4). Debulking is a temporary measure and typically gives palliation for weeks rather than months.

Palliative embolization and image-guided ablation

There is an emerging role for minimal access and imaging-guided minimally invasive surgery to debulk tumours. The use of percutaneous direct puncture therapeutic embolization (DPTE) of hypervascular neoplasms is a relatively new technique aimed at tumour devascularization. It can be used to supplement other techniques such as surgical debulking.[48] In addition to CO_2 laser, interstitial tumour therapy (ITT) has been successfully applied for the treatment of recurrent, non-resectable, local, and/or metastatic head and neck carcinomas.[49] It is a technique whereby a source of energy such as laser, radio-frequency, ultrasonic, or cryoenergy is directly applied into tumours at various depths under ultrasound or magnetic resonance imaging. Several authors have reported their experience with interstitial Nd:YAG laser phototherapy for palliative treatment[50,51] or the use of intratumour injection of gel implants containing the drug followed by interstitial Nd:YAG laser hyperthermia.[52]

Photodynamic therapy

There has been a lot of interest in the use of photodynamic therapy for palliation, particularly in the management of cutaneous neck lesions or large-area superficial mucosal recurrences.[53,54] Photodynamic therapy consists of the selective destruction of tumours using a combination of a photosensitizer administered systemically (dihematoporphyrin ether) and an argon dye-pumped laser. The treatment is associated with morbidity and the place of photodynamic therapy in the future will depend in part on the specificity of the photosensitizing agents.

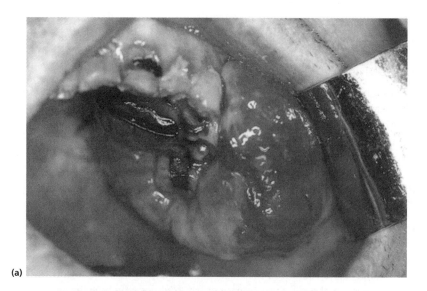

(a)

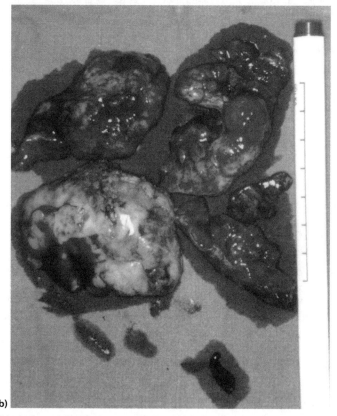

(b)

Fig. 10.4 Debulking of a rapidly growing intraoral tumour. Figure **a** shows the extent of the tumour arising from the left maxillary antrum and extending intraorally. The bulk of the tumour caused the patient severe oral and respiratory compromise and was debulked under local anasthesia with sedation (figure **b**). Debulking provided satisfactory palliation for the few weeks that remained.

Cryosurgery

Liquid nitrogen cryo-ablation has been used for many years[55] and works by rapid freezing and coagulation necrosis. It does have a place in the management of debulking cutaneous neck recurrence, but poor healing and uncontrolled underlying disease limits its value because the treatment poses an increased risk of carotid blow-out.

Tumour ablation

Surgical resection for loco-regional recurrence is an appropriate consideration in a selected group of patients. The postoperative morbidity of surgery will be greater than seen in previously untreated patients undergoing similar procedure.[31,56] There is often no clear-cut distinction between what may constitute 'palliative' or 'curative' treatment in advanced tumours[57,58] and the place of radical surgery is controversial. In such cases the term 'radical palliative surgery with curative intent' has been coined, expressing the reality that although there is little chance of cure, palliation should be accomplished. Careful selection with full and frank discussion with the patients and carers is essential.

The reported lengths to which patients and surgeon will go in an attempt to effect a cure is remarkable[46] and the literature is scattered with examples of 'heroic surgery'.[59] Examples include circumferential pharyngolaryngectomy with total oesophagectomy and free jejunal microvascular anastomosis,[60] transhiatal gastric transposition with pharyngogastric anastomosis for reconstruction of pharyngoesophageal defects,[61] total glossectomy,[62] or total glossolaryngectomy. Carotid artery resection has been described and although it may prolong the disease-free interval,[63,64] it may not increase survival because of the severity of resulting complications.[65] Extra-anatomic carotid bypass[66] or replacement[67] has been reported but the value of such extensive surgery in terms of quality of life and survival remains contentious.

Myocutaneous pedicle

Pedicled flaps have, for much of the last century, been the standard method of reconstruction. Although there has been a shift towards microvascular free tissue transfer, particularly for primary reconstruction, pedicled flaps still have a definite role in palliation. They provide bulk to cover vital structures and their speed of harvest makes them suitable in compromised patients. Specific indications for pedicled flaps include the replacement of neck skin, closure of fistulae, bulk cover following radical neck dissection, and the control of bleeding.[46] Various pedicled flaps are described and examples include pectoralis major (Figure 10.5), deltopectoral, and contralateral bilobed trapezius myocutaneous flap for closure of large defects of the posterior neck.[68]

Microvascular free tissue transfer

Free tissue transfer offers a versatile and reliable reconstruction (Figure 10.1). A combination of skin, muscles, nerves, tendons, and bone can be harvested in a one-stage procedure (Box 10.3). Their place in head and neck surgery is established,[30,69] but their role in palliative surgery has yet to be adequately defined. There are several sources of free tissue available and for the palliation of extensive fungating tumours where bulk is required, the latissimuss dorsi or scapula flaps are favoured. These flaps also have the advantage of providing multiple paddles based on one arterial and venous system. Though patients with skin involvement from head and neck cancer have a poor prognosis, Stavrianos *et al.* (2000)[22] reported that palliation was extended to a mean survival of 23 months following surgical resection, free microvascular flap reconstruction, and

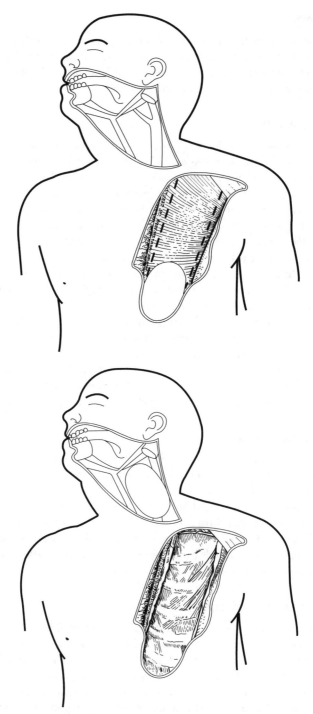

Fig. 10.5 Pectoralis major myocutaneous pedicled flap used following wound breakdown following a radical neck dissection. The flap covers the carotid vessels.

planned postoperative radiotherapy. Despite the emergence of free tissue transfer, the less major procedures remain the keystone of palliative treatment (Ball *et al.* 1999).[47]

Arrest of haemorrhage

'Carotid blow-out' usually occurs when the vessels are left unprotected, for example following radical neck dissection after previous radiotherapy.[47] In spite of well-designed flaps, wound breakdown does occur and consideration must be given to the replacement of skin by pedicled (Figure 10.5) or free tissue transfer. This should be undertaken at the time of neck dissection before wound dehiscence occurs. Carotid blow-out is one of the most feared terminal events and 'herald bleed' can sometimes warn of the pending catastrophe. If time permits, vessels supplying the area such as the external carotid can be ligated; however it may be more appropriate to relieve anxiety and distress by prescribing intravenous sedative preparations.[70]

Dental considerations in general palliative care

The importance of establishing and maintaining oral health in palliative care is readily appreciated.[71] For patients with incurable disease, dentally based specialities can give support in various ways which include ensuring comfort, eliminating sites of infection or potential infection, enhancing oral function, appearance, and self-esteem.[72] The dental team can assist in the diagnosis and management of orofacial pain. Dental caries can be managed by temporary fillings or, where indicated, tooth extraction. Such treatment does not usually require elaborate facilities or equipment and can be performed under local anaesthesia. Dry mouth (xerostomia) is a particular problem, especially in patients who have had radiotherapy to the head and neck.[73] The mucosa is susceptible to infection and the most common organisms are yeasts (candida). The presence of low-grade infection leads to mucositis which tends to be sore and causes difficulties in talking, eating, and denture wearing. The mainstay of treatment is topical antifungal medication, saliva substitutes, and mouth rinses. Dry mouth is also associated with poor periodontal health, gingival bleeding, and halitosis. Relatively simple oral hygiene measures are valuable such as optimal tooth brushing, regular visits to the hygienist, and mouthwash preparations (e.g. chlorhexidine). Patients can find problems with their mouth most distressing but fortunately relatively simple measures are often effective.

Conclusions

Palliative surgery for patients with head and neck cancer is challenging. Radial surgery can lead to poor function and 'quality of life', often without any clear survival benefit. The role of surgery is controversial and relatively simple surgical interventions remain the foundation.

Acknowlegement

The Department of Clinical Photography and Medical Illustration, University Hospital, Aintree.

References

1. Langdon, J.D., and Henk, J.M. (1995). *Malignant tumours of the mouth, jaws, and salivary glands.* Edward Arnold, London.

2. British Association of Otorhinolaryngologists, Head and Neck Surgeons (2000). *Effective head and neck cancer management second consensus document 2000*, p. 4. Royal College of Surgeons of England, London.

3. Woolgar, J.A., Rogers, S.N., West, C.R., Errington, R.D., Brown, J.S., and Vaughan, E.D. (1999). Survival and patterns of recurrence in 200 oral cancer patients treated by radical surgery and neck dissection. *Eur. J. Cancer Oral Oncol.*, **35**, 257–65.

4. Coleman, M.P., Babb, P., Damieck, P., Grosclaude, P., Honjo, S., Jones, J., *et al.* (1999). *Cancer survival trends in England and Wales 1971–1995: deprivation and NHS region.* Office for National Statistics, The Stationery Office Publications Centre, London.

5. Johnson, N.W., and Warnakulasuriya, K.A. (1993). Epidemiology and aetiology of oral cancer in the UK community. *Dental Hlth,* **10** (1), 13–29.

6. Cawson, R.A., Binnie, W.H., Speight, P., Barrett, A.W., and Wright, J.M., (1998). *Lucas's pathology of tumours of the oral tissues* (5th edn). Churchill Livingstone, London.

7. Hermanek, P., and Sobin, L.H. (ed.) (1997). *TNM classification of malignant tumours: UICC International Union against Cancer,* (5th edn). Springer-Verlag Berlin and Heidelberg GmbH & Co, KG.

8. Pashley, N.R. (1980). Practical palliative care for the patient with terminal head and neck cancer. *J. Otolaryngol.,* **9**, 405–11.

9. Goodwin, W.J. Jr., and Chandler, J.R. (1976). Hypercalcemia in epidermoid carcinoma of the head and neck. *Am. J. Surg.,* **132**, 444–8.

10. Olsen, K.D., and Creagan, E.T. (1991). Pain management in advanced carcinoma of the head and neck, [Review.] [19 refs.] *Am. J. Otolaryngol.,* **12**, 154–60.

11. Ventafridda, V., Ripamonte, C., Sbanotto, A., and De Conno, F. (1999). Mouth care. In: *Oxford textbook of palliative medicine* (2nd edn) (ed. D. Doyle, G.W.C. Hanks and N. MacDonald), pp. 691–701. Oxford University press, Oxford.

12. Spaeth, J., Andreopoulos, D., Unger, T., Beckman, J., Ammon, J., and Schlondorff, G. (1997). Intra-operative radiotherapy: 5 years of experience in the palliative treatment of recurrent and advanced head and neck cancers. *Oncology,* **54**, 208–13.

13. Schleicher, U.M., Phonias, C., Spaeth, J., Schlondorff, G., Ammon, J., and Andrepoulos, D. (2001). Intraoperative radiotherapy for pre-irradiated head and neck cancer. *Radiother. Oncol.,* **58**, 77–81.

14. Eckardt, A., and Kelber, A. (1994). Palliative, intra-arterial chemotherapy for advanced head and neck cancer using an implantable port system. *J. Oral Maxillofacial Surg.,* **52**, 1243–6.

15. Eckardt, A., Kelber, A., and Pytlik, C. (1995). Palliative intra-arterial (i.a.) chemotherapy with carboplatin (CBDCA) and 5-FU in unresectable advanced (stage III and IV) head and neck cancer using implantable port-systems. *Eur. J. Surg. Oncol.,* **21**, 486–9.

16. Hughes, R.S., and Frenkel, E.P. (1997). The role of chemotherapy in head and neck cancer. [Review.] [130 refs.] *Am. J. Clin. Oncol.,* **20**, 449–61.

17. Burris, H.A. III, Vogel, C.L., Castro, D., Mishra, L., Schwarz, M., Spencer, S., *et al.* (1998). Intratumoral cisplatin/epinephrine-injectable gel as a palliative treatment for accesible solid tumors: a multicenter pilot study. *Otolaryngol. Head Neck Surg.,* **118**, 496–503.

18. Kowalski, L.P., and Carvalho, A.L. (2000). Natural history of untreated head and neck cancer. *Eur. J. Cancer,* **36**, 1032–7.

19. Jones, A.S. (1995). The untreated patient with squamous carcinoma of the head and neck. *Am. J. Clin. Oncol.,* **18**, 363–8.

20. Burns, L., Chase, D., and Goodwin, W.J. (1987). Treatment of patients with stage IV cancer: do the ends justify the means? *Otolaryngol. Head Neck Surg.,* **10**, 160–7.

21. Cole, R.D., and McGuirt, W.F. (1995). Prognostic significance of skin involvement from mucosal tumors in head and neck. *Arch. Otolaryngol. Head Neck Surg.,* **121**, 1246–8.

22. Stavrianos, S.D., Ragbir, M., McLean, N.R., Kelly, C.G., and Soames, J.V. (2000). Head and neck skin involvement by non-cutaneous head and neck cancers: free flap reconstruction. *Eur. J. Surg. Oncol.,* **26**, 594–8.

23. Epstein, J.B., Robertson, M., Emerton, S., Phillips, N., and Stevenson-Moore, P. (2001). Quality of life and oral function in patients treated with radiation therapy for head and neck cancer. *Head Neck*, **23**, 389–98.

24. Bjordal, K., Hammerlid, E., Ahlner-Elmqvist, M., de Graeff, A., Boysen. M., Evensen, J.F., *et al.* (1999). Quality of life in head and neck cancer patients: validation of the European Organization for Research and Treatment of Cancer Quality of Life Questionnaire – H&N 35. *J. Clin. Oncol.*, **17**, 1008–19.

25. de Graeff, A., de Leeuw, J.R., Ros, W.J., Hordijk, G.J., Blijham, G.H., and Winnubst, J.A. (1999). A prospective study on quality of life patients with cancer of the oral cavity or oropharynx treated with surgery with or without radiotherapy. *Oral Oncol.*, **35**, 27–32.

26. Rogers, S.N., Lowe, D., Brown, J.S., and Vaughan, E.D. A prospective quality-of-life study in patients treated with primary surgery for oral cancer. *Head Neck*, **21**, 394–401.

27. Magne, N., and Marcy, P.Y. (2001). Concomitant twice-a-day radiotherapy and chemotherapy. *Head Neck*, **23**, 678–82.

28. MacDougall, R.H., Munro, A.J., and Wilson, J.A. (1999). Palliation in head and neck cancer. In: *Oxford textbook of palliative medicine* (2nd edn) (ed. D. Doyle, G.W.C. Hanks, and N. MacDonald), pp. 677–89. Oxford University Press, Oxford.

29. Leitner, C., Rogers, S.N., Lowe, D., and Magennis, P. (2001). Death certification in patients treated by primary surgery for oral and oro-pharyngeal carcinoma: 1992–1997. *Br. J. Oral Maxillofacial Surg.*, **39**, 204–9.

30. Rogers, S.N. (2001). Surgical principles and techniques for functional rehabilitation after oral cavity and oropharyngeal oncologic surgery. *Curr. Opin. Otolaryngol. Head Neck Surg.*, **9**, 114–19.

31. Adelstein, D.J. (1994). The community approach to salvage therapy for advanced head and neck cancer. [Review.] [41 refs.] *Seminars Oncol.*, **21**, 52–7.

32. Shedd, D.P., Carl, A., and Shedd, C. (1980). Problems of terminal head and neck cancer patients. *Head Neck Surg.*, **2**, 476–82.

33. Aird, D.W., Bihari, J., and Smith, C. (1983). Clinical problems in the continuing care of head and neck cancer patients. *Ear Nose Throat J.* **62**, 10–30.

34. Droughton, M.L. (1990). Difficult cases: head and neck carcinomas. *J. Pall. Care*, **6** (4), 43–6.

35. Forbes, K. (1997). Palliative care in patients with cancer of the head and neck. *Clin. Otolaryngol.*, **22**, 117–22.

36. Lovel, T. (2000). Palliative care and head and neck cancer. *Br. J. Oral Maxillofacial Surg.*, **38**, 253–4.

37. Ridge, J.A. (1993). Squamous cancer of the head and neck: surgical treatment of local and regional recurrence. [Review.] [143 refs.] *Seminars Oncol.*, **20**, 419–29.

38. Watson, J.C., and Ridge, J.A. (1998). Surgical management of local and regional recurrent head and neck squamous cell carcinoma. [Review.] [71 refs.] *Curr. Opin. Oncol.*, **10**, 207–12.

39. Eckardt, A. (1999). Palliative therapy, terminal care and counselling. In: *Maxillofacial surgery* (vol. 1) (ed. P. Ward Booth, S.A. Schendel, and J.E. Hausamen) pp. 823–31. Churchill Livingstone, London.

40. Rosser, J.C. Jr., Rodas, E.B., Blancaflor, J., Prosst, R.L., Rosser, L.E., and Salem, R.R. (1999). A simplified technique for laparoscopic jejunostomy and gastrostomy tube placement. *Am. J. Surg.*, **177**, 61–5.

41. Price, D.G. (1983). Techniques of tracheostomy for intensive care unit patients. *Anaesthesia*, **38**, 902–4.

42. Malata, C.M., Foo, I.T., Simpson, K.H., and Batchelor, A.G. (1996). An audit of Bjork flap tracheostomies in head and neck plastic surgery. *Br. J. Oral Maxillofacial Surg.*, **34**, 42–6.

43. Aadahl, P., and Nordgard, S. (1999). Percutaneous dilatational tracheostomy in a patient with thyroid cancer and severe airway obstruction. *Acta Anaesthesiol. Scand.*, **43**, 483–5.

44. Kidder, T.M. (1997) Symptom management for incurable head and neck cancer. *Wisconsin Med. J.*, **96** (4), 19–24.

45. Smit, M., Balm, A.J.M., Hilgers, F.J.M., and Tan, I.B. (2001). Pain as sign of recurrent disease in head and neck squamous cell carcinoma. *Head Neck*, **23**, 372–5.

46. Fortunato, L., and Ridge, J.A. (1995). Surgical palliation of head and neck cancers. [Review.] [110 refs.] *Curr. Prob. Cancer*, **19**, 153–65.

47. Ball, A.B.S., Baum, M., Breach, N.M., Shepherd, J.H., Shearer, R.J., Thomas, M.J., *et al.* (1999). Surgical palliation. In: *Oxford textbook of palliative medicine* (2nd edn) (ed. D. Doyle, G.W.C. Hanks, and N. MacDonald), pp. 283–4. Oxford University Press, Oxford.

48. Chaloupka, J.C., Mangla, S., Huddle, D.C., Roth, T.C., Mitra, S., Ross, D.A., *et al.* (1999). Evolving experience with direct puncture therapeutic embolization for adjunctive and palliative management of head and neck hypervascular neoplasms. *Laryngoscope*, **109**, 1864–72.

49. Castro, D.J., Saxton, R.E., Soudant, J., Calcaterra, T., Lufkin, R., Nyerges, A., *et al.* (1994). Minimally invasive palliative tumor therapy guided by imaging techniques: the UCLA experience. *J. Clin. Laser Med. Surg.*, **12**, 65–73.

50. Paiva, M.B., Blackwell, K.E., Saxton, R.E., Calcattera, T.C., Ward, P.H., Soudant, J., *et al.* (1998). Palliative laser therapy for recurrent head and neck cancer: a phase II clinical study. *Laryngoscope*, **108**, 1277–83.

51. Blackwell, K.E., Castro, D.J., Saxton, R.E., Nyerges, A., Calcaterra, T.C., Schiller, V., *et al.* (1993). MRI and ultrasound-guided interstitial Nd:YAG laser phototherapy for palliative treatment of advanced head and neck tumors: clinical experience. *J. Clin. Laser Med. Surg*, **11**, 7–14.

52. Graeber, I.P., Eshraghi, A.A., Paiva, M.B., Paek, W.H., Castro, D.J., Jovanovic, S., *et al.* (1999). Combined intratumor cisplatinum injection and Nd:YAG laser therapy. *Laryngoscope*, **109**, 447–54.

53. Keller, G.S., Doiron, D.R., and Fisher, G.U. (1985). Photodynamic therapy in otolaryngology head and neck surgery. *Arch. Otolaryngol.*, **111**, 758–61.

54. Gluckman, J.L. (1991). Hematoporphyrin photodynamic therapy: is there truly a future in head and neck oncology? Reflections on a 5-year experience. *Laryngoscope*, **101**, 36–42.

55. Goode, R.L., Breitenbach, E.E., and Cox, D. (1974). Cryosurgical treatment of recurrent head and neck malignancies – a comparative study. *Laryngoscope*, **84**, 1950–8.

56. Wax, M.K., and Briant, T.D. (1993). Surgery and postoperative radiotherapy in the management of extensive cancer of the cervical lymph nodes from an unknown primary. *J. Otolaryngol.*, **22**, 34–8.

57. Shaw, H.J. (1986). Palliation in head and neck cancer: discussion paper. *J. Roy. Soc. Med.*, **79**, 84–6.

58. Lucente, F.E. (1994). Treatment of head and neck carcinoma with non-curative intent. [Review.] [13 refs.] *Am. J. Otolaryngol.* **15**, 99–102.

59. Tucker, H.M., Rabuzzi, D.D., and Reed, G.F. (1973). Massive surgery of palliation in malignancy of the head and neck. *Laryngoscope*, **83**, 1635–43.

60. Elias, D., Cavalcanti, A., Dube, P., Julieron, M., Mamelle, G., Kac, J., *et al.* (1998). Circumferential pharyngolaryngectomy with total esophagectomy for locally advanced carcinomas. *Ann. Surg. Oncol.*, **5**, 511–16.

61. Azurin, D.J., Go, L.S., and Kirkland, M.L. (1997). Palliative gastric transposition following pharyngolaryngoesophagectomy. *Am. Surg.*, **63**, 410–13.

62. Bakamjian, V.Y., Cervino, L., Miller, S., and Hentz, V.R. (1973). The concept of cure and palliation by surgery in advance cancer of the head and neck. *Am. J. Surg.*, **126**, 482–7.

63. Nayak, U.K., Donald, P.J., and Stevens, D. (1995). Internal carotid artery resection for invasion of malignant tumors. *Arch. Otolaryngol. Head Neck Surg.*, **121**, 1029–33.

64. Okamoto, Y., Inugami, A., Matsuzaki, Z., Yokomizo, M., Konno, A., Togawa, K., *et al.* (1996). Carotid artery resection for head and neck cancer. *Surgery*, **120**, 54–9.

65. Maves, M.D., Bruns, M.D., and Keenan, M.J. (1992). Carotid artery resection for head and neck cancer. *Ann. Otol. Rhinol. Laryngol.*, **101**, 778–81.

66. Hagood, C.O. Jr., Mozersky, D.J., and Fite, F.W. (1974). Staged palliative resection of recurrent carcinoma of the neck using an extra anatomic carotid bypass. *Surgery*, **76**, 671–3.

67. Karam, F., Schaefer, S., Cherryholmes, D., and Dagher F.J. (1990). Carotid artery resection and replacement in patients with head and neck malignant tumors. *J. Cardiovasc. Surg.*, **31**, 697–701.

68. Horch, R.E., and Stark, G.B. (2000). The contralateral bilobed trapezius myocutaneous flap for closure of large defects of the dorsal neck permitting primary donor site closure. *Head Neck*, **22**, 513–19.

69. Shestak, K.C., Myers, E.N., Ramasastry, S.S., Jones, N.F., and Johnson, J.T. (1993). Vascularized free tissue transfer in head and neck surgery. [Review.] [34 refs.] *Am. J. Otalaryngol.*, **14**, 148–54.

70. UK Medicines Information (2001). *Palliative care prescribing*. Drug information letter no. 117, p. 64. North West Medicines Information Service and Aintree Hospital NHS Trust, Pembroke Place, Liverpool.

71. Regnard, C., Allport, S., and Stephenson, L. (1997). ABC of palliative care. Mouth care, skin care and lymphoedema. [Review.] *B.M.J.*, **315**, 1002–5.

72. Chiodo, G.T., Tolle, S.W., and Madden, T. (1998). The dentist's role in end-of-life care. *Gen. Dentist.*, **46**, 560–5.

73. Sweeney, M.P., Bagg, J., Baxter, W.P., and Aitchison, T.C. (1998). Oral disease in terminally ill cancer patients with xerostomia. *Oral Oncol.*, **34**, 123–6.

Chapter 11

The surgical relief of the symptomatic chest

Bill Nelems

Thoracic surgeons have a unique 'worldview' of illness, fashioned not only by the nature of their work but also because they are often the first amongst specialists to enter the patient's journey with thoracic illnesses.

Eighty per cent of the caseload encountered by thoracic surgeons relates to malignant disease, and 80% of those patients will not survive the illnesses for which they seek our services.[1] Most of these maladies are 'lifestyle' induced. What better case could one make for disease prevention programmes and for augmented palliative care services?

Lung cancer is by far the commonest single condition that we treat, followed closely by malignant diseases from other thoracic tumour sites, and from distant locales that require surgical management by virtue of the all-too-common thoracic metastases.

Even the benign conditions that we treat such as gastro-oesophageal reflex, emphysema, trauma, thoracic outlet syndrome, and the like are fraught with technical difficulties and complex psychosocial parameters.

Who else in the profession is faced with the front-end management of the commonest cause of cancer death amongst both women and men? Who else is confronted with the front-end care of the most treatment-refractory tumour ever known to mankind? Who else is burdened with the front-end 'breaking of bad news' to the extent that it occurs in thoracic surgical practice? Who is the first to gaze down the mediastinoscope or the bronchoscope and to recognize that illness is both serious and potentially life ending? Who else peers first into the open thorax to view the extent of the pathology and to estimate the potential for outcome? The thoracic surgeon does indeed have a unique window into important and interesting facets of health care.

Arguably, the biggest challenge that all of medicine faces is the development and deployment of truly comprehensive standards of care. In trying to provide all patients with 'access to a uniformly high quality of care in the community or hospital wherever they may live and to ensure maximum possible cure rates and best quality of life',[2] one could well use lung cancer as the 'proxy' condition for developing thoracic surgical standards.

First, I have chosen to embrace some of the broad perspectives in discussing the philosophical changes that our profession must confront as we move from biomedicine to psychosociology, from terminal palliative philosophies to supportive care paradigms.

Second, the specific thoracic palliative procedures are well described in the thoracic surgical literature. These will be discussed in table form below.

To date, thoracic surgeons, like most of conventional medical practitioners, have been focused on diseases and their potential cure. It's time now to broaden our perspectives.

The Society of Academic Surgeons and the Surgical Research Society claims that 'the majority of patients who are cured of cancer are cured by surgery alone'.[3] The Pelican Centre claims 'the largest variable in outcome is the [training and accreditation of the] surgeon undertaking the surgery'.[3,4]

In tabling its 44 recommendations and conclusions with respect to comprehensive standards of care for cancer patients, the Calman–Hine Report acknowledged the value of surgical treatment and the appropriate training and accreditation of surgeons.[2]

Be certain that we the thoracic surgical community will remain focused on surgical treatment and accreditation.

The Calman–Hine Report, first published by the Chief Medical Officers for England and Wales in 1995, is now in various stages of implementation within Great Britain. This report provides a blueprint for the world community.

We know that lung cancer, our thoracic surgical proxy condition, is an anxiety-producing state, one that raises high levels of patient concern and fear.[5,6] Patients fear that pain or other potentially disabling symptoms will not be adequately addressed. Patients have also come to believe that they cannot discuss their existential issues regarding spirituality and the meaning of life with physicians.[7] It's time to embrace these aspects of patient care.

As I conduct 'end-of-life' narrative interviews with my patients, I have come to learn that for the patient the journey with illness is often more important than the disease itself or its treatment. Grateful as the patient may be for therapy, their journey is consistently more important than the role played by their surgeon. When conventional treatments are withdrawn, it matters not what particular disease leads to death, or what treatments could or should have been used at earlier stages. Impending death sets its own imperatives. What matters most to the patient at the end of life is whether or not their symptoms will receive adequate palliation, and whether or not they have time to reconcile their spiritual journey and to gather their family and loved ones to their bedside. As a thoracic surgeon now comfortable with end-of-life narrative counselling, I am humbled by these insights, never taught at medical school nor role-modelled during surgical training.

We know that over time the costs associated with the investigation and treatment of lung cancer have escalated exponentially without being matched by better outcomes.[8] It's time to work with governments and health authorities to generate research data that will improve outcomes, improve patient quality of life, and to use health care money more efficiently.

Randomized controlled studies have shown that the deployment of living wills or advance directives has the power to significantly reduce health costs without sacrificing mortality or quality.[9] More importantly, the meticulous fulfilment of patient wishes is a measure of respect and dignity. No published population-based data exists to indicate if living wills have been systematically deployed with lung cancer patients at the time of diagnosis. It's time to spearhead such a study.

We know that lung cancer, for the most part, is a preventable disease.[10] It's time for us to use our influence more effectively in developing primary prevention and early detection screening programmes, and in developing strategic research partnerships.

So what does it mean for thoracic surgeons to broaden their perspectives? As I pondered the content of this book chapter entitled 'The Surgical Relief of the Symptomatic Chest', I began to realise that the modern thoracic surgeon, like a pupa too long incubated in its cocoon, has the potential to emerge as a butterfly of change. It takes courage to change, and the thoracic surgeon is a courageous risk-taker. It seems that we have to become first-rate qualified and accredited surgeons, teachers, palliative care physicians, researchers, prevention experts, administrators, psychologists, and existential humanists to provide 'surgical relief for the symptomatic chest'. I am confident that my colleagues will meet the challenge.

The winds of change are gusting strongly with respect to the ways in which health care is being delivered in many jurisdictions around the world. 'Carpe diem' was not only 'The Dead Poet's Society' motto, but it was also the motto of my old boarding school. It seems now as if this old slogan is a siren calling us to arms.

In British Columbia, the Thoracic Surgical Chest Surgery Association and the Ministry of Health's Provincial Health Service Authority are collaborating in the development of a provincial thoracic surgery programme that will establish exemplary standards of care for the four million citizens that live scattered within a large geographical zone several times the size of Texas. Many of our patients have to travel great distances and at considerable personal expense to obtain treatment. They also have to navigate the challenges of mountainous terrain and severe seasonal winter conditions.

In time, the programme will meet all of the recommendations of the Calman–Hine Report, with a few other evidence-based research initiatives thrown in for good measure. We also have new opportunities to embrace technologies not available to previous generations of surgeons.

The programme will involve 13 thoracic surgeons, located at four different geographic locations within the province, based at host hospitals with immediate access to regional cancer centres. All surgeons will be qualified and accredited by the Royal College of Physicians and Surgeons of Canada.

All patients will commence treatment within two weeks of family doctor referral. Calman–Hine recognized the need of a fast-track system, indicating that it must be matched by the provision of greater capacity in radiology and pathology.[2] Our programme in British Columbia will also recognize the need for fast-track provision for enhanced respiratory services, for anaesthesia, intensive care, and operating room resources, as well as the provision of greater capacity in radiology and pathology.

All patients on entry to the programme will be provided with information pertaining to their illnesses. This entry point will also provide an opportunity to introduce the notion of advance directives in a more comprehensive manner than the current informed consent process. We favour the Sheffield Supportive Care Model whereby the term 'palliative care' is replaced by 'supportive care', and emotional support becomes available for all patients from the time of first diagnosis to cure, or from first diagnosis to death, as the patient's journey dictates.[11] Supportive care resources are mandated by Calman–Hine.[2]

Research is considered an essential standard of care.[12] In British Columbia we are fortunate in having a comprehensive and provincially based tumour registry. Since all patients with lung cancer will be enrolled in the programme, population-based research outcomes will be an actual reality rather than a theoretical target. Advance directives research will ask questions regarding both quality of life and fiscal accountability. All patients are potential candidates for clinical trials.

The Calman–Hine Report encourages increased use of research and clinical nurses and the use of volunteers. The report also favours research initiatives into the links between ethnicity, socio-economic conditions, and cancer incidence and survival. We believe that there is abundant opportunity to deploy advanced practitioner nurses and counsellors within our programme. We have significant challenges in supporting the needs of our First Nations people and our immigrant population.

The programme will facilitate both interdisciplinary undergraduate teaching and postgraduate thoracic surgery residency training.

Table 11.1 lists thoracic conditions that commonly require palliation, provides literature references as to investigation or treatment options, and I have provided my own comments as to my preferences for therapy. Potentially curative therapies will not be included.

We believe that future generations of thoracic surgeons will be more comprehensively trained, that they will indeed have the broader perspectives needed to provide more all-embracing care than we, their teachers, have been able to provide. We also believe that our experiences in enhancing population-based research, advance directives, and supportive care paradigms will have contributed to the paradigm shifts that will evolve.

Table 11.1 Thoracic conditions that commonly require palliation: investigation/treatment options

Thoracic condition	Investigation/treatment literature citation	Author's comments
Malignant oesophageal obstruction	Brachytherapy[13] External beam radiotherapy[14] Chemotherapy[15] Intubation[16] Palliative resection[17]	Generally speaking, I do not favour palliative oesphophageal resection. The use of modern stenting devices is preferred.
Tracheo-bronchial obstruction	External beam radiotherapy[14] Brachytherapy[13] Laser treatments[18] Photo-dynamic therapy[19] Stenting[20]	Airway obstruction is one of the most taxing conditions to manage. All of the modalities listed are valuable in individual cases.
Malignant pleural effusions	Pleurodesis[21] Pleuro-peritoneal shunt[22]	Talc pleurodesis is the preferred technique. Shunting has benefit in managing the 'trapped lung' syndrome.
Superior vena cava (SVC) obstruction	Mediastinoscopy[23] Radiotherapy[14] Endovascular shunt[24]	Mediastinoscopy is not contraindicated in SVC obstruction. Radiotherapy most often suffices to control symptoms. In treatment refractory cases, endovascular stenting is helpful.
Haemoptysis	Radiotherapy[14] Photo-dynamic therapy[19]	Controlled in most cases with radiotherapy.
Major pulmonary haemorrhage	Bronchial embolization[25] Resection[26]	Generally speaking, embolization is preferred to resection. Resection in the presence of major haemoptysis can tax the best of surgeons.
Metastatic chest wall recurrences	Resection[27] Radiation[14]	Clinical judgement on a case-by-case circumstance.
Cerebral metastases	Radiation[14] Neurosurgery[28]	Short-term relief occurs in 70–90% of cases.

Table 11.1 (continued) Thoracic conditions that commonly require palliation: investigation/treatment options

Thoracic condition	Investigation/treatment literature citation	Author's comments
Bone metastases	Radiation[14]	90% of patients with symptomatic bone pain obtain relief with low-dose brief course radiotherapy.[14] Lytic lesions should be treated prophylactically.
Mesothelioma	Extrapulmonary pneumonectomy[29] Pleurectomy/decortication[30] Clinical trials[31]	We await better outcomes from trial results. Considering complication rates and poor outcomes with all treatments, I believe that cases should be referred to clinical trials wherever possible.
Malignant pericardial effusion	Sub-xiphoid pericardial window[32] Thoracotomy with window[33] Pericardiocentesis with sclerosis[34]	The pros and cons of these methods have been well argued in the literature. My preference is for limited left anterior 4th interspace thoracotomy without rib spreading, pericardial window formation, and talc ablation of pericardial and left pleural spaces.

References

1. Cartman, M.L., Hatfield, A.C., Muers, M.F., Peake, M.D., Haward, R.A., and Forman, D. (2002). Lung cancer: district active treatment rates affect survival. *J. Epidemiol. Comm. Hlth.*, **56** (6), 424–9.

2. http://www.doh.gov.uk/cancer/calmanhine.htm A policy framework for commissioning cancer services. A report by the Expert Advisory Group on Cancer to the Chief Medical Officers of England and Wales. *Guidance for purchasers and providers of cancer services*, April 1995.

3. The United Kingdom parliament website: http://www.parliament.the-stationery-office.co.uk/pa/cm199900/cmselect/cmsctech/332/33205.htm#n31.

4. McArdle, C.S., and Hole, D. (1991). The impact of variability among surgeons on postoperative morbidity and mortality and ultimate survival. *B. M. J.*, **302**, 1501–5.

5. Sarna, L., Padilla, G., Holmes, C., Tashkin, D., Brecht, M.L., and Evangelista, L. (2002). Quality of life of long-term survivors of non-small-cell lung cancer. *J. Clin. Oncol.*, **20** (13), 2920–9.

6. Rawl, S.M., Given, B.A., Given, C.W., Champion, V.L., kozachik, S.L., Barton, D., *et al.* (2002). Intervention to improve psychological functioning for newly diagnosed patients with cancer. *Oncol. Nurses Forum*, **29** (6), 967–75.

7. Ugoalah, P.C. (2002). The use of unconventional therapies among cancer patients: implications for nursing practice. *Can. Oncol. Nurs. J.*, **12** (2), 118–24.

8. Evans, W.K., Will, B.P., Berthelot, J.M., and Wolfson, M.C. (1996). The economics of lung cancer management in Canada. *Lung Cancer*, **14** (1), 19–29

9. Molloy, D.W., Guyatt, G.H., Russo, R., Goeree, R., O'Brien, B.J., Bedard, M., *et al.* (2000). Systematic implementation of an advance directive program in nursing homes: a randomized controlled trial. *J.A.M.A.*, **283** (11), 1437–44.

10. Hecht, S.S. (2002). cigarette smoking and lung cancer: chemical mechanisms and approaches to prevention.[Review.] *Lancet Oncol.*, **3** (8), 461–9.

11. Seymour, J., Clark, D., and Marples, R. (2002). Palliative care and policy in England: a review of health improvement plans for 1999–2003. *Pall. Med.*, **16** (1), 5–11.

12. Davis, S., Wright, P.W., Schulman, S.F., *et al.* (1985). Participants in prospective randomised clinical trials for resected non-small-cell lung cancer have improved survival compared with non-participants in such trials. *Cancer*, 56, 1710–18.

13. Sur, R.K., Levin, C.V., Donde, B., Sharma, V., Miszczyk, L., and Nag, S. (2002). Prospective randomized trial of HDR brachytherapy as a sole modality in palliation of advanced esophageal carcinomav – an International Atomic Energy Agency study. *Int. J. Radiat. Oncol. Biol. Phys.*, **53** (1), 127–33.

14. Hoegler, D. (1997). Radiotherapy for palliation of symptoms in incurable cancer. [Review.] *Curr. prob. Cancer*, **21** (3), 129–83.

15. Blom, D., Peters, J.H., and DeMeester, T.R. (2002). Controversies in the current therapy of carcinoma of the esophagus. *J. Am. Coll. Surg.*, **195** (2), 241–50.

16. Christie, N.A., Buenaventura, P.O., Femando, H.C., Nguyen, N.T., Weigel, T.L., Ferson, P.F., *et al.* (2001). Results of expandable metal stents for malignant esophageal obstruction in 100 patients: short-term and long-term follow-up. *Ann. Thorac. Surg.*, **71** (6), 1797–801.

17. Mitani, M., Kuwabara, Y., Shinoda, N., Sato, A., Mitsui, A., Kato, J., *et al.* (2002). The effectiveness of palliative resection for advanced esophageal carcinoma: analysis of 24 consecutive cases. *Surg. Today*, **32** (9), 784–8.

18. Chella, A., Ambrogi, M.C., Ribechini, A., Mussi, A., Fabrini, M.G., Silvano, G., *et al.* (2000). Combined Nd-YAG laser/HDR brachytherapy versus Nd-YAG laser only in malignant central airway involvement: a prospective randomized study. *Lung Cancer*, **27** (3).

19. Hopper, C. (2000). Photodynamic therapy: a clinical reality in the treatment of cancer. [Review.] *Lancet Oncol.*, **1**, 212–9.

20. Wood, D.E. (2001). Airway stenting. [Review.] *Chest Surg. Clin. North Am.*, **11** (4), 841–60.

21. Reeder, L.B. (2001). Malignant pleural effusions. *Curr. Treat. Options Oncol.*, **2** (1), 93–6.

22. Genc, O., Petrou, M., Ladas, G., and Goldstraw, P. (2000). The long-term morbidity of pleuroperitoneal shunts in the management of recurrent malignant effusions. *Eur. J. Cardiothorac. Surg.*, **18** (2), 143–6.

23. Little, A.G., Golomb, H.M., Ferguson, M.K., Skosey, C., and Skinner, D.B. (1985). Malignant superior vena cava obstruction reconsidered: the role of diagnostic surgical intervention. *Ann. Thorac. Surg.*, **40** (3), 285–8.

24. Shah, R., Sabanathan, S., Lowe, R.A., and Mearns, A.J. (1996). Stenting in malignant obstruction of superior vena cava. *J. Thorac. Cardiovasc. Surg.*, **112** (2), 335–40.

25. Fernando, H.C., Stein, M., Benfield, J.R., Link, D.P. (1998). Role of bronchial artery embolization in the management of hemoptysis. *Arch. Surg.*, **133** (8), 862–6.

26. Jougon, J., Ballester, M., Delcambre, F., MacBride, T., Valat, P., Gomez, F., *et al.* (2002). Massive hemoptysis: what place for medical and surgical treatment. *Eur. J. Cardiothorac. Surg.*, **22** (3), 345.

27. Downey, R.J., Rusch, V., Hsu, F.I., Leon, L., Venkatraman, E., Linehan, D., *et al.* (2000). Chest wall resection for locally recurrent breast cancer: is it worthwhile? *J. Thorac. Cardiovasc. Surg.*, **119** (3), 420–8.

28. Moazami, N., Rice, T.W., Rybicki, L.A., Adelstein, D.J., Murthy, S.C., DeCamp, M.M., *et al.* (2002). Stage III non-small-cell lung cancer and metachronous brain metastases. *J. Thorac. Cardiovasc. Surg.*, **124** (1), 113–22.

29. Sugarbaker, D.J., Flores, R.M., Jaklitsch, M.T., Richards, W.G., Strauss, G.M., Corson, J.M., *et al.* (1999). Resection margins, extrpleural nodal status, and cell type determine postoperative long-term survival in trimodality therapy of malignant pleural mesothelioma: results in 183 patients. *J. Thorac. Cardiovasc. Surg.*, **117** (1), 54–63.

30. Soysal, O., Karaglanoglu, N., Demiracan, S., Topcu, S., Tastepe, I., Kaya, S., *et al.* (1997). Pleurectomy/decortication for palliation in malignant pleural mesothelioma: results of surgery. *Eur. J. Cardiothorac. Surg.*, **11** (2), 210–3.

31. Girling, D.J., Myers, M.F., Qjan, W., and Lobban, D. (2002). Multicenter randomized controlled trial of the management of unresectable malignant mesothelioma proposed by the British Thoracic Society and the British Medical Research Council. [Review.] *Semin. Oncol.*, **29** (1), 97–101.

32. Decamp, M.M., Jr., Mentzer, S.J., Swanson, S.J., and Sugarbaker, D.J. (1997). Malignant effusive disease of the pleura and pericardium *Chest*, **112** (4), S291–S295.

33. Olson, J.E., Ryan, M.B., and Blumenstock, D.A. (1995). Eleven years' experience with pericardial-peritoneal window in the management of malignant and benign pericardial effusions. *Ann. Surg. Oncol.*, **2** (2), 165–9.

34. Girardi, L.N., Ginsberg, R.J., and Burt, M.E. (1997). Pericardiocentesis and intrapericardial sclerosis: effective therapy for malignant pericardial effusions. *Ann. Thorac. Surg.*, **64** (5), 1422–7.

Chapter 12

Surgery for the control of symptoms in the abdomen

Alan G. Johnson

The gastrointestinal (GI) tract (including the liver) is the commonest site of primary malignancy in the world. In the West, a combination of gastric, oesophageal, pancreatic, and colorectal cancers outweigh those from breast or prostate; and in the East, primary hepatocellular carcinoma has a huge incidence. In addition, the abdomen is the site of ovarian carcinoma, which is also the second commonest cancer in women, and the liver is the commonest site of secondary tumours from GI tract, breast, and lung.

Whereas in other sites cancers spread by lymphatics and the bloodstream, in the abdomen transperitoneal spread is common, e.g. from ovaries or stomach leading to multiple tumour deposits which are impossible to resect and lead to intestinal obstruction and ascites.

The most difficult benign conditions to manage are: (a) cirrhosis of the liver which leads to portal hypertension, haemorrhage, and ascites and (b) chronic pancreatitis which can give chronic, severe pain.

Decision making

All decisions need wise judgement and a careful balancing of risks and probabilities. It is important that the palliative care team is involved early in the disease process rather than being brought in at the end when the options for management are severely limited. Terms can be confusing and the word 'inoperable' has two distinct meanings. The first is that a tumour is incurable but may be locally resectable and surgery may play a major part in controlling or relieving the symptoms. Secondly, the word can mean that no resection, bypass of obstruction, or palliative measure is possible. Just because a tumour is incurable by surgery it does not mean that 'nothing further can be done'. The option of surgery should always be considered but a small degree of palliation may not justify the discomfort of major surgery. When weighing up the benefits of surgery, the time taken to recover from the operation must be balanced against the prolongation of life and duration of symptom relief.

Box 12.1 shows the main symptoms that require palliation. Each may have several causes.

Gastrointestinal obstruction

The predominance of one symptom or another depends on the level of the obstruction. A benign or malignant stricture of the oesophageal wall can cause dysphagia whereas a malignant stricture of the sigmoid colon will give constipation followed by increasing distension and

Box 12.1 Abdominal symptoms requiring palliation

- Obstruction of the gastrointestinal tract, including dysphagia and vomiting
- Haemorrhage – acute or chronic
- Ascites – malignant or due to portal hypertension
- Jaundice – itching
- Pain
- Tumour bulk, including secondaries

later vomiting (if the iliosecral valve is incompetent). There are six ways of managing chronic intestinal obstruction:

1 resection and anastomosis;
2 bypass with side-to-side anastomosis;
3 proximal stoma;
4 laser destruction of tumour in the lumen;
5 stenting;
6 reduction of secretions.

Resection

It is sometimes argued that there is little point in resecting a carcinoma of the stomach or colon if there is evidence of distant metastases; but this argument is spurious because the secondaries are often asymptomatic and it is the primary that is giving or will give severe symptoms. The problem is that the palliative resection can be nearly as big an operation as a potentially curative resection, e.g. for carcinoma of the oesophagus, stomach, or colon. Sadly the majority of potential curative operations for carcinoma of the stomach and oesophagus are, indeed, palliative. Therefore, the general condition of the whole patient needs to be considered and the risks of the operation weighed against its probable short-term benefits. Because resection of the oesophagus, for example, means opening the chest and the patients may be elderly with chronic lung or heart problems, it is rarely justified unless there is a chance of both long-term palliation or potential cure.

Prophylactic resections

Surgeons may frequently be faced with a patient who has a GI cancer with clear signs or peritoneal or other metastases and where the primary tumour is not yet obstructing. Should it be resected prophylactically to prevent future symptoms? The difficult judgement is whether it is likely to obstruct before the patient dies from the metastases. Any resection must be through normal tissue because an attempt to anastomose malignant tissue can lead to anastomotic breaking down: an intestinal fistula is no palliation!

Bypass with side-to-side anastomosis

When compared with resectional surgery a bypass may just involve a small and quick procedure. Obstruction, especially of the small intestine, may be due to multiple peritoneal deposits with several sites of obstruction. The judgement is about how much bowel to bypass, thinking of possible newer symptoms such as diarrhoea. The alternative is several small bypasses at different levels which prolongs the operation. Side-to-side anastomoses are very *un*likely to leak because the blood supply is not dissected and disturbed. Some decisions are straightforward, e.g. an inoperable (unresectable) carcinoma of the caecum is easily bypassed by ileotransverse colostomy without producing side-effects of diarrhoea because the left side of the large bowel is intact and functioning. A second common situation in which bypass surgery is required is obstruction of the pylorus or duodenum with an antral or pancreatic carcinoma. A gastroje-junostomy is often quite straightforward: it should be placed well away from the tumour so that it is not obstructed within a few weeks by local spread and if possible it should be on the dependent part of the greater curve of the stomach, not anteriorly, so that it empties effectively. In the presence of a pancreatic carcinoma the small intestine should be brought up in front of the colon (antecolic), not behind, to keep it away from the unresected pancreatic tumour.

A third example is when a carcinoma of the pancreas obstructs the second or third part of the duodenum. A gastrojejunostomy is appropriate and the biliary system can either be bypassed surgically or stented (see below). A laparotomy for widely disseminated intra-abdominal malig-nancy always has the risks of implanting malignant cells in the wound, but these do not usually cause symptoms in the time-scale that is envisaged.

Proximal stoma

If a resection or bypass is not possible and there is a 'frozen' pelvis obstructing the rectum then a proximal stoma is the right option. A left iliac colostomy if carefully placed, can be managed relatively easily by patients or their carers. It should protrude a little above the skin to enable the bag to fit well and should not be placed close to a skin fold or bony prominence. Depending on the patient's abdominal shape, it may sometimes be more convenient to place the stoma in the upper abdomen. An ileostomy is usually placed in the right iliac fossa and needs to have a generous 'spout' above the skin to minimize leakage because the contents are liquid. An end stoma with the bowel divided usually functions best but a decision needs to be taken about the obstructive part of the bowel distal to the stoma. This cannot just be closed off unless it is very short because secretions will accumulate and lead to distension of the bowel and even rupture of the suture line. A mucous fistula where the distal limb is brought to the surface in a separate place is one possibility or the stoma itself can be made 'double-barrelled' with both proximal and distal limbs emptying into the bag side by side. This is relatively easy with a small ileostomy but a double-barrelled colostomy can be bulky and need a large bag.

Although there is a natural dislike of a colostomy, it is far easier to manage than rectal incon-tinence and is therefore particularly indicated for unresectable anal or rectal carcinomas that have destroyed the anal sphincter.

The management of ileostomies and colostomies is far easier than it used to be a few years ago due to the experienced stoma nurses and a whole variety of bags and apparatus that suit individual patients. Whenever a stoma is anticipated the surgeon should agree with the patient and the stoma therapist the best possible sites for the stoma: these need to be checked with the patient lying, sitting, and standing because a stoma site that may look ideal with the patient lying down can be right across a crease when the patient sits up.

'Laser' destruction of tumours

When tumours can be reached with an endoscope, e.g. oesophagogastric or rectal, laser photoco-agulation can be used to destroy part of the tumour and open up the lumen. It is also useful for control of bleeding (see below). It is more difficult and dangerous if the lumen is completely obliterated because the extent of the tumour cannot be visualized. The depth of penetration of the laser treatment is important and the procedure must be done with great care to avoid perforation of the organ. The most common use of laser obliteration is for oesophageal tumours that are unresectable in order to relieve the dysphagia.[1] The treatment may need to be repeated after a number of weeks depending on the speed of growth. Argon beam coagulation[2] or photo-dynamic therapy[3,4] in which the tissue is sensitized to light of a certain wavelength, are alternatives.

Stenting

Dysphagia is a most distressing symptom, especially when it becomes so severe that the patient cannot swallow his saliva. The standard way to keep the oesophagus open through an unresectable carcinoma is to put in a stent.[5] The word 'stent' is named after a Stent's composition – a plastic resin-like material that sets very hard and is used for making moulds. They are now made of plastic or more recently of expandable metal mesh[6] and the actual type may be named after the designer, e.g. Atkinson. Some stents, e.g. Celestin, are inserted and fixed in the stomach as part of a laparotomy and are used when a patient is unexpectedly found to have an unresectable carcinoma during an operation. This, however, should be an increasingly rare event as the quality of imaging and laparoscopic staging of the tumour improves and therefore, most are now inserted endoscopically. Stenting can be combined with dilatation or laser treatment but there is always a risk of rupture of the oesophagus when the stent is pushed through, particularly if the shape of the lower oesophagus is distorted. The problem with any oesophageal stent is that food gets stuck because there is no peristalsis through this segment. The meals have to be liquidized. They are, therefore, only an advantage if the patients have reached the stage where they cannot swallow liquids. Other complications include the tumour growing over the proximal end of a plastic stent or through the mesh of a metal stent and blocking it again because the stent has a shoulder which rests on the upper border of the tumour. This can be treated with laser or argon beams.[2] A third complication is that gastric contents can reflux up into the mouth because the lower oesophageal sphincter is no longer functioning. Stents can also be used in the rectum to overcome obstruction by an inoperable tumour, and expandable metal stents are being placed endoscopically for gastric oulet obstruction.[7] Different endoscopic techniques are appropriate for different situations and may be used one after the other.[8]

Reduction of secretions

If intestinal obstruction cannot be overcome, symptoms can be relieved by reducing the secretions pharmacologically. Atropine-like drugs were commonly used in the past but they can produce unpleasant symptoms of dry mouth and eyes. Proton pump inhibitors can reduce the gastric acid secretion very greatly and somatostatin analogues (e.g. octreotide) help with biliary, pancreatic, and intestinal secretions. They can be injected subcutaneously by a patient or carer, and long-acting forms are now available which require an injection only once a mouth.[9]*

Feeding in the presence of GI obstruction

When the obstruction cannot be bypassed, treated with laser, or stented, a difficult decision has to be made about if and how to feed the patient. This will depend on the patient's alertness and general condition, the amount of tumour spread, other symptoms, and likely prognosis. Hydration

* This is a non-licensed indication at the time of going to press.

can be maintained by intravenous infusion and nutrition can even be given intravenously, but this may be inappropriate in the management of terminal disease. It is important not to allow artificial feeding and dehydration to prolong distress and dying and the ethical and legal aspects are important.[10] Intravenous administration has the added disadvantage of limiting the patient's mobility. Fluid and liquidized food may be introduced into the GI tract in three ways:

1 *a fine-bore nasogastric* tube which has the disadvantage of being visible on the face. It is appropriate for oesophageal obstruction or other conditions when this patient cannot swallow, e.g. neurological problems;

2 *a percutaneous endoscopic gastrostomy*(PEG) is particularly used for patients with dysphagia after strokes and other chronic conditions in which swallowing is difficult. It may not be possible with advanced oesophageal or pharyngeal cancer because the endoscope cannot be introduced through the tumour (although sometimes the stomach can be inflated with a fine tube). The procedure is not without its complications: if it slips out before the stomach has become adherent to the abdominal wall, peritonitis can develop;

3 *a feeding gastrostomy or jejunostomy* which may be fashioned surgically. A feeding jejunostomy is often created as part of a major upper GI cancer resection for feeding during the immediate postoperative period. It is a small operation to do later if a patient develops obstruction from a local spread or secondaries. Usually a Foley catheter is inserted with the balloon only partly inflated to avoid obstruction to the jejunal lumen. It should be placed as high up the jejunum as possible to allow maximum length of intestine for absorption. The advantage of both the PEG and a feeding jejunostomy or gastrostomy is that the tube is concealed beneath the clothing and other people are unaware of it.

Whenever a procedure is seen to be 'minimally invasive' there is a risk of overuse.[11] There has been a tendency to insert PEGs shortly before patients die, which is inappropriate. The timing is difficult and the decision to embark on artificial feeding, of any kind, needs to be taken sympathetically and carefully. Ideally, the patients should decide in consultation with their carers and the multidisciplinary health care team, according to agreed national guidelines.[12]

Haemorrhage

The second distressing symptom that often requires surgical treatment is haemorrhage, which can be either acute or chronic. Box 12.2 shows the primary causes.

Chronic haemorrhage usually comes from primary gastric or colonic cancers which become ulcerated – indeed, anaemia is a common presenting symptom. Even if the tumour is incurable because of secondary spread, anaemia and recurrent blood transfusions can be prevented by local palliative resection. Carcinoma of the caecum is a good example, where local resection can be very worthwhile, even in the presence of inoperable metastases. However, it is important not to assume that the bleeding is coming from the tumour because other benign treatable causes can also be present.

Primary tumours that cause bleeding are cancers of the stomach and the colon, including polyps and sometimes the oesophagus. A primary carcinoma of the pancreas may erode into the duodenum and bleed and an ampulllary carcinoma may give the exotically named 'silvery stools' – a combination of steathorrea and melaena! Secondary deposits in the intestinal wall, although not common, may come from primary sources such as melanoma of the skin, choriocarcinoma, and other rare cancers.

Box 12.2 Causes of gastrointestinal haemorrhage

Malignant

- Primary carcinomas
- Other tumours eroding from outside the intestinal wall
- Secondary deposits in the intestinal wall
- Haemobilia

Benign

- Peptic ulceration
- Acute erosions (stress ulcers)
- Oesophageal and gastric varices
- Angiodysplasia of the colon
- Diverticular disease of the colon

Acute or chronic peptic ulceration may arise independently of other inoperable disease or as a consequence of chemotherapy, steroids, or non-steroidal anti-inflammatory drugs used for pain control.[13] The Cox-II inhibitors have greatly reduced this risk.[14] Therefore, prophylactic measures such as acid suppression with H_2 receptor antagonists or proton pump inhibitors and/or mucosal protection with drugs such as sucralphate are preferable to more complicated therapeutic measures once a patient has bled. Haemobilia is rare but comes from a tumour or abscess in the liver eroding into a bile duct. The classic symptoms are upper-right quadrant pain, jaundice, and melaena.

Angiodysplasia of the colon (usually caecum) is a benign condition occurring in older patients and causing a brisk heavy rectal bleed of altered blood rather than melaena.[15] Diverticular disease is a very common condition in older patients and a diverticular bleed, usually giving a brisk fresh blood loss from the left colon rather than chronic loss. It usually stops spontaneously.

Management

It is important to appreciate that in a patient with malignant disease even severe haemorrhage can be due to a benign cause and stopped by relatively simple, minimally invasive methods.

Endoscopic techniques

Bleeding peptic ulcers can be diagnosed and the bleeding stopped in over 80% of cases by injection with adrenaline alone or with a heat probe through the gastroscope.[16] Similarly, angiodysplasia of the caecum can be diagnosed and treated with localized diathermy at colonoscopy, although angiography is sometimes needed to make the diagnosis. Antral erosion with multiple smaller ulcers are easily diagnosed by gastroscopy but difficult to treat endoscopically because there are so many of them. Oesophageal and sometimes gastric varices are treated by endoscopic sclerotherapy or banding.[17] This is worthwhile even if the portal hypertension is associated with an unresectable primary hepatocellular carcinoma. Bleeding from primary unresectable malignancies of the oesophagus and stomach and rectum can also be treated endoscopically using argon beam coagulator[2] and this can be repeated as necessary if the bleeding recurs. One of the disadvantages is that it has to be done every few weeks to keep a fungating tumour under control.

Resection

If a bleeding gastro or duodenal ulcer fails to respond to injection or if antral erosions fail to respond to acid-blocking drugs, then resection or under sewing at open operation is required. In the same way, angiodysplasia or a bleeding diverticulum in the colon can be treated by local resection without a major disturbance to the patient.

The difficulty with diverticular disease is to discover which of the many diverticula is bleeding: if they are limited to the sigmoid colon it can be resected but they may be distributed throughout the colon. A total colectomy is difficult to justify as palliation. Elderly patients in particular stand a quick operation far better than recurrent hypotension and large blood transfusions. Obviously the effect of an operation must be carefully weighed against the patient's condition and prognosis from the underlying disease, but it is very distressing for a patient to die of uncontrolled haemorrhage.

Secondary deposits in the bowel wall can often be resected by a simple wedge resection or small full-width resection when the small bowel is involved. This may be a quick and simple procedure.

Exclusion and bypass

The most difficult situation facing the surgeon is when a fixed unresectable tumour (e.g. of the pancreas) is eroding into the bowel wall. Occasionally, the area can be excluded by closing either side (this can be done quickly with staples) and then continuity of the gut restored by a side-to-side bypass. For example, if a carcinoma of the pancreas is eroding into the third part of the duodenum, this can be excluded either side of the bleeding point and the proximal jejunum anastomosed onto the second part of the duodenum, or the stomach, to drain the gastric contents, bile, and pancreatic juice. The lumen of the small excluded segment can be packed with haemostatic sponge. A similar technique can be used on the right side of the colon. A long length of bowel, however, should not be excluded at both ends because it will distend with secretions. Sometimes just removing the bleeding area from the gastric acid stream or faecal contents can reduce or stop the bleeding – at least for the few weeks or months that may be all that is required.

Embolization

A lesion of the liver causing haemobilia can be embolized at arteriography, but embolization of the wall of the bowel is usually dangerous because it leads to localized gangrene and perforation.

Ascites

A moderate amount of ascites may produce no symptoms apart from some distension and a dragging sensation. When the abdomen becomes more tense, it can be very uncomfortable and in particular produce marked anorexia by compressing the stomach, leading to poor nutrition. Both malignant ascites (exudate) and ascites due to portal hypertension (transudate) are treated initially by spirinolactone and sodium restriction. Malignant ascites can be treated by intermittent paracentesis, but if drains are left in they will continue to drain as the fluid is continually formed by either transudation or exudation. Repeated paracentesis alone in the presence of portal hypertension leads to even further depletion of the albumin as the ascites rapidly reforms. Intravenous, low-sodium albumin must be given at the same time to replace the protein intravenously.

Any incision into the peritoneal cavity should be avoided if at all possible because it will leak fluid, even if carefully sutured. The surgeon must resist the temptation to repair a bulging (but not strangulated) umbilical or inguinal hernia.

Surgery can be particularly helpful in really intractable cirrhotic ascites in the form of a peritoneo-venous shunt. This enables the ascitic fluid to recirculate into the venous system and preserve the leaking albumen. The shunt has a one-way valve lying subcutaneously over the abdomen and a tube is burrowed subcutaneously up the chest and inserted with a purse-string suture into the internal jugular vein and down into the superior vena cava. The tip must be intrathoracic, not just in the neck, so that the negative pressure of the chest in relation to the abdomen causes the fluid to flow continually with respiration (flow can be checked by Doppler ultrasound). They can last unblocked for several years. More recently, transjugular intrahepatic porta systemic shunts (TIPSS), which are used to lower portal hypertension, have also been found to help with refractory ascites.[18]

Shunts for malignant ascites are not so long-lasting because they more easily become blocked with cancer cells, protein, debris, and omentum. They are, of course, only used when there is already disseminated cancer so that allowing cancer cells to flow into the major veins does not matter. Two commonly used models of shunts are the Leveen and Denver, the latter having the theoretical advantage that the valve can be pumped by pressure over it to encourage flow in the early stages and thereby prevent the tube from blocking.

Jaundice

Jaundice is an unpleasant symptom because it is unsightly, gives anorexia, and causes itching. Friends and relatives of deeply jaundiced patients are repelled by their appearance and this compounds their feeling of isolation. When the jaundice is obstructive it should be relieved by surgical, endoscopic, or radiological means unless the patient already has irreversible liver failure and a very short prognosis.

Surgical bypass

If the biliary system is obstructed at the level of the common bile duct, bile can be drained into a jejunal Roux loop anastomosed to the common hepatic duct or the gall bladder. When, as with a pancreatic carcinoma, the tumour is likely to spread up the duct then the higher up the anastomosis can be the better. The cystic duct may join quite low down the common hepatic duct so an anastomosis onto the gall bladder is only used when the gall bladder joins clearly above the obstruction and the patient's life expectancy from other causes is short. The higher obstructions, e.g. gall bladder cancer or hilar cholangiocarcinoma (provided the right and left main ducts are in communication and not obstructed where they join), can be treated by a bypass onto the duct of segment III. The segment III duct is easily accessible in the base of the falciform fissure deep to where the round ligament joins and when obstructed is a good size for a satisfactory anastomosis.

Stents

The biliary system is another area where stents are particularly valuable because they can be put in either *endoscopically* at ERCP (endoscopic retrograde pancreaticocholangiography) or

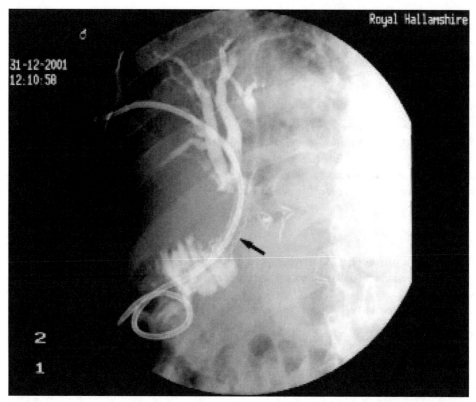

Fig. 12.1 Patient with recurrent carcinoma of the gall bladder at the porta hepatis. Internal/external plastic stent inside a previously blocked metal stent (arrow) draining a segment of the liver (which was sufficient to maintain adequate liver function). The patient was mobile and at home.

percutaneously across the liver. They are often used temporarily to drain the liver before resectional or bypass surgery on the ducts, but they can also be a 'permanent' solution to an obstructed biliary system. In general, ERCP is used for lower bile duct lesions such as carcinoma of the pancreas and transhepatic stents for higher lesions such as hilar cholangiocarcinoma and carcinoma of the gall bladder. The stents are up to 8 French gauge with side holes and are kept from falling into the duodenum by flanges or a curled end ('pig tail'). They are often named after their designer (e.g. Carey-Coons). Metal (e.g. Wall stents) have a greater diameter when fully expanded because they expand in position after insertion (Figure 12.1). An internal/external stent is one that is placed through a bile duct lesion but also has its proximal end protruding from the patient's side into a drainage bag. This enable it to be flushed or if it is blocked, for bile to drain out retrogradially into a bag. As a last resort, if the biliary obstruction cannot be negotiated a purely external drain can be used to drain the upper biliary system and reduce the jaundice. This is kept in place by a pig tail which can be straightened before removal and by tapes and plaster to the skin. Patients or carers can learn to empty the bile bag regularly without too much trouble.

Complications

Biliary stents can be obstructed by tumour growth but have the added problem of being blocked by concretions and 'sludge' and the bile being deposited on the surface. A narrow plastic stent may need to be changed every three months or so but this is not a difficult manoeuvre at ERCP (if the stent protrudes into duodenum) because there is already a channel through the tumour. The expandable metal stents remain patent longer and if they do become blocked a plastic stent can be placed through the middle of them, but they themselves cannot be removed because they become embedded in the tissues.

Itching

Itching can be a very distressing symptom in patients with jaundice (who often have little pain). Piriton and cholestyramine are the first-line drugs but are not always effective. Rifampicin is worth trying as a second-line treatment – and ultraviolet light can be helpful. New evidence suggests that itching may be due to endogenous opiates and opiate antagonists may be used, provided opiates are not needed for pain relief.

Pain

Surgery has a part to play in the relief of pain from abdominal organs but only when other methods have failed. Pancreatic pain is very difficult to manage and there are two surgical options:

1 resection;
2 splanchnicectomy.

Resection

Palliative resection of carcinoma of the pancreas is seldom justified because the time to recover from such a major procedure often does not match well with prognosis. The pain is often due to a direct invasion of the posterior abdominal wall. Chronic pancreatitis on the other hand is a benign, incurable disease which produces severe pain, sometimes leading to long-term opiate addiction. Chronic pancreatic pain may be due either to multiple blockages of the duct system giving pain after eating, or due to involvement of the posterior abdominal wall and nerves in the inflammatory process. For the first problem the operation of opening the duct longitudinally and anastomosing small bowel to it en route (Puestow procedure) can be useful, but for inflammatory pain resection may be the only option.[19] It will require a total pancreatectomy and lead to a brittle diabetes (even if the patient is not already diabetic). Pancreatic islet transplantation, with the patient's own islets isolated from the resected specimen, looks a promising solution to this complication.[20]

Splanchnicectomy

Coeliac axis block percutaneously is a possible intervention for malignant pancreatic pain. Because of its risks some pain specialists are reluctant to use it for benign disease. Recently, dividing the splanchnic nerves (sympathetic afferents) just above the diaphragm has become popular again because it can be done with minimal access using the thoracoscope: unfortunately, the effect is usually only temporary.[21] The most important place of surgery in the management of pain is anticipation and prevention by resection or bypass before it occurs. Prevention of future pain is one of the key aims of palliative surgery.

Reduction of tumour bulk

In the old days, surgeons were taught not to excise only part of a tumour but to remove it completely or not at all. This policy was based on the belief that partial resection would merely disseminate the tumour without any benefit. This had some justification before effective radio-therapy and chemotherapy were available. Nowadays for radio- or chemo-sensitive tumours, reduction of tumour bulk can be a considerable aid to treatment. If most of an intra-abdominal radio-sensitive tumour can be removed, the remaining area can be marked with surgical clips to help target radiotherapy later. Sometimes surgeons are asked to remove residual tumour bulk *after* treatment, e.g. para-aortic lymph nodes from testicular tumours. Carcinoid syndrome with multiple liver secondaries is a good example of the value of surgical debulking and the more of the liver secondaries that can be removed, the less the patient has the unpleasant side-effects of flushing and diarrhoea. This is especially important in this condition because the long-term prognosis may be quite good.

Debulking is an important part of the management of advanced ovarian cancer before chemotherapy is started.

Embolization

Arterial embolization is used to slow growth in some vascular tumours and to cause temporary necrosis of tumours in the liver. This is an alternative to resection for neuroendocrine tumours, but there is always a danger of massive release of hormones as the tumour necroses. Very vascular tumour may be embolized before resection to reduce both vascularity and bulk.

Cryosurgery

This is used effectively for small tumours and skin lesions but it has proved disappointing for liver secondaries. It is difficult to cool the lesion sufficiently and safely very deep in the liver close to the inferior vena cava and it is difficult to be sure that all the tumour has necrosed. It has been used in conjunction with resection, where resection of all tumour would leave insufficient functioning liver.

Radiofrequency ablation

This is becoming popular for irresectable primary or secondary liver tumours.[22] The degree of temperature change is far less than with cryosurgery and the probe can be introduced percutaneously or via a laparoscope. This is proving particularly useful in primary hepatocellular carcinoma in a cirrhotic liver where anything but a small resection would compromise liver function because liver function and regeneration is greatly reduced.

Resection of metastases

Only a few years ago many clinicians would have smiled at the suggestion of resecting metastases in the liver, yet thoracic surgeons have resected lung secondaries and neurosurgeons brain secondaries from tumours that are either slow growing or relatively sensitive to drug therapy, e.g. prostatic carcinoma, choriocarcinoma, and some types of carcinoma of the lung. Increasingly, palliation has been achieved in carefully selected patients. In the abdomen, liver metastases create the greatest challenge because they are so common. Since resection of secondaries from colorectal cancer was first performed ten or so years ago, there are a number of centres in the world achieving 30–40% five-year survival after major hepatic

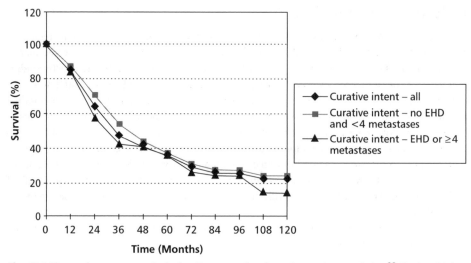

Fig. 12.2 Five and ten-year survival after liver resection for colorectal secondaries.[23] Kaplan–Meier plot. (EHD = Extra-hepatic disease)

resection in the absence of secondaries elsewhere.[23] Modern scanning techniques make it much easier to exclude other secondary spread. Even when cure is not achieved there is worthwhile palliation and extension of life, and it is cost-effective.[24] Figure 12.2 shows an example of the survival figures. So far this is only proven for colorectal metastases yet in principle it may be beneficial for patients after radical resection of gastric or pancreatic carcinoma who then develop liver secondaries alone. Unfortunately, however, from these primary sites transperitoneal spread, local recurrence, and other distant metastases nearly always accompany liver secondaries. Liver resection was until recently a dangerous operation with heavy blood loss, but now in experienced hands the operative mortality is down to less than 4% with 60% of patients not needing any blood transfusion thanks to technical advances such as ultrasonic dissectors and argon beam coagulators as well as a new understanding of the segmental structure of the liver.

Conclusion

Abdominal surgeons have a major role to play in palliative care. Great improvements in recent years in surgical safety, anaesthetic techniques, postoperative pain control, and general care, together with new attitudes to postoperative mobilization, mean that surgery is not necessarily the traumatic intervention that it has often seemed. This is well illustrated by the standard inguinal hernia repair where the postoperative stay has changed from three weeks to less than 24 hours over the last 40 years without any change in fundamental surgical technique. Many palliative care physicians have not been in an operating theatre for very many years and are still plagued by memories of traumatic inductions, massive blood loss, and postoperative pain, vomiting and multiple complications. Patients must not be denied the benefit of surgery – often quite simple and quick – because of old-fashioned prejudices; and they must not be denied the possibility of cure of their secondaries by ignorance of modern surgical achievements. But when surgical intervention is not possible or advisable, the surgeon still has the responsibility and privilege of listening, supporting, and comforting.

Acknowledgement

I am grateful to Dr. R. Peck for Figure 12.1.

References

1. Pietrafitta, J.J., and Dwyer, R.M. (1986). Endoscopic laser therapy of malignant esophageal obstruction. *Arch. Surg.*, **121**, 395–400.
2. Robertson, G.S.M., Thomas, M., Jamieson, J., Veitch, P.S., and Dennison, A.R. (1996). Palliation of oesophageal carcinoma using argon beam coagulator. *Br. J. Surg.*, **83**, 1769–71.
3. Dougherty, T.J., Gomer, C.J., Henderson, B.W., Jori, G., Kessel, D., Korbelik, M., *et al.* (1998). Photodynamic therapy. *J. Natl. Cancer Inst.*, **90**, 889–905.
4. Lightdale, C.J. (2000). Role of photodynamic therapy in the management of advanced esophageal cancer. *Gastrointest. Endosc. Clin. North Am.*, **10**, 397–408.
5. Boyce, H.W. (1993). Stents for palliation of dysphagia due to esophageal cancer. *N. Engl. J. Med.*, **329**, 1345–6.
6. Cowling, M.G., Hale, H., and Grundy, A. (1998). Management of malignant oesophageal obstruction with self-expanding metallic stents. *Br. J. Surg.*, **85**, 264–6.
7. Shand, A.G., Grieve, D.C., Brush, J., Palmer, K.R., and Penman, I.D. (2002). Expandable metallic stents for palliation of malignant pyloric and duodenal obstruction. *Br. J. Surg.*, **89**, 349–50.
8. Ponec, R.G., and Kimmey, M.B. (1997). Endoscopic therapy of esophageal cancer. *Sur. Clin. North Am.*, **77**, 1197–217.
9. Sandostatin Lar (2002) S.P.C. Novartis Pharmaceuticals
10. Lennard-Jones, J.E. (1999). Giving or withholding fluid and nutrients: ethical and legal aspects. *J. Roy. Coll. Phys. London*, **33**, 39–45.
11. Tham, T.C.K., Taitelbaum, G., and Carr-Locke, D.L. (1997). Percutaneous endoscopic gastrostomies: are they being done for the right reasons? *Q.J.M.*, **90**, 495–6.
12. Rabeneck, L., McCullough, L.B., and Wray, N.P. (1997). Ethically justified, clinically comprehensive guidelines for percutaneous endoscopic gastrostomy tube placement. *Lancet*, **349**, 496–8.
13. Hawkey, C.J., Karrasch, J.A., Szczepanski, L., Walker, D.G., Barkun, A., Swannell, *et al.* (1998). Omeprazole compared with misoprostol for ulcers associated with non-steroidal anti-inflammatory drugs. *N. Engl. J. Med.*, **338**, 727–34.
14. Emery, P., Zeidler, H., Kvien, T.K. Guslandi, M., Naudin, R., Stead, H., *et al.* (1999). Celecoxib versus diclofenac in long-term management of rheumatoid arthritis: randomised double-blind comparison. *Lancet*, **354**, 2106–11.
15. Richter, J.M., (1989). Angiodysplasia: natural history and efficacy of therapeutic interventions. *Dig. Dis. Sci.*, **34**, 1542–6.
16. Chung, S.C.S., Lau, J.Y.W., Sung, J.J.Y., Chan, A.C.W., Lai, C.W., Ng, E.K.W., *et al.* (1997). A randomized comparison of adrenaline injection alone and adrenaline plus heat probe treatment for actively bleeding peptic ulcers. *B.M.J.*, **314**, 1307–11.
17. Gimson, A.E.S., Ramage, J.K., Panos, H.Z. Hayllar, K., Harrison, P.M., Williams, R., *et al.* (1993). Randomised trial of variceal band ligation versus injection sclerotherapy for bleeding esophageal varices. *Lancet*, **342**, 391–4.
18. Lebrec, D., Giuily, N., Hadengue, A., Vilgrain, V., Moreau, R., Poynard, T., *et al.* (1996). Transjugular intrahepatic porta systemic shunt S: comparison with para-centesis in patients with cirrhosis and refractory ascites: a randomised trial. *J. Hepatol.*, **25**, 135–44.
19. Beger, H.G., Buckler, M., Bittner, R., Oettinger, W., and Roscher, R. (1989). Duodenum preserving resection of the head of the pancreas in severe chronic pancreatitis: early and late results. *Ann. Surg.*, **209**, 233–8.

20. Teuscher, A.U., Kendall, D.M., Smets, Y.F., Leone, J.P., Sutherland, D.E., and Robertson, R.P. (1998). Successful islet autotransplantion in humans. *Diabetes*, **47**, 324–30.

21. Buscher, H.C.J.L., Jansen, J.B.M.J., van Dongen, R., Bleichrodt, R.P., and van Goor, H. (2002). Long-term results of bilateral thoracoscopic splanchnicetomy in patients with chronic pancreatitis. *Br. J. Surg.*, **89**, 158–62.

22. Solbiati, L., Livraghi, T., Goldberg, S.N., Ierace T., Meloni, F., Dellamore, M., *et al.* (2001). Percutaneous radio-frequency ablation of hepatic metastases from colorectal cancer: long-term results in 117 patients. *Radiology*, **221**, 159–66.

23. Scheele, J., Stang, R., and Altendorf-Hofmann, A. (1995). Resection of colorectal liver metastases. *World J. Surg.*, **19**, 59–71.

24. Beard, S.M., Holmes, M., Price, C., and Majeed, A.W. (2000). Hepatic resection of colorectal metastases in Sheffield (1997–1999). A cost-effective analysis. *Ann. Surg.*, **232**, 763–76.

Chapter 13

Symptom control in urological malignancy

Alan P. Doherty and Joe M. O'Sullivan

Introduction

Urological cancers represent a disparate group of diseases with some common ground with regard to carcinogenesis and symptomatology. Symptom control in advanced urological cancers presents some unique challenges for the surgeon and oncologist. Many of the severe symptoms are debilitating physically, mentally, and socially. Patients are often embarrassed to admit to urinary difficulties, especially incontinence and haematuria, and this can lead to unnecessary suffering. Pain, especially in prostate cancer patients, is often underreported or underestimated. This chapter will discuss the symptoms of urological malignancies and surgical and oncological interventions to palliate them. In addition, a brief review of the literature on 'adjunctive nephrectomy', palliative cystectomy, and radical prostatectomy for locally advanced disease is included.

Clearly, the control of symptoms is paramount in helping patients maintain a good quality of life in the face of advanced malignancy. However, another important aspect of care in terminally ill patients is the use of interventions in order to prevent or delay the onset of symptoms and in some cases even prolong survival. Relatively asymptomatic patients with metastatic urological cancer are increasingly common, probably due to increasing use and sophistication of modern imaging and other diagnostic techniques. It is therefore important for those involved in the care of such patients to be aware of the various interventions now available.

Palliative care is both a multimodality and multidisciplinary process. The psychological, social, and somatic needs of a patient are all equally important. Similarly, correction of anaemia, nutritional status, and support for family are essential. These aspects of palliative care are not included in this chapter.

Symptoms of advanced urological malignancy

Urological cancers can cause a variety of symptoms. The combination of symptoms depends on the nature of the primary tumour. However, many urological malignancies have several features in common in the advanced disease situation. Symptoms include pain, bleeding, obstruction, infection, fistula, renal failure, debility and weakness, change in bowel habit, lower urinary tract symptoms (LUTS), and lymphoedema (Table 13.1).

Pain

Pain in urological malignancy is occasionaly seen secondary to obstruction of the urinary tract. Neuropathic pain syndromes in pelvic malignancy are not infrequent. This sort of pain is often not responsive to opiates alone and usually requires the use of tricyclic antidepressants such as

Table 13.1 Symptoms of advanced urological malignancy

Symptom	Possible causes	Impact on patient
Pain	Nerve compression/invasion Bone metastases Obstruction of hollow viscus Capsular fascial stretch	Immobility Loss of confidence Fatigue
Haematuria	Tumour, infection, chemotherapy	Severe: anaemia/shock/clot retention
General features of malignancy	Loss of weight, cachexia	Depression, disfigurement
Recurrent UTI	Fistula	Antibiotic resistance
Peripheral oedema	Low albumin/pelvic malignancy/IVC compression	Immobility, pain, disfigurement
Bladder outflow obstruction	Acute-on-chronic urinary retention with overflow incontinence/obstructive nephropathy	Pain, uraemia, anuria, oliguria,
Urinary incontinence	Fistula	Social isolation, embarrassment
Diarrhoea	Fistula	Social isolation, embarrassment
Dyspnoea	Lung metastases	Immobility
Lower urinary tract symptoms	Urge, frequency, nocturia, incomplete emptying, straining, poor flow, hesitancy, post-micturition dribbling	Reduced social interaction, pain

UTI = urinary tract infection; IVC = inferior vena cava

amitryptiline, and non-steroidal anti-inflammatory drugs. Uncontrolled local pelvic disease frequently presents with a constant dull dragging pain that radiates to the lower back. Involvement of the lumbo-sacral spine may similarly cause pain in the lower back that radiates down the leg and into the buttock. Involvement of the perineal nerve roots will cause a burning perineal pain that can be exacerbated by sitting. Such patients appear to be unable to keep stil, constantly shifting their position in an attempt to gain respite from their discomfort. These pains are extremely difficult to control and reinforce the need to prevent local disease recurrence. Ano-rectal involvement can cause tenesmus, with patients complaining of the constant urge to defaecate, which in turn leads to worsening of the pain.

Haematuria

Recurrent attacks of haematuria can cause clot retention and symptomatic anaemia. There are a number of potential causes of haematuria in patients with advanced urological malignancy. Investigation should include urine microscopy and culture as well as cystoscopy. Cystoscopy can be both diagnostic and therapeutic. Haematuria can also be the result of treatment with cyclophosphamide or radiotherapy.

When simple irrigation fails, treatment options include palliative pelvic radiotherapy as well as formalin intravesical irrigation. Before formalin is used, ureteric reflux must be out-ruled. Life-threatening haemorrhage rarely occurs from haemorrhagic cystitis or uncontrolled bladder tumours.[1] If fulguration, laser treatment, or intravesical instillations fails to control the haemorrhage, it may be necessary to perform trans-femoral percutaneous internal iliac embolization. Embolization unfortunately rarely succeeds and palliative cystectomy may be necessary as a last resort. As an alternative, urinary diversion, either through surgical or percutaneous routes, has been effective in anecdotal situations in stopping haemorrhagic cystitis from non-malignant causes. The use of radiotherapy in the treatment of haematuria secondary to bladder tumours is well established and is discussed later. It is also important to remember that infection can exacerbate haematuria and this should be excluded as a cause.

Urinary incontinence and fistulae

Disruption of the sphincter mechanism can occur with locally advanced tumours. Bladder dysfunction can also follow pelvic radiotherapy. It is important to exclude reversible causes such as urinary tract infection and overflow incontinence. Intermittent self-catheterization (ISC) or permanent catheterization can be helpful.

Fistulae involving the urinary tract can be distressing and frightening. Locally advanced bladder cancers can infiltrate the bowel in males and either the bowel or vagina in females, leading to persistent leakage of urine. Less commonly, involvement of skin can lead to the leakage of urine through the abdominal wall. Active palliative therapy of a malignant fistula can lead to considerable improvement in quality of life. The standard surgical approach of excision of the fistula and repair is often impossible in these patients. The aim of treatment is to limit the extent of leakage, minimizing the effects of continual perineal irritation. Thus urinary catheters, or less commonly, vaginal tampons are often of help. Alternatively, patients with a reasonable life expectancy can try urinary diversion with percutaneous nephrostomy tubes or formation of an ileal conduit.

Lower urinary tract symptoms

Uncontrolled locally advanced bladder tumours can cause supra-pubic discomfort, frequency of micturition, nocturia, urgency, and incontinence. If radiotherapy has been used the bladder may be of small capacity. In these cases, palliative diversion or catheterization are the only effective interventions. If symptoms are due to tumour bulk or trigone irritation, it may be possible to reduce tumour mass with transurethral resection of tumour or with radiotherapy.

Leg oedema

Leg, perineal, and abdominal oedema are a frequent complication of locally advanced bladder cancer. The usual causes in advanced pelvic malignancy are pelvic venous obstruction, thrombosis, and obstruction to pelvic lymphatics.

Symptoms from renal cell carcinoma (RCC)

The heterogeneity of renal cell carcinoma and its variable natural history defy diagnostic and therapeutic generalizations. Nevertheless, symptoms from RCC are rare in early disease but common in locally advanced and metastatic disease. Most commonly encountered are pain, haematuria, paraneoplastic syndromes, and compression of adjacent viscera. The classic triad is pain, haematuria, and flank mass. Pain can indicate invasion of the posterior abdominal wall, nerve roots or paraspinous muscles. Gastrointestinal symptoms are rare although invasion of tumour into the large bowel, mesentery, and colon is sometimes seen. Likewise, liver involvement is usually from metastases and not from direct invasion. Stauffer's syndrome is non-metastatic hepatic dysfunction. These patients have abnormal liver function tests, white blood cell loss, fever, and areas of hepatic necrosis.[2]

Haematuria occurs when the collecting system is breached. Clot colic often causes loin to groin pain. Weight loss, fever, night sweats, and sudden development of a varicocoele in a male patient are not uncommon findings. Hypertension is due to segmental renal artery occlusion or to elaboration of renin or renin-like substances. Paraneoplastic symptoms occur because the kidney is involved in the production of prostaglandins, 1,25 dihydroxycholecalciferol, renin, and erythropoietin. In malignancy, other hormones such as parathyroid-like factors, glucagons, human chorionic gonadotropin, and insulin can be produced.

Surgical interventions for palliation of urological cancers (Table 13.2)

Palliative diversion for metastatic upper tract (ureteric) obstruction

There are many options for diversions for malignant ureteric obstruction. Retrograde ureteral stenting refers to a ureteric stent being inserted through the bladder. Percutaneous drainage is performed by inserting a tube directly into the kidney from the skin. This is usually done with ultrasound

Table 13.2 Palliative surgical procedures

Procedure	Aim
Suprapubic catheter	Relief of urethral obstruction/control of urinary incontinence
Nephrostomy	Relief of ureteric obstruction
Ileal conduit	Urinary diversion
Palliative cystectomy	Control of bleeding, prevention of LUTS
Palliative nephrectomy	Survival benefit
Clean intermittent self catheterization 'CISC'	Relief of urethral obstruction
Ureteric stents	Relief of ureteric obstruction
'Channel' TURP	Relief of urethral obstruction
Perineal urostomy	Urinary diversion
Cutaneous ureterostomy	Urinary diversion
TURBT and cystodiathermy	Tumour debulking and control of haematuria
Formalin/allum bladder irrigation	Control of haematuria
Indwelling urethral catheter	Relief of urethral obstruction or control of incontinence
Spinal decompression	Prevent pressure damage to spinal cord
Closure of fistula	Treat effect of fistula, thus depending on type, e.g. skin excoriation, diarrhoea, recurrent sepsis, etc.
Radical penectomy	Control of fungating lesion
Pelvic exenteration	Rarely a palliative procedure

LUTS = lower urinary tract symptoms; TURP = transurethral resection of the prostate; TURBT = transurethral resection of bladder tumour guidance. This tube can subsequently be converted into an indwelling ureteric tube inserted via this percutaneous tract, so-called antegrade ureteric stenting. Open surgical diversions include ureteral exploration with intraoperative ureteric stent insertion, open nephrostomy tube, or ileal conduit. These are occasionally necessary. If only one ureter is obstructed, it may be divided and the upper end anastamosed to the unobstructed ureter (trans-uretero-ureterostomy – TUU). Supra-pubic diversion for patients with very poor prognosis is best achieved with a cutaneous ureterostomy (with TUU to avoid two stomas). Ileal conduit is sometimes needed if the unobstructed ureteric segments are short. Ileal conduits are particularly useful when the bladder is either removed in a palliative cystectomy, or when the bladder is non-functioning (defunctioning ileostomy). An alternative to the ileal conduit following palliative cystectomy is the ureterosigmoidostomy.

Novel diversion techniques have been proposed. Many authors have described their experience with expandable metallic wallstents.[3,4] Further innovations have included extracorporeal[5] and subcutaneous techniques.[6] These techniques have the advantage of negating the need for a nephrostomy tube and an external appliance. These techniques have not been widely adopted, largely due to their relative complexity and lower success rates when compared to the ureteric stent or the nephrostomy.

A common clinical dilemma is choosing the best form of diversion. The main options are retrograde ureteric stenting and percutaneous nephrostomy tube insertion. Factors to consider include the technical feasibility, effectiveness in bypassing the obstruction, complications, and patient satisfaction.

Retrograde ureteric stenting usually is performed under general anaesthetic while percutaneous nephrostomy is a local anaesthetic procedure. In cases when the anaesthetic risk is high, percutaneous nephrostomy tube insertion is favoured. For both procedures, preliminary dialysis is occasionally needed when serum potassium is dangerously high. When the underlying disease process is near the ureteric orifices, making them difficult to identify, a percutaneous approach is again favoured. This latter situation is often seen with malignancies involving the bladder in the region of the trigone. Of course, percutaneous nephrostomy tube insertion can be subsequently attempted where retrograde stenting has failed and this is successful in about 75% of patients.[7] Thus, although percutaneous nephrostomy is an excellent form of diversion, cystoscopy with an attempt at retrograde pyelography and stent insertion as an initial step is an attractive alternative as this offers the ability to confirm the malignant nature of the obstruction in addition to obtaining biopsy for histology.

Palliative diversion for metastatic ureteral obstruction has been reviewed by Abraham.[8] In this retrospective cohort from the Philippines, 96 such patients were identified. Seventy-two had either surgical diversion, retrograde stenting, or percutaneous nephrostomy tube insertion (with or without antegrade stenting). The cause was cervical carcinoma in 39%, bladder cancer in 16%, colorectal in 14.5%, prostate in 12.5%, uterine in 4.1%, breast and testes 3.1%, lymphoma and gastric 2%, and ovarian 1%. Obstruction was bilateral in 44% of cases and this reflects the high proportion of cervical cancers. The authors concluded that the most successful diversion (in terms of improvement in renal function and resolution of symptoms) was percutaneous nephrostomy (75%). Complications of urinary diversions were seen in 31% of cases. Of those who had a percutaneous nephrostomy (n = 55), 15% fell out, 9% had an infection, 7% had a urine leak, and 5% blocked.

Acute renal failure is a relatively common urological emergency. As many as one-third of all patients considered for a diversion procedure are new presentations of advanced malignancy. In such circumstances, the decision on whether to intervene to relieve the effects of obstructive uropathy can be difficult given the dreadful mean survival rates of these patients. In a study of 77 patients undergoing percutaneous nephrostomies and their survival,[9] the authors suggest that palliative diversion be carried out only after a resonable expectation of prolonged survival is judged to be feasible, or in other words, if further therapeutic interventions are possible. This is usually the case for undiagnosed cases. In other circumstances, such as when patients progress while on treatment, or in the presence of other life-threatening co-existent morbidity, poor performance status, or uncontrolled pain, intervention should be resisted with the consent of the patients and relatives. Thus, although urinary diversion is possible using percutaneous nephrostomies followed by antegrade ureteric stents, a peaceful death from uraemia is occasionally a more humane alternative.

The role of urinary diversion has been investigated in a prospective study of 42 patients who presented with renal failure secondary to malignant obstructive nephropathy.[10] Obstructive nephropathy was relieved in 33 of the 42 patients with percutaneous nephrostomies. The median survival for the entire group was 133 days (range 7–712 days). Survival of six months or more was seen in 17 patients, nine of whom had bladder cancer. However, five patients died within 30 days of undergoing urinary diversion, three of whom had bladder cancer. Patients who had had many therapeutic modalities prior to urinary diversion had the shortest median survival.

It must be remembered that long-term nephrostomy is difficult for patients to manage at home and can make terminal care nursing almost impossible. Although the improvement in renal function is best achieved with nephrostomy, it should be performed only as a last resort in the dying patient.

Palliative procedures for malignant bladder outflow obstruction

Emptying the bladder with catheterization is probably the most common method by which bladder outflow obstruction is circumvented. Other interventional approaches include transurethral resection of prostate (TURP) for cases with obstructing prostate cancer. In women, bladder outflow obstruction is seen in cases of locally advanced pelvic malignancy.

Catheterization

An indwelling catheter can be placed either urethrally or supra-pubically. An indwelling catheter should be a last resort type of therapy for long-term bladder drainage. Virtually all patients develop bacteriuria after a short period of time. A contracted fibrotic bladder may be the ultimate result. Bladder stones may form on the catheter balloon. The catheter can dilate and erode the bladder neck. This results in the inability to retain the balloon. Bladder spasms can be problematic, resulting in bypass and thus incontinence.

A supra-pubic catheter is more comfortable and obviates the urethral and bladder neck complications of a urethral catheter. However, the use of a supra-pubic catheter does not prevent urinary leakage due often to detrusor contraction. When blockage occurs, nurses and even junior medical staff are reluctant to change this type of catheter. The long-term risk of carcinoma of the bladder secondary to catheterization is not a relevant complication in the patient with advanced malignancy. Supra-pubic catheters should be avoided in cases of bladder cancer for risk of wound infiltration by tumour.

A more recent advance has been the development of intermittent self-catheterization (ISC). This is an effective way of avoiding a long-term catheter.[11] The technique requires a cooperative and motivated patient or even willing family member. The patient must have adequate hand control and be able to gain access to their urethra. Community specialist nurses are usually available to help patients learn the technique. Many patients are initially reluctant to perform this procedure. A clear and thorough explanation that it is simple and offers considerable advantages must be given. For adult patients a 14 or 16 French catheter is used. Usualy these are made of plastic and some are lined with hydrophilic coatings (Lofric). Catheters can be reused and need only be kept clean, not sterile. Complications that can occur include false passages, bladder perforation and bacteriuria; however, symptomatic urinary tract infection is rare.

'Channel' TURP

The term 'channel TURP' is used to describe the procedure of endoscopically removing malignant prostate tissue that is causing bladder outflow obstruction. Usually this group of patients has locally advanced as well as metastatic disease. Often they have gone into acute urinary retention and have an indwelling catheter, or suffer severe, bothersome lower urinary tract symptoms such as nocturia, urge, poor flow, and dribbling.

The method of resection is identical to a TURP for benign disease, but the extent of resection may differ. Some surgeons continue to resect to the prostate capsule, while others stop as soon as they have resected enough tissue to allow the passage of urine.

The results from surgical intervention are very good. In a review of 41 patients undergoing channel TURP, all were able to void following the procedure.[12] Incontinence is an increased risk in patients having a channel TURP compared to a TURP for benign disease. In Mazur's series, two patients had a resection that was carried through the external urinary sphincter because it had been invaded by tumour and consequently they were incontinent postoperatively.

Some surgeons argue that channel TURP should be reserved for cases in acute retention that have not responded to hormone ablation. This view is supported by a randomized study comparing channel TURP and bilateral orchidectomy with bilateral orchidectomy alone in patients with acute urinary retention secondary to prostate carcinoma, in whom hormonal manipulation was thought appropriate.[13] Ten of the 12 patients were voiding well one month following bilateral orchidectomy alone. Only two patients in this group required TURP. The authors concluded that channel TURP conferred extra morbidity and therefore should be held in reserve for those patients unable to void after hormonal manipulation.

Prostatic stents

A variety of prostate stents have been used in an attempt to overcome bladder outflow obstruction in malignant as well as benign disease. The Urolume was one of the first to be used for benign prostatic hyperplasia (BPH) in high-risk patients in acute urinary retention (AUR).[14] It was effective with nearly all patients able to void spontaneously after insertion. However, severe irritative symptoms were seen in the majority of patients and the stents were prone to encrustation, and this was associated with the development of a urinary infection.

The thermo-sensitive Nitinol mesh stent (Memotherm, Bard/Angiomed, Germany) can be easily installed and removed. Treatment of high-risk patients with bladder outflow obstruction despite androgen ablation from advanced prostatic carcinoma using this sort of stent has recently been reported.[15] After inserting the stent, 33 (94%) of the 35 patients were able to void spontaneously. The authors conclude that for high-risk patients with bladder outflow obstruction caused by prostatic carcinoma, the insertion of a permanent metal stent system offers a useful alternative treatment to transurethral resection. Nevertheless, the indwelling catheter probably remains the most common method used to overcome bladder outflow obstruction in unfit patients.

For patients fit for channel TURP, permanent stents have not become popular. This is largely because of the problems of migration, infection, and encrustation. For patients in whom hormone therapy has yet to be given a chance to take effect, temporaroy bio-absorbable stents have caught the imagination in the treatment of AUR for malignant disease and BPH.[16]

Palliative nephrectomy/excision of renal bed recurrence

Nephrectomy in patients with locally advanced or metastatic disease is indicated for reasons other than control of symptoms. Adjuvant nephrectomy, in other words, in combination with immunotherapy, is believed to prolong survival in this group. The role of nephrectomy in this setting is discussed later (p. 00). Symptoms of renal carcinoma occur late. It is often difficult in advanced disease to clear the renal bed and para-aortic lymph nodes of all macroscopically visible disease. The prognosis in this group is particularly poor. Only 12% of patients who underwent incomplete excision of locally extensive tumour were alive at 12 months.[17] Thus, the indications for palliative nephrectomy for the purpose of control of symptoms are not clear-cut. The potential benefits from nephrectomy have to be balanced against the operative mortality and morbidity as well as the dismal natural history.

When local symptoms occur, it is sometimes due to local infiltration of other organs. In palliative operations, complete excision of the tumour, including excision of involved bowel, spleen, or abdominal wall muscles, can be undertaken. However, palliative nephrectomy for pain control is not always effective.

Renal cell carcinoma extension into the inferior vena cava can cause symptoms of vena-caval obstruction (Budd–Chiari syndrome). Surgery is indicated for symptom relief and for survival benefit. Long-term survival is more likely for patients undergoing radical nephrectomy and vena-caval thrombectomy when the tumour thrombus involves the infra-hepatic IVC than for extensions above the hepatic veins when very few long-term survivors are described. This is changing to some extent, due to the advent of immunotherapy. In a report of radical surgery with adjuvant immunotherapy for patients with inferior vena cava invasion and co-existent distant metastases, long-term survival benefit was described.[18] Of the 31 cases of metastatic renal cell cancer with extensive disease and vena cava extension, 80% underwent the full course of surgery and postoperative immunotherapy. At a mean follow-up of 18 months, 26% of the patients were alive. Actuarial overall five-year survival of the group was 17%. Tumour thrombus level did not correlate with overall survival, while immunotherapy, tumour grade, and metastatic site provided significant prognostic information. Patients with an isolated pulmonary metastasis had a five-year survival rate of 43%, while in those with low-grade tumours it was 52%. The authors conclude that in contrast to the poor results of surgery only in patients with renal cell carcinoma and concurrent inferior vena caval invasion, reasonable five-year survival may be achieved after combined aggressive surgery and immunotherapy. Patients in whom metastasis was limited to the lungs and those with grade 1–2 tumours had a better prognosis.

Surgical intervention is sometimes indicated for renal cell carcinoma recurrence in the renal bed after nephrectomy. The outcome of 30 cases with isolated recurrence was recently described.[19] The incidence of isolated renal bed recurrence among T1-3 (with negative nodes and no metastases) renal cell carcinomas treated with unilateral nephrectomy was just under 2% at five years. Sixty per cent presented with symptoms related to the recurrent tumours. Overall long-term survival with locally recurrent renal cell carcinoma was 28% survival rate at five years. Calculating survival among symptomatic and asymptomatic patients revealed no discernible difference in outcome. Three treatment groups were identified: observation (n = 9), therapy excluding surgical extirpation (n = 11), and complete surgical resection alone or in conjunction with additional therapy (n = 10). The five-year survival rate with surgical resection was 51% compared to 18% treated with adjuvant medical therapy and only 13% with observation alone. This study suggests that select patients may benefit from an aggressive surgical approach.

Palliative cystectomy

Patients with incurable bladder cancer may or may not develop severe local symptoms from the primary tumour or may have these symptoms controlled with conservative measures, such as transurethral resection of bladder tumour (TURBT) or radiation therapy. It is conceivable that many such patients could retain their bladders even though they may ultimately die from metastatic disease. Thus, in patients with gross nodal metastases (usually visible on preoperative imaging studies), or distant metastases, systemic therapy should probably be initiated before considering extensive local management such as palliative cystectomy or radiation therapy (p. 00). The latter two modalities should probably be withheld unless there is complete or nearly complete response to systemic chemotherapy, when surgical resection of limited metastases (and the primary tumour) can render the patient free of apparent disease.

Palliative cystectomy is indicated for persistent troublesome bleeding, but fortunately this is relatively rare. Radiation haemorrhagic cystitis is relatively common but usually controlled by simple measures such as cystodiathermy and/or formalin irrigation.

Following radiotherapy for pelvic malignancy, bladders can end up small and contracted, causing incontinence and bothersome lower urinary tract symptoms. Cystectomy in these patients can significantly improve quality of life.

Palliative interventional radiology

Although details of the indications, benefits, and risks of interventional radiology are outside the scope of this chapter, it is worth noting the highly effective nature of such interventions. For example, in report of percutaneous embolization of the internal iliac arteries in 108 patients with uncontrollable haemorrhage due to pelvic neoplasms (urinary bladder in 50, uterus in 39, ovary in 16, and prostate in three), complete control of the haemorrhage was achieved in 74 patients, partial control in 23, and no control in 11. Seventy patients experienced post-embolization syndrome (nausea, vomiting, gluteal pain, and fever due to tissue necrosis), and three had transient acute tubular necrosis caused by the contrast medium.[20] The authors stress that it is important for success that the embolization be bilateral and that the embolic agent used be a permanent one.

Multimodality urological procedures in advanced disease: 'adjunctive surgery'

Adjunctive nephrectomy

Metastatic renal cell carcinoma is often seen without local symptoms. This accounts for the fact that although approximately 30% of patients have metastases at the time of diagnosis, far fewer than this present with severe symptoms. Nephrectomy under these circumstances is generally performed in an attempt to prolong survival, not to prevent the onset of symptoms, although this is an added potential benefit. This sort of nephrectomy has been called adjunctive nephrectomy, since it is used in combination with immunotherapy.

Nephrectomy in the presence of metastases has a long history in surgical practice. This is mainly due to early reports that suggested removal of the primary lesion induced spontaneous regression of the metastases.[21] This concept was widely believed and palliative nephrectomy was performed for both control of symptoms and regression of the metastatic sites. However, spontaneous regression of metastases following nephrectomy probably is not a reality. At best, regression occurs in renal tumours only rarely, in perhaps 0.4% of patients.[22] Others report no regression at all.[23] Reports that support spontaneous regression were either based on studies that were restricted to the use of chest radiography for the assesment of regression or were performed in selected patients with good performance status.[24]

Nevertheless, evidence does exist to support adjunctive nephrectomy, not for spontaneous regression but for survival benefit. Preliminary results of the South West Oncology Group (SWOG) Trial 8949 were reported at the American Urological Association meeting in 2000. A total of 245 patients were randomized to either immediate interferon or radical nephrectomy followed by interferon. There was a four months median survival advantage for the group who had nephrectomy. It seems likely, therefore, that nephrectomy prior to systemic therapy yields a survival benefit. The European Organization for the Research and Treatment of Cancer (EORTC) have presented similar data using the same protocol as SWOG. There were five comlete responses for nephrectomy and interferon compared to none in the interferon-alone group. Improvement in survival was 10 months. It is worth noting that as many as 20% are unable to have immunotherapy after tumour nephrectomy. This is due to the toxicity of immunotherapy. Side-effects include fever, chills, malaise, nausea, vomiting, diarrhoea, and other constitutional symptoms. The most serious side-effects are primarily renal and cardio-vascular. Interleukin-2 induces pre-renal failure with hypotension, fluid retention, respiratory distress syndrome, and oliguria.

In these studies, no account was taken of the general morbidity after nephrectomy. Improved survival must be tempered by the fact that recovery may take up to eight weeks, which means that improved survival in quality-of-life terms may only be two months. It is possible to spend the whole of the terminal period having treatment. It is also noteworthy that there was no nephrectomy-alone arm to these studies. It might be that the survival benefit is accured from the nephrectomy alone. Unfortunately there is no randomized control trial to compare nephrectomy versus no nephrectomy in the presence of metastases. Some early case–control studies showed no survival advantage.[17] Nevertheless, the advent of immunotherapy may be changing the previously held belief that surgery was the only effective alternative. A combination of the two is becoming standard practice in patients with good performance status and low-volume metastatic disease.

Even more aggressive surgical management includes excision of solitary metastases in addition to the renal primary. Five-year survival is improved with excision of solitary renal metastasis.[25] In patients with good performance status and solitary resectable pulmonary metastasis, the five-year survival is 30% in combination with immunotherapy.

Adjuvant cystectomy

Radical cystectomy remains the most effective means to cure invasive transitional carcinoma of the bladder. Cure is most likely in early-stage disease. However, even in the small proportion of patients with microscopic nodal disease, radical cystectomy with pelvic node dissection may be curative. Five-year survival in the 30% range has been reported for such patients by several groups.[26] Others have published less optimistic results.[27] In one report nearly all patients with metastatic bladder cancer die within two years.[28]

Radical cystectomy provides excellent local pelvic control. Local pelvic recurrence rates for even stage T3b and T4 disease are routinely under 12% and are considerably lower for Stage T2 and T3a lesions. Given that overall approximately 35% of patients with bladder cancer die from recurrent disease, it follows that most deaths due to TCC occur due to metastases in the absence of local pelvic recurrence. Moreover, almost all the patients with pelvic recurrence have concomitant or soon to appear metastases as well. Indeed, it is interesting to note that it is probably because of the low pelvic recurrence rate that pre-cystectomy radiotherapy does not improve survival over cystectomy alone.[29]

Because of the significant failure rates as a result of distant metastases, attempts at combining cystectomy with preoperative (neoadjuvant) or postoperative (adjuvant) chemotherapy have been advocated. Thus, as mentioned above, in patients with gross nodal metastases or distant metastases, systemic chemotherapy should probably be initiated before considering radical cystectomy or radical radiation therapy. In the presence of a complete or nearly complete response to systemic chemotherapy, then surgical resection of limited metastases (and the primary tumour) can render the patient free of apparent disease.

Adjuvant prostatectomy

Whether radical prostatectomy confers a benefit in terms of survival or quality of life in patients with locally advanced prostate cancer is not known. Most centres do not offer radical prostatectomy in clinically locally advanced disease and prefer instead to offer radiotherapy and/or hormonal manipulation. Sometimes locally advanced disease is identified as an unexpected finding after radical surgery. Non-organ-confined disease can be treated with prostate bed adjunctive radiotherapy. Whether or not such a combined approach has a survival or quality of life benefit is being addressed by the EORTC trial 22911. This is a phase III randomized study of postoperative external radiotherapy (60 Gy) versus no immediate further treatment in patients with pT3 pN0 prostatic adenocarcinoma. The study aims to compare local recurrence rates, acute and late morbidity, overall survival, disease-free survival, and cancer-related survival in these two groups. If this study shows a benefit for the combined approach, asymptomatic patients with locally advanced prostate cancer may soon be offered adjunctive radical prostatectomy.

Oncological interventions for palliation of urological cancers

In this section we will attempt to address the oncological management of the symptoms of advanced urological cancers. Each of the major cancers will be discussed separately from the point of view of symptoms involved and available treatments. This text is not meant as an in-depth discussion of the technical aspects of radiotherapy or chemotheraphy but as a broad outline of the options available.

Prostate cancer

Prostate cancer was the second most common cancer diagnosed in men in the UK in 1997,[30] representing 17% of male malignancy. In the US it is the most common male non-dermatological cancer, accounting for 29% of new cancer diagnoses.[31] Twelve per cent of male cancer deaths in the UK in 1999 were due to prostate cancer. Predominantly, cancer of the prostate is a disease of elderly men characterized by initial responsiveness to androgen suppression either surgically by castration or more commonly by luteinizing hormone-releasing hormone agonist injections. Symptom control in advanced prostate cancer is usually good while responding to first-line hormone manipulation, however the length of response is variable with a median duration of 18 months. Once this strategy has failed, second-line treatments including corticosteroids, anti-androgens, diethylstilbesterol and cytotoxic chemotherapy, including estramustine, have only limited success in preventing disease progression with short-lasting, subjective responses in approximately 30% of patients. They can be effective, however, in reducing suffering and improving quality of life.

Bone pain

Bone is the most common site of prostate cancer metastases. Between 80 and 100% of patients who die of the condition have metastatic spread to the skeleton. In the UK up to 65% of patients with prostate cancer have bone metastases at diagnosis.[32] The most common sites of bone metastases are the well-vascularized areas of the skeleton with the vertebral column and the pelvic bones being affected most commonly. Prostate cancer bone metastases are usually osteoblastic in nature, however evidence suggests that bone resorption may play a significant part in the establishment of metastatic lesions.[33]

Up to 75% of these patients experience pain at some stage of the illness with as many as 50% reporting inadequate analgesia.[34] Bone pain has a multifactorial aetiology with stimulation of nociceptors by cytokines, e.g. substance P, serotonin, PGE_1 and PGE_2, involvement, compression, or stretching of nerves, vasculature and periostium, increased intramedullary pressure, and pathological fractures all playing a role. From the oncological point of view, the most useful tool in reducing bone pain is ionizing radiation. This can be delivered in two ways: external beam radiotherapy and unsealed source radiotherapy (radionuclides).

External beam radiotheraphy

External beam radiotherapy has long been shown to be effective in the palliation of painful bone metastases. Response rates in the order of 80% have been documented. The treatment offers a quick and well-tolerated method of improving pain control with little or no morbidity. Radiation is delivered using mega-voltage linear accelerators or Cobalt machines. Most commonly, parallel opposed fields with simple conventional planning are used. In general, it is better to simulate patients as this provides a record of the treated area for future reference in case the patient requires retreatment. The treated area should also be tattooed using a tiny amount of Indian ink as this provides a future reference when planning further irradiation in previously treated areas. Toxicity from the treatment depends on the area treated. Nausea commonly occurs when abdominal or pelvic areas are irradiated using large fractions. This can easily be prevented using standard anti-emetics. Patients can feel tired but this is generally short-lasting.

A wide range of fractionation schedules and doses have been used and controversy exists with regard to the optimum. In the UK, single fractions of 8 Gy are most commonly given. This reduces hospital visits and frees up machine time in order that more patients can be treated. The use of single large fractions is well established and has been shown to be as effective as multiple fractions with regard to pain relief.[35–37] Some oncologists favour the use of multifractionated higher-dose schedules, claiming a dose response effect.[38,39]

Pain relief in prostate cancer bone metastases can occur between two days and six weeks post-radiation. The mechanism of action undoubtedly includes tumour cell kill, but the occasional rapidity of response leads to the conclusion that other factors may be involved. Theories include killing of osteoblast and fibroblasts.

Hemi-body irradiation

When large areas of the skeleton are involved by prostate cancer, pain can be difficult to manage. One radiotherapeutic technique used in this situation is hemi-body irradiation. Pain relief is achieved in the order of 71–89% of patients and maintained until death in approximately two-thirds of them.[40,41] The usual doses are 6 Gy for the upper half of the body and 8 Gy for the lower half of the body. The main potential toxicities are nausea and vomiting, and lethargy. Patients are premedicated with steroids the night before the treatment. In some centres patients are admitted overnight. Full blood counts need to be checked in the weeks following the radiation. Blood count nadirs occur at 10–14 days. A gap of about two weeks should be left between treatment of both halves of the body.

Unsealed source radiotherapy

Bone-seeking radionuclides, including strontium-89-chloride (^{89}SrCl), phosphorous-32-orthophosphate (^{32}P), rhenium-186-hydroxyethylene diphosphonate (^{186}Re-HEDP), and samarium-153 (^{153}Sm) have been used for many years in the palliation of bone metastases in prostate cancer.[42,43] The isotopes are attracted to areas of osteoblastic reaction, which is characteristic of bone metastases from prostate cancer. Pain responses in the order of 70% have been reported with the most commonly used isotopes, ^{89}SrCl,[44] ^{153}Sm, and ^{186}Re-HEDP.

Strontium is a calcium analogue which concentrates in osteoblastic bone metastases. The isotope may remain in bone for 100 days and is excreted renally. Strontium is a beta-emitter with a range in tissue of 1.4 mm. The half-life is 50.5 days. Normal bone takes up a very small proportion of administered activity and bone marrow depression is transient with a nadir occurring at approximately four weeks. The usual administered activity is 150 MBq. An isolation room is not necessary and treatment is given as an outpatient by intravenous infusion. The major contraindications are marrow suppression and uncontrolled incontinence (because the isotope is excreted in urine and may cause contamination). Treatment with ^{89}S-Cl has been shown to be equivalent, from the point of view of pain relief, to hemi-body irradiation.[45]

Rhenium-186 has also gained popularity as a therapeutic isotope. Gamma rays are emitted as well as the therapeutic beta rays. This allows for scintigraphic imaging of the isotope distribution. The usual administered activity of ^{186}Re-HEDP is between 1100 and 2500 MBq. Excretion is renal and the dose limiting toxicity is thrombocytopenia. Contraindications are as with strontium. Samarium-153 mirrors the distribution of technetium when injected. As with ^{186}Re-HEDP, ^{153}Sm also emits gamma rays. The physical and chemical properties are shown in Table 13.3. Bone-seeking radionuclides are underutilized in the treatment of painful bone metastases because of perceived lack of cost-effectiveness and limited availability. However, this treatment strategy has been clearly shown to be economical.[46,47]

Table 13.3 Properties of commonly used radionuclides

Radionuclide	Pharmaceutical	Half-life (days)	β max. energy	Max. range in tissue (mm)	γ-photon
Rhenium 186	HEDP	3.8	1.07	4.7	137(9)
Samarium 153	EDTMP	1.95	0.8	3.4	103(28)
Strontium 89	Chloride	50.5	1.46	6.7	0

Chemotherapy for advanced prostate cancer

Cytotoxic chemotherapy can provide symptom palliation in advanced prostate cancer. The most commonly used drugs include mitoxantrone, docetaxel, paclitaxel, estramustine, etoposide, and vinblastine.[48] Improved pain control and quality of life have been demonstrated using mitoxantrone and prednisolone in a randomized controlled trial.[49] Benefit must be balanced against risk of toxicity, bearing in mind the elderly population involved.

Bladder cancer

Bladder cancer represented 5% of new cancer diagnoses in the UK in 1997 and 3% of cancer deaths in 1999.[30] The most common sites of metastases are pelvic lymph nodes, lung, liver, and bone. Patients with advanced disease are frequently elderly and frail and unfit for major intervention. Therefore treatment stategies are tailored for these needs. Haematuria and pelvic pain are the most common symptoms needing palliation in advanced bladder cancer, and radiotherapy and chemotherapy have useful roles in their management.

Radiotherapy

Palliative local radiotherapy can be used in the palliation of pelvic pain and haematuria resulting from local recurrence or persistence of bladder cancer. Various fractionation schedules are used depending on physician preference and performance status of the patients. For patients with poor performance status, particularly if travel to and from the treatment centre is difficult, single fractions of 6–8 Gy to the bladder can be used. This can reduce haematuria dramatically and also potentially improve pain control. The treatment can be repeated. The technique generally uses a parallel pair set up with conventional planning. Ideally the patient is simulated with the aid of a cystogram, however for expediency in a busy department the fields can be designed simply while the patient is on the treatment machine. The usual treatment fields are 10×10 cm in dimension. The most common acute toxicities are nausea, cystitis, and occasionally diarrhoea. Patients also report tiredness.

Hypo-fractionation involves the use of larger than usual fractions (>2 Gy) of radiotherapy. In advanced bladder cancer patients with poor performance status, this approach has been shown to be of benefit using a schedule of once-weekly fractions of 6 Gy for five to six weeks.[50–52] This delivers a total dose of 30–36 Gy and local control rates approaching 25%. The most common acute toxicity is increased urinary frequency and the potential exists for significant late toxicity. However, it is a satisfactory palliative regimen for patients with advanced bladder cancer who cannot tolerate standard radical radiotherapy.

Other palliative radiotherapy schedules include 30 Gy in 10 fractions over two weeks, and 20 Gy in five fractions in one week. The bladder plus pelvic nodes can be irradiated with tolerable toxicity, producing improved pain control and decreased haematuria. Radiotherapy can also be used to palliate pain from bladder cancer metastatic to bone, soft tissues, or lung.

Chemotherapy

Chemotherapy can be a useful addition to the palliation of advanced bladder cancer and can in selected cases deliver prolonged survival and potentially cure. Combination chemotherapy is used with the most well-established regimen being methotrexate, vinblastine, adriamycin, and cisplatin (MVAC). This combination has shown response rates in the order of 65%.[53,54] Patients require reasonable renal function in order to tolerate cisplatin. Treatment usually requires an overnight stay in hospital for every cycle. The usual duration of treatment is six cycles. Other useful drugs include paclitaxel, carboplatin, and 5-flourouracil. Recently, gemcitabine plus cisplatin has shown equal benefit compared to MVAC, with potentially less toxicity and fewer hospital admissions.[55]

Renal cell cancer

The role of radiotherapy in advanced renal cell cancer is essentially limited to the treatment of bone and brain metastases. Compared to bone metastases from other sites, it is thought that higher doses of radiation are needed to achieve pain control in renal cell cancer.[56] Doses in the order of 40–50 Gy in 1.8–2 Gy fractions are used.

Whole-brain radiotherapy can be used to palliate brain metastases and reduce the need for steroids for symptom control. In the case of solitary brain metastases, surgical excision may be feasible and provide potential cure. Local irradiation of the primary tumour bed can provide analgesic benefit but acute toxicity rates, especially nausea, can be high and most centres avoid this treatment where possible.

Testis cancer

Testicular cancer is a highly curable condition. Even in very advanced stages, cure is possible with a combination of chemotherapy, radiotherapy, and surgery. Most patients are keen to participate in clinical trials once conventional treatments have failed. However, it is important not to lose sight of symptom control when considering treatment strategies. In general, seminomas are highly responsive to radiotherapy and excellent palliation can be achieved even with relatively low doses. Relief from brain, lung, and bone metastases is possible using radiotherapy. Teratomas are less radio-responsive than seminomas; however, radiotherapy may help in pain control.[57]

Other urological cancers

For cancers of the penis, ureter, and female urethra, irradiation may be palliative for the primary tumour, regional adenopathy, and bone metastases. The usual schedules for soft-tissue masses are 30 Gy in 10 fractions, while single fractions of 8 Gy are useful for bone pain. Cytotoxic chemotherapy can also give some palliative benefit, especially in penile cancer.[58]

Conclusion

There is a welcome trend towards anticipating symptoms and trying to prevent them, rather than treating them once they have occurred. However, even if this policy is unsuccessful, palliation by medical or surgical means is often effective.

References

1. Fair, W. (1974). Formalin in the treatment of bladder haemorrhage. Techniques, results, and complications. *Urology*, **3** (5), 573–6.
2. Boxer, R.J., Waisman, J., Lieber, M.M., Mampaso, F.M., and Skinner, D.G. (1978). Non-metastatic hepatic dysfunction associated with renal carcinoma. *J. Urol.*, **119** (4), 468–71.
3. van Sonnenberg, E., D'Agostino, H.B., O'Laoide, R., Donaldson, J., Sanchez, R.B., Hoyt, A., *et al.* (1994). Malignant ureteral obstruction: treatment with metal stents – technique, results, and observations with percutaneous intraluminal US. *Radiology*, **191** (3), 765–8.
4. Pauer, W., and Lugmayr, H. (1992). Metallic wallstents: a new therapy for extrinsic ureteral obstruction. *J. Urol.*, **148** (2, Pt. 1), 281–4.

5. Tomooka, Y., Yokoyama, M., and Takeuchi, M. (1994). Extracorporeal urinary bypass for malignant ureteral obstruction. *Urology*, **43** (6), 878–9.

6. Lingam, K., Paterson, P.J., Lingam, M.K., Buckley, J.F., and Forrester, A. (1994). Subcutaneous urinary diversion: an alternative to percutaneous nephrostomy. *J. Urol.*, **152** (1), 70–2.

7. Harding, J.R. (1995). Percutaneous antegrade ureteric stent insertion in malignant disease. *Clin. Radiol.*, **50** (1), 68.

8. Abraham, J. (1998). Palliative diversion for metastatic ureteral obstruction. http://members.tripod.com/nktiuro/paper1.htm

9. Lau, M.W., Temperley, D.E., Mehta, S., Johnson, R.J., Barnard, R.J., and Clarke, N.W. (1995). Urinary tract obstruction and nephrostomy drainage in pelvic malignant disease. *Br. J. Urol.*, **76** (5), 565–9.

10. Harrington, K.J., Pandha, H.S., Kelly, S.A., Lambert, H.E., Jackson, J.E., and Waxman, J. (1995). Palliation of obstructive nephropathy due to malignancy. *Br. J. Urol.*, **76** (1), 101–7.

11. Lapides, J., Diokno, A.C., Silber, S.J., and Lowe, B.S. (1972). Clean, intermittent self-catheterization in the treatment of urinary tract disease. *J. Urol.*, **107** (3), 458–61.

12. Mazur, A.W., and Thompson, I.M. (1991). Efficacy and morbidity of 'channel' TURP. *Urology*, **38** (6), 526–8.

13. Thomas, D.J., Balaji, V.J., Coptcoat, M.J., and Abercrombie, G.F. (1992). Acute urinary retention secondary to carcinoma of the prostate. Is initial channel TURP beneficial? *J. Roy. Soc. Med.*, **85** (6), 318–19.

14. Williams, G., Coulange, C., Milroy, E.J., Sarramon, J.P., and Rubben, H. (1993). The urolume, a permanently implanted prostatic stent for patients at high risk for surgery. Results from five collaborative centres. *Br. J. Urol.*, **72** (3), 335–40.

15. Gottfried, H.W., Gnann, R., Brandle, E., Bachor, R., Gschwend, J.E., and Kleinschmidt, K. (1997). Treatment of high-risk patients with subvesical obstruction from advanced prostatic carcinoma using a thermo-sensitive mesh stent. *Br. J. Urol.*, **80** (4), 623–7.

16. Isotalo, T., Talja, M., Hellstrom, P., Perttila, I., Valimaa, T., Tormala, P., *et al.* (2001). A double-blind, randomized, placebo-controlled pilot study to investigate the effects of finasteride combined with a biodegradable self-reinforced poly L-lactic acid spiral stent in patients with urinary retention caused by bladder outlet obstruction from benign prostatic hyperplasia. *B. J. U. Int.*, **88** (1), 30–4.

17. Dekernion, J.B., Ramming, K.P., and Smith, R.B. (1978). The natural history of metastatic renal cell carcinoma: a computer analysis. *J. Urol.*, **120** (2), 148–52.

18. Naitoh, J., Kaplan, A., Dorey, F., Figlin, R., and Belldegrun, A. (1999). Metastatic renal cell carcinoma with concurrent inferior vena caval invasion: long-term survival after combination therapy with radical nephrectomy, vena caval thrombectomy, and postoperative immunotherapy. *J. Urol.*, **162** (1), 46–50.

19. Itano, N.B., Blute, M.L., Spotts, B., and Zincke, H. (2000). Outcome of isolated renal cell carcinoma fossa recurrence after nephrectomy. *J. Urol.*, **164** (2), 322–5.

20. Pisco, J.M., Martins, J.M., and Correia, M.G. (1989). Internal iliac artery: embolization to control hemorrhage from pelvic neoplasms. *Radiology*, **172** (2), 337–9.

21. Silber, S.J., Chen, C.Y., and Gould, F. (1975). Regression of metastases after nephrectomy for renal cell carcinoma. *Br. J. Urol.*, **47** (3), 259–61.

22. Montie, J.E., Stewart, B.H., Straffon, R.A., Banowsky, L.H., Hewitt, C.B., and Montague, D.K. (1977). The role of adjunctive nephrectomy in patients with metastatic renal cell carcinoma *J. Urol.*, **117** (3), 272–5.

23. Myers, G.H., Jr., Fehrenbaker, L.G., Kelalis, P.P. (1968). Prognostic significance of renal vein invasion by hypernephroma. *J. Urol.*, **100** (4), 420–3.

24. Marcus, S.G., Choyke, P.L., Reiter, R., Jaffe, G.S., Alexander, R.B., Linehan, W.M., *et al.* (1993). Regression of metastatic renal cell carcinoma after cytoreductive nephrectomy. *J. Urol.*, **150** (2, Pt. 1), 463–6.

25. O'Dea, M.J., Zincke, H., Utz, D.C., and Bernatz, P.E. (1978). The treatment of renal cell carcinoma with solitary metastasis. *J. Urol.*, **120** (5), 540–2.

26. Grossman, H.B., and Konnak, J.W. (1988). Is radical cystectomy indicated in patients with regional lymphatic metastases? *Urology*, **31** (3), 214–16.

27. Zincke, H., Patterson, D.E., Utz, D.C., and Benson, R.C., Jr. (1985). Pelvic lymphadenectomy and radical cystectomy for transitioal cell carcinoma of the bladder with pelvic nodal disease. *Br. J. Urol.*, **57** (2), 156–9.

28. Loehrer, P.J., Sr., Einhorn, L.H., Elson, P.J., Crawford, E.D., Kuebler, P., Tannock, I., *et al.* (1992). A randomized comparison of cisplatin alone or in combination with methotrexate, vinblastine, and doxorubicin in patients with metastatic urothelial carcinoma: a cooperative group study. *J. Clin. Oncol.*, **10** (7), 1066–73.

29. Crawford, E.D., Das, S., and Smith, J.A., Jr. (1987). Preoperative radiation therapy in the treatment of bladder cancer. *Urol. Clin. North Am.*, **14** (4), 781–7.

30. Cancer Research Campaign (2001). Cancer statistics. www.cancerresearchuk.org

31. Landis, S.H., Murray, T., Bolden, S., and Wingo, P.A. (1999). Cancer statistics, 1999. *C. A. Cancer J. Clin.*, **49** (1), 8–31.

32. Pisters, L.L. (1999). The challenge of locally advanced prostate cancer. *Semin. Oncol.*, **26** (2), 202–16.

33. Charhon, S.A., Chapuy, M.C., Delvin, E.E., Valentin-Opran, A., Edouard, C.M., and Meunier, P.J. (1983). Histomorphometric analysis of sclerotic bone metastases from prostatic carcinoma with special reference to osteomalacia. *Cancer*, **51** (5), 918–24.

34. Bonica, J.J. (1987). Importance of effective pain control. *Acta Anaesthesiol. Scand.* **85** (Suppl.), 1–16.

35. Price, P., Hoskin, P.J., Easton, D., Austin, D., Palmer, S.G., and Yarnold, J.R. (1986). Prospective randomized trial of single and multifraction radiotherapy schedules in the treatment of painful bony metastases. *Radiother. Oncol.*, **6** (4), 247–55.

36. Price, P., Hoskin, P.J., Easton, D., Austin, D., Palmer, S., and Yarnold, J.R. (1988). Low-dose single fraction radiotherapy in the treatment of metastatic bone pain: a pilot study. *Radiother. Oncol.*, **12** (4), 297–300.

37. Cole, D.J., (1989). A randomized trial of a single treatment versus conventional fractionation in the palliative radiotherapy of painful bone metastases. *Clin. Oncol.*, **1** (2), 59–62.

38. Blitzer, P.H. (1985). Reanalysis of the RTOG study of the palliation of symptomatic osseous metastasis. *Cancer*, **55** (7), 1468–72.

39. Arcangeli, G., Micheli, A., Giannarelli, D., La Pasta, O., Tollis, A., Vitullo, A., *et al.* (1989). The responsiveness of bone metastases to radiotherapy: the effect of site, histology and radiation dose on pain relief. *Radiother. Oncol.*, **14** (2), 95–101.

40. Hoskin, P.J., Ford, H.T., and Harmer, C.L. (1989). Hemibody irradiation (HBI) for metastatic bone pain in two histologically distinct groups of patients. *Clin. Oncol.*, **1** (2), 67–9.

41. Salazar, O.M., Rubin, P., Hendrickson, F.R., Komaki, R., Poulter, C., Newall, J., *et al.* (1986). Single-dose half-body irradiation for palliation of multiple bone metastases from solid tumors. Final Radiation Therapy Oncology Group report. *Cancer*, **58** (1), 29–36.

42. Lewington, V.J. (1996). Cancer therapy using bone-seeking isotopes. *Phys. Med. Biol.*, **41** (10), 2027–42.

43. Porter, A.T., and Davis, L.P. (1994). Systemic radionuclide therapy of bone metastases with strontium-89. *Oncology*, **8** (2), 93–6; discussion 96, 99–101.

44. Mertens, W.C., Stitt, L., and Porter, A.T. (1993). Strontium 89 therapy and relief of pain in patients with prostatic carcinoma metastatic to bone: a dose response relationship? *Am. J. Clin. Oncol.*, **16** (3), 238–42.

45. Dearnaley, D.P., Bayly, R.J., A'Hern, R.P., Gadd, J., Zivanovic, M.M., and Lewington, V.J. (1992). Palliation of bone metastases in prostate cancer. Hemibody irradiation or strontium-89? *Clin. Oncol.*, **4** (2), 101–7.

46. Quilty, P.M., Kirk, D., Bolger, J.J., Dearnaley, D.P., Lewington, V.J., Mason, M.D., *et al.* (1994). A comparison of the palliative effects of strontium-89 and external beam radiotherapy in metastatic prostate cancer. *Radiother Oncol.*, **31** (1), 33–40.

47. Maxon, H.R., Schroder, L.E., Hertzberg, V.S., Thomas, S.R., Englaro, E.E., Samaratunga, R., *et al.* (1991). Rhenium-186(Sn)HEDP for treatment of painful osseous metastases: results of a double-blind crossover comparison with placebo. *J. Nucl. Med.*, **32** (10), 1877–81.

48. Kelly, W.K., Curley, T., Slovin, S., Heller, G., McCaffrey, J., Bajorin, D., *et al.* (2001). Paclitaxel, estramustine phosphate, and carboplatin in patients with advanced prostate cancer. *J. Clin. Oncol.*, **19** (1), 44–53.

49. Tannock, I.F., Osoba, D., Stockler, M.R., Ernst, D.S., Neville, A.J., Moore, M.J., *et al.* (1996). Chemotherapy with mitoxantrone plus prednisone or prednisone alone for symptomatic hormone-resistant prostate cancer: a Canadian randomized trial with palliative end-points. *J. Clin. Oncol.*, **14** (6), 1756–64.

50. Jose, C.C., Price, A., Norman, A., Jay, G., Huddart, R., Dearnaley, D.P., *et al.* (1999). Hypofractionated radiotherapy for patients with carcinoma of the bladder. *Clin. Oncol.*, **11** (5), 330–3.

51. Srinivasan, V., Brown, C.H., and Turner, A.G. (1994). A comparison of two radiotherapy regimens for the treatment of symptoms from advanced bladder cancer. *Clin. Oncol.*, **6** (1), 11–13.

52. McLaren, D.B., Morrey, D., and Mason, M.D. (1997). Hypofractionated radiotherapy for muscle-invasive bladder cancer in the elderly. *Radiother. Oncol.*, **43** (2), 171–4.

53. Logothetis, C.J., Dexeus, F.H., Finn, L., Sella, A., Amato, R.J., Ayala, A.G., *et al.* (1990). A prospective randomized trial comparing MVAC and CISCA chemotherapy for patients with metastatic urothelial tumors. *J. Clin. Oncol.*, **8** (6), 1050–5.

54. Sternberg, C.N., Yagoda, A., Scher, H.I., Watson, R.C., Geller, N., Herr, H.W., *et al.* (1989). Methotrexate, vinblastine, doxorubicin, and cisplatin for advanced transitional cell carcinoma of the urothelium. Efficacy and patterns of response and relapse. *Cancer*, **64** (12), 2448–58.

55. Vogelzang, N.J., and Stadler, W.M. (1999). Gemcitabine and other new chemotherapeutic agents for the treatment of metastatic bladder cancer. *Urology*, **53** (2), 243–50.

56. DiBiase, S.J., Valicenti, R.K., Schultz, D., Xie, Y., Gomella, L.G., and Corn, B.W. (1997). Palliative irradiation for focally symptomatic metastatic renal cell carcinoma: support for dose escalation based on a biological model. *J. Urol.*, **158** (3, Pt. 1), 746–9.

57. Horwich, A., Huddart, R., and Dearnaley, D. (1998). Markers and management of germ-cell tumours of the testes. *Lancet*, **352** (9139), 1535–8.

58. Dexeus, F.H., Logothetis, C.J., Sella, A., Amato, R., Kilbourn, R., Fitz, K., *et al.* (1991). Combination chemotherapy with methotrexate, bleomycin and cisplatin for advanced squamous cell carcinoma of the male genital tract. *J. Urol.*, **146** (5), 1284–7.

Chapter 14

Wound and reconstructive problems in advanced disease

Thomas J. Krizek

Introduction

A surgical colleague and I were discussing the importance of listening to patients with advanced disease. He asked whether I thought that wounds could speak to us and whether it was important to listen to them. Of course he is correct – listening takes many forms, not merely sounds but signs and other non-auditory ways of communicating. We need to listen to wounds and, particularly, the patients who happen to have the wounds as part of their advanced disease.

Wound management and reconstruction in patients with advanced disease would seem, on the very face of it, to be an oxymoron. And yet I shall try to persuade you that plastic and reconstructive surgery is an integral and important part of managing patients with advanced disease and is intrinsic to palliative care. *Plastic*, as in *plastic* surgery, is a term derived from the Greek word *plastikos* and refers to shape or form. Many, perhaps, consider plastic surgery to involve only shape or form, and equate it conceptually only with cosmetic surgery; surgery on essentially normal tissue undertaken for the primary purpose of changing appearance. However, although this is important work, the bulk of our work involves the management of acute and chronic wounds and reconstructing the often disfiguring and deforming consequences of the healing process itself.

The terms 'wounds' and 'wound healing' apply to all tissues whose integrity is disturbed by physical injury, including surgical procedures, or by disruption from infection, tumours, or radiation. For purposes of this review I shall largely limit the discussion to skin and soft tissues even though the healing of fractures or regeneration of the liver after infection, for example, may be just as important in other contexts.

Wound management

Gertrude

Gertrude was a 68-year-old patient with an advanced carcinoma of her breast. After a modified radical mastectomy and postoperative radiation she developed a painful, ulcerating recurrence of her tumour within the radiated field on her chest wall. The ulceration progressed to involve several of the underlying ribs. It was determined that she had metastatic disease. There was legitimate concern about the affects of chemotherapy on an open, contaminated wound.

Gertrude is a paradigm for this chapter. She has advanced disease and, whether or not chemotherapy moderates the progression of her disease, she has entered a phase of her illness where any surgical procedure would be considered palliative rather than curative. Gertrude is but one of many who, as they get older, will experience 'wounds' as one of the problems of ageing. Because of age and accompanying diseases, including malignancy, many patients are in the last year of their lives and, for many, the wound is a particularly debilitating and painful part of the dying process; although not the cause of death, it may be a major feature of the last months and days.

Scope of the problem

In a recently published, marvellous review of the biology of wounds, Robson and colleagues put some numbers on the scope of the problem we are facing in the U.S.A.[1] Between the ages of 45 and 64 years, the incidence of chronic ulcerated wounds of all kinds is 120 per 100 000 persons and increases to 800 per 100 000 persons at age 75 years and older. These wounds include pressure sores, venous ulcers, and arterial and diabetic neuropathic ulcers. Pressure ulcers alone are reported to affect 11% of all hospitalized patients and 24% of nursing-home patients. Venous ulcers occur in 1% of the population and diabetic ulcers are found in 15% of the 16 million diabetics; each year 50 000 will undergo amputation of a limb. Of the 7 million persons receiving home health care each year, one-third are being seeing for the treatment of wounds, at a cost of $42 billion per year. In addition to these chronic wounds, there are approximately 50 million surgical procedures performed each year, many on the older population, including those with advanced disease.

In order to understand the problems of acute and chronic wounds and to determine the feasibility and propriety of addressing such wounds, it is necessary to understand some of the biology of healing.

Wound healing

For purposes of discussion it is necessary to divide wounds into two categories, acute and chronic.

Acute wounds

The acute wound refers to a surgical procedure or acute injury. The management imperative is to close the wound successfully. The biological goal of healing of skin and soft tissue is to re-establish the structural continuity of the tissue and have it regain the maximum strength that it can achieve. Strength in skin and soft tissue is a function of the fibrous protein, collagen, which is produced by fibroblasts and then remodelled by the the body in response to stress. Deficient fibroplasia results in deficient strength, while exuberant fibroplasia will result in large and unsightly scars or keloids, and stress of poorly oriented wounds can lead to distortion and limitation of motion. For fibroplasia to occur the wound must first be closed.

The first response to injury is blood clotting which prevents exsanguination. This is almost immediately accompanied by inflammation which is the body's initial defence against noxious intruders, mechanical, chemical, and biological in the form of micro-organisms. The inflammatory response varies in its intensity and duration depending on whether foreign bodies remain or micro-organisms reach critical levels. Ultimately, the defining conclusion of inflammation is marked by successful closure of the wound.

Wound closure in the surgical wound is accomplished by co-apting the wound edges as accurately as possible by sutures or tape and epithelialization will then functionally close the wound, often within hours. When edges cannot be easily approximated, more complex techniques are employed to rotate or advance tissue from adjacent areas or to transplant tissue from other areas of the body, either by skin grafts or more complex microsurgical tissue transfers. The goal remains to close the wound. When wounds remain open, the body will spontaneously attempt to close the wound by encouraging epithelial cells to migrate along the surface and by contracting from the margins so that, like a shrinking picture frame, the open area will gradually diminish. It is obvious that this latter process is slow, painful, and when areas are large or in areas that do not easily contract, the wound may simply never close itself. In areas where the tissue is very pliable, such as the cheek, contraction is efficient. Other areas, such as the scalp, the heel, or the sternal area simply do not contract efficiently.

Wound healing is such a biological necessity that the processes of wound healing will take percedence over almost any other biological process. There are some impediments to healing that, in the chronically ill patient, are worth noting. They can be divided into general and local factors.

General factors

Nutrition It is obvious that many elderly or ill patients are not well nourished. Such people will often simply lose their appetites and the perceived sensations of hunger that drive most of us to the cupboard or dining room. I have watched my elderly mother-in-law who, when in an assisted-living facility would simply not feel like going to the dining room, until she became almost so weak she could not walk. This occured even while we visited regularly and believed she was getting top-notch care. When we brought her to live with us, we had to transport her in a wheelchair. Almost a year and a half later she is now walking everywhere with a walker for steadiness, but with a vigour and strength which surprises us. The multiple ssmall sores she had on her feet and the inevitable abrasions which peeled away layers of skin have healed. She still does not recognize hunger but, when offered food on a regular basis, eats heartily.

Wound healing is one of the body's true imperatives and, short of oedema from malnutrition, patients are usually nutritionally capable of healing. The objective tests for nutritional depletion are not as accurate as we should wish. Serum albumin is only a gross indicator. Transferrin levels are, perhaps, more indicative in acutely ill patients such as those with burns. Weight loss may also be suggestive but we often do not have serial weights to indicate any trends.

Vitamins Rare is the adult who is not taking vitamins. Of course, scurvy was one of the first vitamin deficiencies to be identified with wound healing when the healed wounds of sailors began to break down. Vitamin C is necessary for the ongoing production of collagen (aids in the hydroxylation of proline). One glass of freshly squeezed orange juice probably offers sufficient vitamin C to cure scurvy, which is why we so rarely, if ever, see a case. Excess of vitamin C may have other values, but with healing, enough is enough. Of course the other vitamins, A, B, D, and E, are also important but easily delivered in sufficient quantity.

Steroids Corticosteroids are known to interfere with healing. These agents moderate and actually diminish the inflammatory process which is necessary to protect the body and the patient. Steroids also influence the process of fibroplasia adversely. Vitamin A will neutralize the local wound effects of systemic steroids but it should be noted that not all ointments labelled 'A & D' actually contain either viatmin A or D; so read the label. A surgical procedure performed on a patient, even on substantial doses of steroids (such as a patient undergoing correction of rheumatoid joints in the hand), will usually heal satisfactorily if the wound is closed properly and no infection occurs. Steroids are, therefore, an issue but not a complete impediment to healing.

Immune deficiency Immune deficiency occurs in many conditions in addition to AIDS. Persons with chronic infection, burned patients, patients with malignancy, and others may have diminished immune capacity. They, like patients on steroids, present a challenge but not a contraindication to appropriate surgical procedures. These patients' wounds are more susceptible to infection and consequent delayed healing. The rest of the healing process occurs satisfactorily. The immune process has many effects on the wound, particularly the chronic wound, in affecting many of the humoral factors that modulate the local wound healing process.

Local factors

Vascularity It is intuitively obvious that vascularity and wound healing have a direct and proportional interrelationship: the better the vascularity, the better the healing. This, however, is only relative since even marginally vascularized areas will also heal acceptably, albeit more slowly or with more challenges for the wound manager. The issue with diabetes, for instance, is threefold. Diabetic patients have more vascular problems in their lower extremity than normal persons which predisposes to wound healing problems. These patients also may be more susceptible to infection, particularly from gram-positive organisms. Finally, they often have neuropathic or partially anaesthetic areas which also make them more susceptible to injury and less able to heal well.

It is sometimes necessary to consider revascularization of an area before a wound can heal. Most often, vascularity is usually adequate, even if diminished, to allow a wound to heal if other factors like infection are controlled.

Radiation Although radiation is not a common wound problem it becomes a most important issue in patients with advanced disease like Gertrude in the case presented. It is commonly thought, mistakenly I believe, that the problem with irradiated wounds is that they are not sufficiently vascular to support healing. Any surgeon who has incised into irradiated tissue will assure you that bleeding is impressive and there must be alternate explanations for wound healing problems. In fact, radiation interferes with the fundamental building blocks of healing, the primitive fibroblast precursors, and the entire process is, to a great extent, lacking much of cellular constituents of collagen production. When this is recognized and taken into consideration, wound healing can be accomplished. For instance, when local bacterial growth is controlled, skin grafts can be successfully applied to open irradiated wounds, and certainly well-vascularized skin and soft tissue, when introduced from non-irradiated areas, will offer means of successful closure.

Bacteria Although I have not mentioned bacterial contamination as a major factor influencing healing until now, I believe it to be one of the most important and certainly the most overlooked problems in managing wounds, Bacteria normally exist in the skin, lodged in hair follicles and glands, and even the most extensive skin preparation prior to surgery does not sterilize the skin. This bacterial flora can be measured and is about 10^3 bacteria per gram of tissue over the entire surface area of the body. Even ultraviolet radiation delivered during the course of an operation, which may sterilize the surface of the operative field, does not affect the rate of infection in wounds. It has been demonstrated that, except for streptococcal organisms which are bad in almost any amount, most organisms must reach levels of 10^5 bacteria per gram of tissue before infection occurs. The problem is related to the degree of contamination inherent in the operation, such as colon contents, which determines infection. This becomes even more of a problem in chronic wounds which, since they are open wounds, easily harbour more than 10^5 organisms per gram, which makes spontaneous closure (epithelialization and contraction) more difficult and often impossible, and may compromise even the most imaginatively designed and elegantly executed surgical closure.

Chronic wounds

A wound that is not successfully closed at the time of surgery or immediately after injury rapidly becomes a 'chronic' wound. The clinical appearance of the inflammatory response, often described as granulation tissue or 'proud flesh', is not something about which the wound care person should be proud since it reflects that the wound has entered a chronic phase. Such chronic wounds may remain open indefinitely until they are surgically closed. Open wounds are often painful, exude tissue fluids, and are nutritionally depleting. Gertrude presents a chronic, irradiated, probably heavily contaminated open wound. It will remain as such unless managed appropriately.

The first step in relieving pain and managing the wound is to reduce the degree of microbial contamination. What I am about to present is almost counterintuitive. Systemically administered antibiotics do not affect local wound bacteria except when the antibiotic is delivered and has an adequate tissue level before the bacteria arrive. When performing elective surgery in which contamination is anticipated, such as colon surgery, it is appropriate to deliver adequate antibacterial coverage to the tissue before the operation and during the time of exposure. It has been repeatedly demonstrated that when systemic antibacterials are administered after the bacteria have had a chance to become lodged in the tissue, usually a period of about three to four hours after contamination, they do not affect the growth of microorganisms.[2] Thus, when we encounter a chronic ulcer, a pressure sore, a gangrenous toe, or an open, contaminated wound such as Gertrude presents, the administration of systemic antibacterials does not alter the local wound flora. These bacteria seem to be isolated from the perfusion of drugs and it has been repeatedly shown, by actually measuring the tissue level of the bacteria, that in order to change the bacterial level it is necessary to approach the wound differently.

Alexis Carrel, Noble Laureate in 1910 for introducing microsurgery, performed some of the most elegant of all wound care experiments near the front lines in France during World War I.[3] He carefully monitored the microbial flora of the wounds by taking samples with a glass rod with a small wire loop and spreading an amount on a glass slide and then counting the microorganisms, much like we do today with quantitative microbiology. He demonstrated that when bacteria were more than one or two on a slide, wounds became purulent and could not heal. When he found only one micro-organism every five slides, he called it 1/5 and correlated it with a healthy wound. Of course, he did not have antibiotics but rather he used topical chemicals to kill the bacteria without injuring the tissue. He criticized the use of saline or plain dry dressings and introduced the Carrel–Dakin method of irrigating wounds with hypochlorite solutions. Since the chemical breaks down rapidly, almost continuous irrigation was required. Many said it was 'bunk' and refused to accept his technique. Many, now almost a century later, will continue to use saline or dry dressings and allow the wound to remain contaminated.

I strongly advocate careful wound evaluation by quantitative microbiology performed on tissue samples (the technique is similar to measuring bacterial levels in the urine and the testing is standard in Hospital Microbiology Procedures books). When levels exceed 10^5 bacteria per gram, wounds will not heal, skin grafts will not predictably 'take', and wounds cannot be assuredly closed. Systemic antibiotics serve no useful purpose in these wounds and only promote the emergence of resistant organisms. Use topical agents such as silver sulfadiazine, monitor progress with bacterial counts, and when the wound has fewer than 10^5 bacteria per gram it may be closed if clinically appropriate.

Wound closure

Although I have repeatedly emphasized the importance of wound closure, some patients with advanced disease do not require closure. Not all wounds need to be closed. Wounds are most often foul smelling because of necrotic tissue and bacterial activity. Wounds are most often painful because of the bacterial growth. These problems can be managed without formal surgical closure.

Debridement is a term which means to 'cleanse'. This can most efficiently be accomplised by surgical removal of necrotic tissue. In open wounds, such tissue is usually without blood supply and is without sensation. Most necrotic tissue can be removed painlessly, without anaesthetic, and usually at the bedside. A trained wound care nurse should be empowered to perform this task. Enzymatic agents and 'wet to dry dressings' encourage the growth of bacteria and are conceptually less effective than mechanical debridement and far less efficient. Adequate debridement eliminates the foreign material and topical antibacterials, monitored by quantitative bacterial studies, will render a wound 'healthy' and pain will often disappear promptly.

There are many patients whose overall condition may be such that efforts at surgical closure are inappropriate. Patients who have had strokes, are suffering neurological deterioration, and cannot be rehabilitated may appropriately be treated by the measures I have outlined. Although textbooks may depict elegant flap closure techniques for pressure sores of the sacrum, ischium, or trochanteric areas, such procedures are often life threatening in the very elderly and the postoperative immobility required for healing may dispose to respiratory and other problems.

The ladder

Any plastic surgeon relishes the opportunity to show off the technical virtuosity which has evolved in the last decades. However, simple is still the best and wounds are to be approached by what has been termed a reconstructive ladder. One begins at the bottom, employing the simplest approach of either leaving the wound open or closing it by approximating wound edges. Sometimes advancing wound edges requires additional incisions to relax or allow rotation and advancement of nearby tissue. Tissue is, fortunately, quite elastic or expansible as many of us have demonstrated with a middle-age spread. It is possible to move large amounts of tissue, often employing transfer of the underlying muscle as the vascular supply of the overlying skin and soft tissue. We have also learned that fairly large amounts of tissue can be transplanted using the vascular pedicle of the tissue of origin which may be attached to recipient vessels at some distant site. These are the fundamentals of reconstructive surgery. As my friend Larry Gottlieb has pointed out, the reconstructive ladder does not require that we take each step from simple to complex; instead it is more a 'reconstructive elevator', in which we skip a couple of inappropriate steps (or floors) and go directly to the most efficient and appropriate procedure.

Reconstructive surgery

Reconstructive surgery is the fundamental characteristic of plastic surgery. Some surgery may be simply constructive, such as congenital deformity where the tissue is absent from the beginning. For patients we are addressing here, however, reconstruction means restoring of lost parts. The history of our speciality, dating back thousands of years, began with efforts to restore lost noses and other visible parts. The significance of appearance, even to those with advanced disease, cannot be underestimated. Let me tell you about Dorothy. Dorothy may be the most memorable patient of my 45-year career in surgery.

Dorothy

When I first met Dorothy in 1968, shortly after my arrival at Yale, she was about a year following a composite resection of a portion of her tongue, mandible, and a radical neck dissection on one side followed by radiation; I was but a couple of years from my residency.

Apparently free from tumour, Dorothy asked that I rebuild her jaw and help her regain an appearance, not of beauty but an appearance of 'normal'. In an era prior to regular use of microsurgery, in the infancy of craniofacial surgery, and at the advent of myocutaneous flap transfer, my efforts were traditional and almost uniformly unsuccessful. A generation of plastic surgery residents came to know and share in Dorothy's care over the next decade. She came to the hospital regularly, since life in her small community consisted of an uncaring husband and unfeeling neighbours who, along with most who encountered her in the mall or grocery store, were put off by her appearance.

Our surgical floor at the Yale-New Haven Hospital became her real home and the nurses, residents, and students became her family. Her deformity blurred and all who knew her looked past it and saw a vibrant, funny, courageous woman known as Dorothy. About seven years into our journey, she commented that her eyelids had become baggy and I performed a blepharoplasty or eyelid 'tuck', for which I won the 'Golden Hand Award' at the annual resident banquet; an award for the most unforgettable (incomprehensible?) operation of the year.

In 1978, we decided to move on to a position at the Columbia-Presbyterian Medical Center. I encouraged Dorothy and my other patients to continue care in New York (she actually lived almost equidistant between New York and New Haven) but she said she couldn't leave her friends at Yale. She was almost despondent over the thought of another surgeon caring for her, despite the fact of, and in the face of, the modest success I had achieved.

About six months before I actually moved, Dorothy presented with a new mass in her neck which was recurrent carcinoma; an almost unprecedented recurrence of such a cancer after almost a decade-long, tumour-free interval. Dorothy already had had a feeding tube for years. She had already had all the radiation she could tolerate and she refused chemotherapy or any further surgery. She came to Yale finally to die. Her death and my departure for New York were almost coincident.

She taught me dignity in the face of disfigurement. She taught me how little I know about the natural progression of cancer. She taught me not how to die with dignity, but how dignified people die.

Her cancer surgery was immensely important since it gave her another decade of life. And yet her deformity deprived her of the acceptance into society which so many of us would feel is truly 'happy' life. Reconstructive surgery, for purposes of improving appearance, is immensely important; appearance has effects which are far more than skin deep. The emotional wounds from deformity and disfigurement, both congenital and acquired, from injury or malignancy, from normal processes of ageing or prematurely from disease, most often go to the core of human emotion and self-recognition.

Dorothy and thousands of others have taught me, other plastic surgeons, and in fact all who deal with disfigurement and deformity that the issues of life and death are not necessarily the most important. Bill Shankly, a coach of the Liverpool football (soccer) team was once quoted as observing that:[4]

Some people think football is a matter of life and death . . .
I can assure them it is much more serious than that.

Surgical palliation is more than life and death and how we die; it is also about how we live until we die. Newspaper writers, reporters, and much of the public are sometimes surprised that people make choices in which life, and therefore death, is secondary. Jehovah's Witnesses accept death rather than blood transfusions; eternity is a more important stake than life. Patients sometimes refuse the amputation of an extremity, even when the alternative may be death. Patients almost uniformly choose less deforming surgery or radiation for many cancers when the survival rates may be less than more extensive procedures. Burned patients may choose to die rather than survive into a prospect of prolonged period of skin grafting and painful rehabilitation. Dax Cowart, a young man who fought to die rather than continue painful skin grafting, presented the paradigm in modern medical ethics to demonstrate informed consent and the concepts of autonomy. The dramatic video of his struggle, *Please let me die*, produced in 1975, is commonly shown to all new medical students[5] and the subsequent essays on the subject were a modern introduction into medical ethics.[6]

This chapter incorporates some of the mental, emotional, psychological, as well as physical aspects of surgical palliative care.

Palliative care

I should ask the reader to push the edge of the envelope with me in addressing the definition of palliative care. We have been adjusted to thinking of palliative care as the terminal care of patients who are dying from incurable disease, most typically malignancy, AIDS, or cardiovascular disease. Of course, that is the focus of much of surgical palliative care. But palliation is a broader concept, even than health and disease. Derived from words meaning cloak or to conceal, it also refers to efforts to reduce the violence of a disease, to help it to abate. I have been on panels where speakers referred to withdrawing life-support from an unconscious person who sustained massive brain injury a few days earlier as palliative care. Some might agree that withdrawing life-support from an elderly person with a total-body, full-thickness burn qualifies as an example of palliative care. The definition also means to moderate the intensity of a disease without eliminating it. As such, the repair of cleft lip moderates the intensity of the deformity; it does not eliminate it. When I reconstructed Dorothy's jaw, I was offering her a cloak to hide her deformity, to conceal it, to 'palliate' the effects of her disease, but without curing it. Even the blepharoplasty offered emotional and mental palliation; few people were ever more pleased to have the bags removed from their eyelids. She had no jaw, could not eat but a few sips, and talked with difficulty but her life was truly enriched by this form of palliative surgery.

Plastic surgery

In a time when health care costs and resources are reaching the limits of what even a generous society can provide in terms of care and services, the era of philosophical pragmatists, utilitarians, and futilitarians is upon us. The futility of prolonging the lives of those with terminal illnesses is being emphasized. This is not a new idea. In mobile societies, the elderly, the severely injured, and the otherwise unproductive were left behind as the band, tribe, or whatever unit involved moved on. It was a matter of practical utility that such persons were to be left behind; the survival of the majority depended on it. I submit that many who are disfigured and deformed by their disease, whether it is cancer or burns, become as incapable of production in our society, as was Dorothy, long before their disease is metastatic or terminal.

Plastic surgeons have been on this ethical cusp for a long time; a history which dates to antiquity when the most awful punishment, short of death, was to have one's nose amputated for a crime – the disfigurement was a public marking of the misdeed. When the term of punishment was theoretically completed, earliest plastic surgeons tried to correct it; to mitigate that the punishment might not be lifetime banishment. Unwanted children were abandoned and, although some healthy appearing infants might be adopted and raised as slaves, the deformed and disfigured faced inevitable death. Throughout most of history, children with cleft lips were left to die and the famous story of Oedipus is part of our vocabulary.* No religion advocates the killing of other human beings without just cause such as self-defence against a potentially mortal attack, individually or as a nation in the form of a just war or, more controversially, capital punishment. Societies which have come to killing infants, the elderly, the mentally defective, or the insane have in general determined that rather than determining just cause, they have determined that a category of humans are not truly human and as such have no right to the respect which human dignity should deserve. This has been a dilemma for plastic surgeons since we have cared for a portion of society, the deformed, who have in many societies been determined to be less than human and less deserving of life itself. One of my teachers observed that 'it is the divine right of man to look human'. Whether it is a child with a cleft lip or an adult with a disfiguring result from a burn or from cancer treatment, a form of palliative care is to endeavour to make the person appear and feel human.

I should like to explore briefly how this form of surgery may be appropriate for wounds and deformity, even for those with advanced disease.

General

Mental/emotional/psychological

The fear of deformity from surgery is often almost as bad as the fear of the disease itself, whether it be cancer or burns or injury. The fear of pain, whether it be in the recovery room, the burn unit, the changing of burn dressings, or the terminal phases of cancer, is almost as bad as the pain itslef. The data hardly need re-emphasis to those involved in these issues but the relief of pain is one of the most poorly understood and taught subjects in nursing and medical schools and residencies. Similarly is the fear of disfigurement or deformity as part of the treatment of cancer, burns, or other life-threatening disease. Surveys of nurses, therapists, students, and others who work in burn centres almost uniformly aver that, were they to be burned and admitted to the burn centre, that they wished to die. Fear of pain was part of it, fear of dressing changes and skin grafts was part of it, but the largest part was the fear of the resulting deformity and what it meant to them as part of continuing acceptance and productivity in an appearance-oriented society. Dax Cowart wanted to die rather than face his disfigurement and deformity from his burns and he sued his doctors to let him die. So too with Dorothy. There was no question that the hospital became the only accepting society in Dorothy's life and times have not changed that much.

....

* When Queen Jocasta learned from the Oracle that the child she was carrying would kill her husband, the king, she disfigured the newborn male by binding and injuring his feet to make them swollen (oedema = swelling and pus or pes = feet) and thus he became named Oedipus or 'swollen feet'. He was adopted anyway and the rest is 'history'.

Several decades ago, patients who had undergone major ablative surgery of the anterior jaw were, like Dorothy, not reconstructed initially. Actually one of these patients who had his jaw removed became very famous when a cartoon character, Andy Gump, was modelled after him. The operation in which the jaw was removed and not reconstructed became known as the 'Andy Gump' operation. I heard it said that no reconstruction, as for Dorothy, should be begun until patients had survived a year and demonstrated that they were free of disease. It is now clear that few, particularly of the ablative surgeons, had the faintest idea how to rebuild these patients. There has been a recent reiteration of this process in the modern approach to breast reconstruction. For decades, no reconstruction after mastectomy was considered appropriate; again, we had little capability to successfully accomplish the recon-struction. Even after techniques were developed, many surgeons advised against reconstruc-tion, or to wait a year to see if there would be recurrence. The evolution has been to less disfiguring surgery, even to the ablation of the primary tumour by ultrasound or directed thermal destruction, without surgery. The driving force was appearance, deformity, disfig-urement, not necessarily the very best odds for survival. The patients were the driving force in these changes, not the surgeons.

At least from a mental, psychological point of view, surgery to minimize or ameliorate defor-mity from treatment or disease is palliative; it 'cloaks' the deformity and makes tolerable the inevitability of death.

Physical

Once the concept of a surgical approach is accepted, it is possible to imagine many surgical procedures which are 'palliative' in the sense that they relieve physical discomfort or limita-tions but which have essentially no effect on the course or outcome of the underlying disease. It would seem obvious that a surgical ablation of, for instance, the eye with the orbit and a portion of the maxilla might appropriately be closed with the rotation of skin or skin-muscle flap rather than leaving an open cavity. Prosthetic devices are part of the armamentarium of the reconstructive surgeon to replace lost parts (noses and ears for instance) when surgical reconstruction is not feasible. A surgical procedure to implant osteo-integrated devices is often useful to make fixation of prosthetics secure and obviate the embarrassment of having an artifical ear, for instance, come loose while swimming or while adjusting glasses.

Scarring is part of healing; from surgery but even from radiation or other ablative techniques. All scars contract and as they do, their length becomes shorter. The shortening of a linear scar may pull on an eyelid or a lip and cause visible distortion and have functional consequences as well. The surgical release of these, even in the face of uncontrolled cancer, may alleviate physical as well as mental distress.

Special procedures

It has been said that plastic surgery is a speciality of 'bed sores and bad sores'. These are special issues regarding palliative care that require some special consideration.

Pressure sores/bed sores

Frederick

Frederick is a 75-year-old man who has experienced several strokes and is now in a chronic care facility. Unable to feed or dress himself, he is only passively aware of his surroundings and does not recognize family members. He has severe spasms in his lower extremities and has developed severe flexion contractures. Although efforts to turn him have been undertaken, he first developed a sacral ulcer and, subsequently, in response to turning to his side has developed ulcers over each greater trochanter. It seems unlikely that Frederick will survive more than a few months, even with excellent nursing care.

Frederick's overall condition and unawareness of the need to spontaneously change position place a sometimes overwhelming burden on health care providers and, despite plaintiff desire that sores be a *res ipsa loquitor*,* not all pressure sores are completely preventable. The physical and nutritional depletion of this patient and other patients with metastatic disease, AIDS, or other pre or terminal illnesses predispose to pressure sores. Pressure sores are the result of unrelieved pressure; a few hours is more than enough to cause a full-thickness loss of tissue. When tissue is compressed, the tissue with the least effective blood supply (fat and muscle) is the first to become ischaemic and the first to become necrotic. As tissue is compressed between bone and an unyielding surface such as a bed, a board, a cast, or an unpadded chair, the skin is the last to become necrotic since it is really the most vascular. When the skin dies and a black eschar appears, the underlying cavity always seems larger than what has been predicted.

Additionally, ischaemic tissue becomes oedematous, and like oedematous burned tissue, is prone to infection, particularly from streptococci. It is one of the indications early in the care of impending pressure sores where systemic antibiotics, with an emphasis on controlling streptococci, are appropriate. Moisture and maceration also dissolve the protective keratinized outer layer of skin and make it additionally prone to infection.

Pressure sores are, therefore, not only fresh wounds but ischaemia and infection both cause inflammation which aggravates discomfort. The approach to pressure sores must recognize these factors.

Treatment involves:

◆ Relieve any further pressure.
◆ Penicillin or other anti-streptococcal agent early.
◆ Prevent maceration and moisture which disposes to infection.
◆ Debride the wound, preferably by excision, to remove necrotic and dying tissue.
◆ Eliminate infection. Measure bacterial levels and employ topical anti-bacterial agents.
◆ Close the wound, maybe!

The first measure is self-evident. The elimination of infection is less intuitive. Infection in pressure sores as in all open wounds, including burns, is the result of a concentration of bacteria within the involved tissue itself. Early use of systemic antibacterials may prevent streptococcal infection. Elegant studies have repeatedly demonstrated that these contaminated wounds soon become isolated from the bloodstream, and antibiotics, administered systemically, fail to reach the tissue in adequate enough amounts to reduce the measured number of micro-organisms in

---

* *Res ipsa loquitor*, translated as 'the thing speaks for itself', implies in legal terms that the situation, here a pressure sore, is obviously the result of negligence and could not, in fact, occur without negligence. If this were accepted by the court, the burden of proof would switch to the defence to prove that the pressure sore was not the result of negligence. This relieves the plaintiff from having to prove negligence through evidence and expert testimony.

the wound. A truly important advance in managing such wounds and burns is the recognition that, to adequately control bacterial growth, the antibacterial must be delivered directly to the wound. Topical antibacterials such as silver sulfadiazine reduce wound contamination, and critically to this situation, reduce pain and promote spontaneous healing.

When it comes to consideration of closing pressure sores in very ill patients, such as Frederick, particularly where the nutritional status is poor, one should recognize that not all wounds need to be closed. Most of the pain is due to inflammation and infection, and when controlled with topical antibacterials becomes less of a problem. Good dressing care, including the use of gels, limits the amount of protein loss through the wound itself. Finally, the closure of pressure sores is more complicated than it would appear. Unless the underlying factors that caused the sore in the first place are completely eliminated, which is very difficult, prompt recurrence after closure can be anticipated. In fact, experience indicates that more than half of all pressure sore closures have broken down within a year. It is surgical truism that 'when one loses sight of the objectives, one has to redouble the efforts'.

When managing pressure sores in the palliative situation, the goal is usually to relieve pain, to reduce the depletion of nutrients through the wound, and render overall management easier. Only when closure of the wound can be done quickly, effectively, and with little morbidity should a surgical procedure be considered as part of the definitive management. Frederick should have his wounds managed by topical antibacterials; no surgical procedure is appropriate.

Other bad sores

Although pressure sores are the most common, there are other wounds that may present in patients with advanced or terminal disease. I remember asking and answering the question as to whether a skin graft would successfully 'take' when applied to an ulcer on the leg caused by a leukaemic infiltrate; it does! Patients with serious and terminal illnesses who are malnourished are subject to all the other problems that other patients experience. A thrombosed haemorrhoid is as uncomfortable and reversible in a terminal patient as in anyone else. Such problems as leg ulcers, abscesses, avulsions, and lacerations may occur in any of these patients and should be definitively managed.

The most important message I wish to convey is that ulcerations from tumours are painful for very much the same reason as in pressure sores. They are oedematous and subject to infection which is much of the reason for the pain. Relief of the inflammation and tissue contamination with the use of topical antibacterials will make the difference.

Gertrude Gertrude, mentioned at the beginning of the chapter, faces the possibility of a painful, necrotic, foul-smelling wound on her chest. The fact that tumour is recurrent in the wound and in underlying ribs places her situation into the category of patient with advanced disease. No surgical procedure would be curative. However, debridement of obviously necrotic tissue, even if it requires an operative procedure under general anaesthetic, should help reduce her pain. I believe much of the pain of these ulcers is due to infection and, once again, I believe in topical antibacterial agents and monitoring of the wound with serial quantitative cultures of the bacterial flora. Whether the wound should be closed depends on the clinical response to the above measures. Often a wound that has been radiated, even one that contains malignancy, will respond to the above measures and become less painful and, in fact, develop granulation tissue onto which a skin graft may be applied successfully. Such a closed wound is usually much less painful, even though recurrence in the wound may occur. The closed wound would minimize infection and allow chemotherapy. More indolent wounds may be closed by the rotation of healthy muscle from the regions such as the latissimus dorsi or rectus abdominis muscles, onto which healthy-muscle skin grafts may be placed.

Gertrude may, in fact, receive her greatest palliation from her advanced disease by thoughtful, scientifically sound wound management.

Burn care

I am hard pressed to identify a surgical condition which seems further away from our concepts of palliative care than burn injury. Burn injury, as with most traumatic events, is unanticipated. Whereas the diagnosis of cancer or AIDS is made, information may be delivered to patient and family with sensitivity and the implications learned and understood on reflection. When the prognosis for survival is thought to be only a matter of months, this information may also be delivered and patient and family supported. Not so with burn injury. Well one moment, in excruciating pain the next. Depending on the patient, the nature of the burn injury (fire, chemical, electrical), the location of the injury (trunk, face, extremities, genitalia, etc.), the depth of the burn (varying from the most superficial to that involving the full thickness of the skin), the size of the burn (measured as a percentage of total body surface [TBSA]), and the associated injuries (inhalation of smoke, falls with fractures, etc.), the severity of the injury is highly variable. It is impossible to generalize about burn injury other than to say that all are painful, and for most serious burns there is the danger of death or, with survival, disfigurement and disability. It is a most difficult time for patient and family alike. The crisis of the situation makes deliberation and reflection all but impossible and the responsibility of the treating surgeon becomes immense.

Bryan

Bryan was an 18-year-old man who sustained incinerating burn injury over about 98% total body surface area when he was trapped in an automobile in an accident in which his fiancée was killed. He was intubated at the scene and arrived in the burn centre within an hour of injury. The depth of his injury was unquestionably full thickness and it was clear to the team that survival would be impossible ('unprecedented') and we so informed his parents. Since Bryan had not sustained major burn to his upper airway and immediate airway obstruction was not likely, I chose to remove the endotracheal tube. As is common among burn patients, no matter how large the burn, the patient was conscious and alert, albeit in pain. Morphine was titrated intravenously and it was possible to share information with Bryan. He had the opportunity to speak to his parents at some length and they had the opportunity to share expressions of love and affection. He had the opportunity to meet with the chaplain and some of his friends.

Intravenous fluids were given to alleviate thirst and he was also allowed to drink fluids. When the burn eschar in the lower chest began to constrict respiration and cause apprehension, escharotomies released the chest wall and provided comfort. Bryan was given adequate morphine so that apprehension and pain relief were adequate during the eight hours that he remained alive. Nothing, including the removal of the endotrachal tube, was done to hasten his death.

Burn management

Bryan, a young man in otherwise good health, would have been an almost ideal prospect for surviving major injury, including burns. It was clear, however, that his situation was hopeless and no effort would have saved his life. He fell into a category of burn injury to which we refer as 'unprecedented survival'. Burn mortality is largely a function of the size of the burn and the age of the patient. At the extremes of life, infants and those over age 60 years have a poor prognosis for almost any burn which involves more than 20% of the TBSA. Some young children have survived burns in excess of 90% TBSA but, in general, burns over 50% TBSA will have an expected mortality of at least 50%.

A burn injury is the ultimate wound management problem. Just like any other open wound, the imperative is to close the wound. Burn wounds must heal either by re-epithelialization of the burned wound itself or by skin grafts. If the burn injury is partial thickness, some of the epidermal elements in the hair follicles and glands allow the wound to resurface itself and heal without skin grafts. This, of course, is the same mechanism that allows healing of the donor sites from which skin grafts are removed. When the wound is full thickness, wound closure can be accomplished only by contraction of the margins or by the application of skin grafts. It is often forgotten or misunderstood that all skin grafts must be from the patient's own skin. Skin obtained from other species (xenografts – usually pig skin) or from cadavers (allografts) provides only temporary coverage and will always be rejected by the patient. Cultured skin may be occasionally used in which small biopsies of the patient's own skin are grown in tissue culture to expand a small sample into many sheets of epithelium. This cultured skin is fragile, requires that there be essentially no contamination, and lacks a substantial dermal network to provide structural support. These techniques are not readily available and may cost hundreds of thousands of dollars for a major burn injury. If more than 50% of the body is burned, the remaining, unburned skin must be the source of skin for covering the open wounds. Much of this unburned skin, however, may be in areas such as the face, the genitalia, the hands or feet, or other areas which are not suitable as donor sites.

Unprecedented survival

Bryan was in this category; no patients with burns of his size and depth, at any age, have survived. It is sometimes possible, as in this case, within minutes of the patient's arrival in the burn centre to determine that the patient has no chance for survival. I have made the diagnosis and determined that prognosis is hopeless only reluctantly. Since his death was inevitable, within hours or, at the most, days, how should he be managed in a 'palliative' fashion?

Intubation

The first consideration in Bryan's case was his endotracheal tube. It is almost a reflex action for Emergency Medical Technicians (EMTs) to insert an endotracheal tube to maintain an airway on burned patients, particularly when the burns are around the face. However, even in patients who have been burned about the face and nose, the pharyngeal tissue and laryngeal and tracheal portion of the airway is almost never burned. The problem with the airway and lungs in burned patients is from smoke and not from heat; the chemical reaction from the smoke often does not develop for 18–24 hours. There is almost no therapeutic reason for maintaining a patient intubated, particularly when we have determined that the patient is not going to survive the injury. The tube, whenever possible, should be removed and the patient allowed to talk. Surprisingly, most patients, even with lethal injuries, can be clear and converse for a period of time. They should be given this opportunity. I removed Bryan's tube and he had the opportunity to talk to his family and to the chaplain.

There were those on my team who indicated that their preference, in this circumstance, would be to receive morphine and remain unconscious until death occurs. This is a balance between death in the situation where one 'never knew what hit him' and the opportunity to say the last farewells.

Resuscitation

Burned patients lose immense amounts of fluid into their tissues and by evaporation. A patient burned over 50% TBSA, who weighs about 70 kg, would be expected to require about 16–18 litres of electrolyte solution in the first 24 hours after injury (half in the first eight hours) to maintain adequate urine output, the usual parameter of successful resuscitation. It is inappropriate to force intravenous fluids on patients whom we have determined will not survive. Rather than striving for some arbitrary urine output, therefore, we should attempt to determine whether the patient is experiencing uncomfortable thirst and, if so, provide adequate hydration. Patients who are aware and thirsty should be given fluids by mouth, even at the risk of some gastric dilatation, which is surprisingly uncommon. It goes without saying that intubation of the gastrointestinal tract is inappropriate; tubes in the nose and mouth are uniformly uncomfortable.

Surgical procedures

It would seem implausible that any surgical procedure in these circumstances would be appropriate but some may be useful. Burn wounds uniformly become oedematous. When the swelling occurs beneath unyielding, full-thickness, charred, burned tissue (eschar), the constriction can be painful and, on occasion, contribute to apprehension, even panic. On occasion, the release of such eschar can be salutary, particularly when the eschar is constricting the chest and limiting breathing. A release of the constricting burn eschar around Bryan's chest made breathing easier and relieved apprehension. Since the eschar is made up of charred skin, nerve fibres have been destroyed and incisions through eschar are usually painless, can be done without even local anaesthetic and at the bedside in an intensive care unit.

Pain relief

The observation that burned patients often have fairly clear mentation, at least initially, places the burn team on the horns of a dilemma. There is, perhaps, no more excruciating pain than burns, particularly large burns. It is medical and surgical imperative that this pain be relieved to the degree possible. Because of the unstable cardiovascular system in the face of the major fluid shifts which accompany burn injury in the first 24–48 hours, all pain medication must be given intravenously and titrated to the patient's degree of relief. Unfortunately, relief can often be achieved only at the expense of complete consciousness.

Patients who have had severe inhalation injury may require intubation, pulmonary assistance with a respirator, and coincidentally the need to induce total somnolence and paralysis. This presents a somewhat different circumstance from Bryan's: communication directly with the patient becomes impossible and the desires of the patient can only be inferred. When the situation is one in which survival would be 'unprecedented', it is usually possible to infer that the patient, if in a position to make a decision, would choose comfort care rather than intrusive manoeuvers that have no chance of success. I would argue that such patients should be given sufficient morphine to relieve all apprehension, even if it is necessary to render the patient unconscious.

Summary

Patients with advanced diseases of many kinds often encounter wounds as either a part of their disease itself or coincidentally with their overall condition. Patients who have undergone major ablative surgery, even if the surgery was not curative, always benefit from successful closure of their operative wounds and, often, reconstructive surgery of accompanying deformity. The biological imperative in wound management is successful wound closure. Many of the general and local factors which adversely affect normal wound healing can be successfully managed, even in people with advanced disease. Special attention has been directed toward reconstructive procedures, wound closure in contaminated wounds, and in the management of pressure ulcers. Management of burn patients with lethal injuries also often involves surgical procedures and attention to their wounds.

References

1. Robson, M.C., Steed, D.L., and Franz, M.G. (2001). Wound healing: biologic features and approaches to maximize healing trajectories. *Curr. Prob. Surg.*, **38** (2), 72–140.

2. Robson, M.C., Edstrom, L.E., Krizek, T.J., and Groskin, M.G. (1974). The efficacy of systemic antibiotics in the treatment of granulating wounds. *J. Surg. Res.*, **16**, 299–306.

3. Carrel, A., and Dehelly, G. (1919). *The treatment of infected wounds*. Paul B. Hoeber, New York.

4. Simon, R.L., (1991). *Fair play: sports, values, and society*. Westview Press, Boulder.

5. Video (1975). *Please let me die*. Interview by Dr Robert, B. White with Dax Cowart. University of Texas Medical Branch film series, Galveston.

6. Klever, L.D. (ed.) (1989). *Dax's case: essays in medical ethics and human meaning*. Southern Methodist University Press, Dallas.

Chapter 15

Neurosurgical palliation

Dennis L. Johnson

Introduction

This text lays the groundwork for a new competence in surgery and a new approach to the way we care for our patients – to care more about healing than curing – to confront human suffering in its totality, rather than just human disease. As our technology advances and the cost of health care continues to escalate, we tend to isolate ourselves from the suffering of patients in order to see more patients and perform more surgery. A 'non-surgical' abdomen begs the question of diagnosis and absolves the surgeon of further responsibility. A neurosurgeon delegates the care of a stroke victim to a neurologist or intensivist when we lack the surgical technology to 'fix' or cure the problem at hand. Eric Cassell has asserted that one of the strange intellectual paradoxes of our time is the separation of the disease that underlies the suffering from both the person and the suffering itself, as though the scientific entity of disease is more real and more important than the person and the suffering.[1]

Caring more about the patients that we are called to serve and stretching our professional lives even thinner is not enough. Attitudes and professional behaviour must change. There is a thin interval that separates our humility from arrogance and our courage from our fear of failure. It is easier to mend bodies with our hands than to explore what is in their hearts and minds.

The definition of palliative surgery and medicine used in this chapter is given scope by a discussion of suffering and how suffering is bound into the patient–physician relationship. The value of the physician's presence in the healing process is emphasized. A discussion of hope and miracles has been included. How do we offer hope when nothing more can be done?

The general principles that follow are applicable to the palliative care of any surgical patient. The section on methodology provides a framework upon which to apply those principles. Even though palliative surgery is hardly another speciality and is something that each of us does every day, the criteria or indications for palliative consultation will provide a greater sense of when to think about palliative care and when a referral is appropriate. The case studies of patients, who suffer benign pain, malignant pain, malignant brain tumours, hydrocephalus, intracranial injury, and intracerebral haemorrhage, bring to focus how, what, why, when, and where palliative care impacts the individual patient with a particular emphasis on the neurosurgical patient.

The chapter will include topics of neurosurgical palliation which are addressed separately and more expertly in other surgical textbooks, such as gamma knife, the surgical treatment of epilepsy, movement disorders, affective disorders, vertigo, spasmodic torticollis, and spasticity.

Definitions

Palliative medicine and surgery is the active, total care of patients who suffer from incurable diseases. The *pall-* of *palliative* care defines the velvet covering which protects the coffin. The image is a flag-draped coffin pulled in a caisson by a team of black horses, followed by the riderless black horse with the dead rider's boots set backwards in the stirrups. It is an honour and privilege to be a *pall* bearer. When you accompany your patients in the journey to the end of their lives – when you walk through the valley of the shadow of death – you may have to carry them. You will become a pallbearer and have the honour and privilege to bring closure.

To separate palliative surgery from palliative medicine is as sophistic as separating medicine from surgery or neurology from neurosurgery. Palliation is a concept which is not new to neurosurgery. The neurosurgeon sees far more incurable diseases than conditions that can be cured. Indeed, the history of surgery and neurosurgery is an imperfect account of how the concept of palliative medicine has developed. Just as armed conflict is a staging ground for many other developments in surgery, the battlefield is also where the surgeon is confronted with untold suffering, engages the many dimensions of pain, and witnesses the urgency of palliation. The wounds of war may be mendable, but they are not curable.

Skill sets in palliative surgery (Box 15.1)

The most important skill in palliative care is the ability to communicate with patients and their families. The skill involves more than the gift of the gab but acknowledges the common ground of our humanity – that we are bidden to care for one another. The common ground can be more tangible in the form of common interests, mutual respect, and shared values. Understanding the patient's values, interests, and spirituality is key to helping the patient make difficult decisions and caring for them during the dying process. Pain management is often referred to the Pain Service but is as much the province of palliative care. There are many dimensions of pain, and the management of pain includes the entire family. Non-pain symptoms such as nausea, dyspnoea, and pruritis can be more disabling than pain. Finally, knowledge of health care plans, health maintenance organizations, Medicare, and hospice benefits as well as the capabilities of local long-term acute care facilities, rehabilitation hospitals, nursing homes, and home care resources are important to helping the patient and family create an enduring plan of care.

Box 15.1 Skill sets in palliative surgery

- Managing the dying process
- Communicating with patients and families
- Psychosocial and spiritual care
- Decision making
- Management of complications of treatment
- Pain management
- Non-pain symptom management
- Venues and systems of care

The dimensions of suffering (Box 15.2)

Soelle has said, 'Unbearable suffering excludes change and learning. The weight of unbearable suffering makes us feel totally helpless; we are stripped of the autonomy to think, speak, and act.'[2] Suffering has many dimensions. The *physical* dimension is displayed by the entrenched soldier with cold, wet feet or the patient with a brain tumour who has an eye-closing headache. The same soldier may fear the night as much as he fears the howl of the aircraft overhead. The brain-tumour patient also feels the separation of what used to be known from what is now uncertain – the *emotional* impact of his illness and the fear. While Sigmund Freud was being treated for cancer of the mandible in 1939, he remarked, 'The people around me have tried to wrap me in a cocoon of optimism: the cancer is shrinking, the reactions to the treatment are only temporary, etc. I don't believe any of it and don't like being deceived.'[3]

Knowing that increasing headache or a worsening gait is a sign of progressive or recurrent malignant brain tumour or understanding that complete paralysis may follow increasing 'malignant' back pain adds yet another '*cognitive*' dimension to suffering, just as knowing that an artillery barrage precedes the next wave of the onrushing army.

The *spiritual* aspects of suffering often revolve around the patients' relationship with their God. The word spirit is derived from the Hebrew root *breath* and from the Latin word *wind*. Thus the theologian Marcus Borg has defined spirituality as the wind around us and the breath within us.[4] Similarly, Dietrick Bonhoeffer spoke of spirituality as 'the beyond amongst us'. War threatens the breath within us and dims the beyond amongst us.[5] The soldier suffers because his God could allow this killing to take place or kills in the name of his God. The sick and dying patient suffers 'Why me?' and 'How could God do this to me?' The dying patient may be suffering retribution for yesterday's sins.

In a Godless world, man is unique and isolated in a tough, hostile environment, and human experience is not explainable. We are who we are and make choices. Spirituality is defined by who we are and what we value – home, family, acres of ploughed fields, a larger salary, and a bright, new car. In a Godless war, the soldier is stripped of his identity and wears the same helmet as all the other soldiers. He is separated from home, family, and loved ones. The hospitalized patient suffers similar losses. The *existential* suffering of the soldier and the dying patient stems from the inexplicability of human experience – and drifting into the final void of nothingness.

Pain and suffering are often considered synonymous. On the other hand, depression can be one of the worst forms of 'unbearable' suffering but have nothing to do with pain. Though they are much alike, pain may be limited to a physical dimension or may have emotional, spiritual, cognitive, and existential dimensions.

The physical dimension of pain can be classified as nociceptive or neuropathic. Nociceptive pain is a normal physiological response to a painful stimulus which avoids injury and is designed

Box 15.2 The dimensions of suffering

- Physical
- Emotional
- Spiritual
- Cognitive
- Existential

to preserve life. Nociceptive pain changes with position and activity. On the other hand, neuropathic pain is an inappropriate, pathological, or uninterpretable response which has no protective or survival value.

Pain can supersede its physical dimension if the pain is seen as divine retribution for past wrongs or sins. The cognitive impact of a pain of unknown origin may weigh heavily when summed with other dimensions of suffering.

The patient–physician relationship

The trust and confidence that a patient derives from the presence of the attending physician and the commitment of the physician to the continuing care of the patient helps sustain him through his illness. More importantly, the dying patient is comforted by the promise of non-abandonment. The strength and substance of such relationships is alluded to by the Judaic philosopher, Martin Buber, who described the relationship between 'Ich' (or 'I') and 'Du' (familiar form of 'You').[6]

The relationship is characterized by mutual acceptance, giving, and understanding. The Venn diagram in Figure 15.1 graphically demonstrates this bond. The two circles that represent the relationship of the two people may be at a distance from one another to represent an acquaintance or social contact, or they may simply touch to indicate a business partner or colleague. The overlapping circles connote a marriage, lasting friendship, brotherhood, or 'blood' tie, which are joined in trust, clarity, and commitment. The degree to which the circles overlap signifies the depth of commitment and trust – the patient–doctor bond. The Venn diagram (Figure 15.2) can be expanded by a third circle that symbolizes the patient's disease or dying. The degree to which the circles of disease and 'I' overlap denotes the degree to which the patient understands their disease; similarly, the overlap of the physician and disease represents the understanding or perspicacity of the physician with the disease. Where the three circles interlock could represent resolution – not cure or antidote, but hope. And what hope is there in dying?

Offering hope when there is nothing more that can be done

Hoping for a miracle cure is the epitome of the great American dream and is the colossal public charade that has driven health care into bankruptcy. Hope becomes the patient's fight for

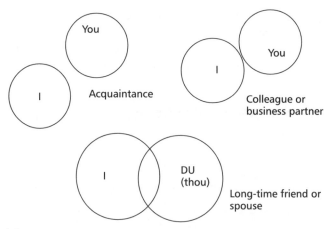

Fig. 15.1 I and thou.

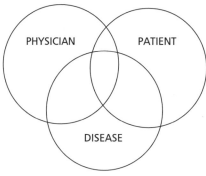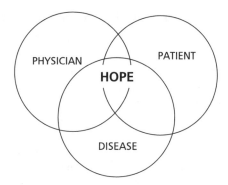

Fig. 15.2 Hope.

life and the family's crusade to find the most hopeful treatment. The 'fight' for life becomes the patient's preoccupation and wastes valuable life time. And what hope is there in dying?

Through the voice of Claudio in *Measure for Measure*, William Shakespeare reminds us that 'The miserable have no other medicine; but only hope.' What hope is there in dying? You cannot give up your fight for life!

'There is nothing more that can be done!' rings hollow to the sick and dying patient. For the interlocking rings of the Venn diagram to separate at this critical point in time is unimaginable; that the physician would abandon his patient is inconceivable. We are drawn back to Eric Cassell's assertion that we cannot separate the disease from the person or the suffering – that they need to be managed as one – and the care extends to death.[1] In the *Compact Oxford Dictionary*, hope is defined as an expectation of something desired, a feeling of trust or confidence, or promise. In Scotland, a *hope* is a small, enclosed valley, branching outward from the main dale and running up to the mountain ranges. The twenty-third Psalm reads, 'yea, though I walk through the *valley* of the shadow of death, I will fear no evil: for thou art with me; thy rod and thy staff comfort me.' We can still assuage suffering even if it means carrying them through a 'small valley' of hope in the final stage of their journey.

So what hope is there in dying? You can't give up the 'fight'! Unfathomable hopes include the hope to be cured, the hope that death can be avoided, and the hope of winning the lottery. Christ's crucifixion and resurrection gives hope of everlasting life. In the small valley, hope is the way home, comfort, freedom from pain, forgiveness, and love. These are fathomable hopes – hopes that we can promise to fulfil. Palliative care gives the hope of dying comfortably, instead of the certainty of dying in agony. Palliative care offers the hope and support of dying at home in place of dying in the hospital. 'There is nothing more that can be done' is replaced by 'Even though your disease does not seem curable, I can still help you, listen to you, comfort you, value you, and care for you until you die'.

But the 'fight' may continue in the mind of the patient and family to hold out against the shame of failure in our culture. Comments like 'She's given up the fight' or 'There's no more fight in him' are dispiriting, derogatory, and demeaning. These statements only perpetrate the myth that you only need to keep trying and fighting to win. Homer in *The Iliad* tells us 'It is not possible to fight beyond your strength, even if you strive.' The comforting or palliative process should begin long before death comes to heal the spirit, to validate the patient's self-esteem, and to prepare closure. There is no fight at the end of life. There is peace.

Of dying and dignity: moving towards death

When all is said and done, taking care of incurable patients is hard work and can dull the senses. When a patient is dying or incurable, we often stop going into the hospital room and prefer to 'round' outside the room. And then we stop rounding. Nurses may similarly 'bottom' the patient on their list of priorities and may stop turning and bathing the patient. 'As needed' medications are not given because the patient is unable to ask, lacks the strength to find the call button, or is simply not seen very often. We hate failure when we suffer loss. We fear death, and we fear dying. The image of 'dust to dust' frightens us.

We are called to relieve suffering. We are bidden to care for one another, and the mitigation of suffering is the enduring goal of medicine and its measure of continuing success. As the patient dies, we should not push them away and drain away our own spirit and 'burn out' our sensitivity. We can draw them to us, comfort them, and carry them if necessary in the last leg of their journey. We absorb their strength and character and become stronger ourselves and more capable of 'carrying on' (Figures 15.3–15.7).

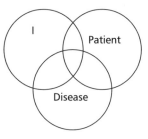

Fig. 15.3 The original Venn diagram describes an intimate bond with the patient and thorough awareness of disease.

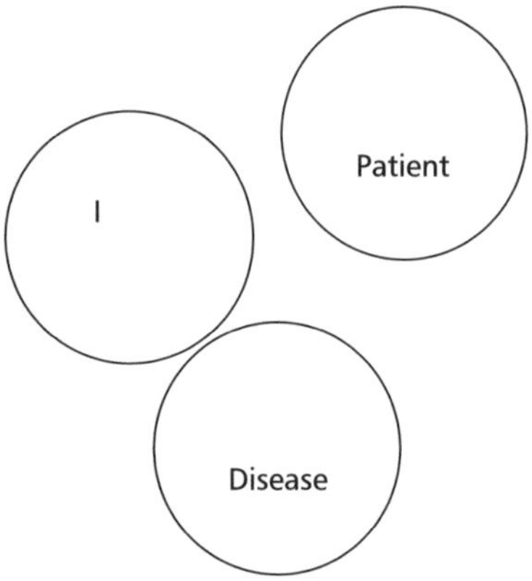

Fig. 15.4 The patient pushed away. As the patient begins to die or has a disease which cannot be cured, we insulate ourselves and push the patient away.

Fig. 15.5 Drawing nigh. We can draw them to us, comfort them, and carry them if necessary. Listening and *presence* become more important than radiographs or the scalpel.

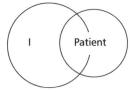

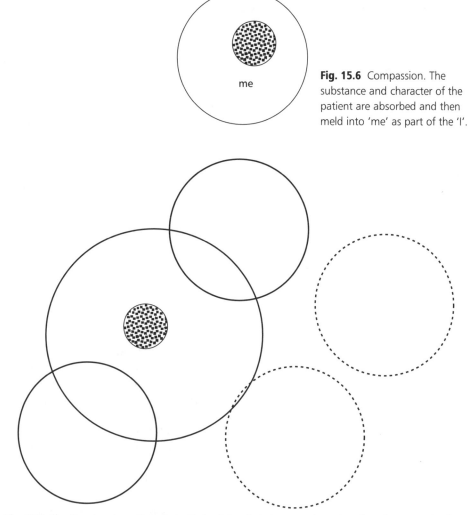

Fig. 15.6 Compassion. The substance and character of the patient are absorbed and then meld into 'me' as part of the 'I'.

Fig. 15.7 The 'I' gains strength and depth (and the circle becomes larger) and carries on to develop other bonds and relationships.

Guiding principles

The simplicity of these principles bears testimony to their validity.

Relieve pain and suffering

Pain and suffering are often considered synonymous. Though they are much alike, pain may be limited to a physical dimension or may also have spiritual and cognitive dimensions. Pain can supersede its physical dimension if the pain is seen as divine retribution for past wrongs or sins. The cognitive impact of a pain of unknown origin may weigh heavily when summed with other dimensions of suffering. On the other hand, depression can be one of the worst forms of 'unbearable' suffering but have nothing to do with pain. Nausea can have no association with pain but may eclipse any sense of comfort or peace. To implement this guideline is no easy task.

Facilitate clarity of thought

Facilitate clarity of thought that is consistent with amelioration of suffering. More can be done for patients than to just 'put them down' with a narcotic drip. Confusion, sundowning, hallucinations, and depression can be successfully managed at the end of life. Demented, agitated, psychotic, and aphasic patients are particularly challenging.

Maximize quality of life

Maximize the quality of the life that remains before death. The interventions that are used are always weighed on a scale of risks and benefits. The treatment of life-threatening illnesses is not a lottery ticket. If you lose the lottery, you only lose the money you invested. If salvage chemotherapy, which was the hope for a cure (winning the lottery), is not effective, the patient's life may be shortened and made more miserable by pain, malaise, asthenia, bone marrow depression, mucositis, and sepsis.

Methodology

The issue is how to mitigate suffering, and the task is how to move from curing to healing (Box 15.3). Look for and find *meaning* in the patient's life outside of suffering. Discover the *origin* of the suffering to focus the management. The next step is to *validate* the meaning of the patient's life for the patient as well as the family, even in the context of suffering. This step is as important as managing the symptoms of illness. Finally, it is important to envision an *end* to suffering. Not only must symptoms of pain, nausea, and dyspnoea be relieved, but the patient often wants to know when death can be expected. Uncertainty breeds anxiety and blocks closure.

Moving from theory to practice often separates the academic who writes textbooks and publishes papers from the clinician who is consumed by the practice of medicine. Though clinicians who love to write are more facile in writing about the practical aspects of medicine or surgery, personal experience is often discounted as anecdotal or paternalistic and put aside. But an anecdotal case of *one* may be the difference between zero and one – the difference between futility and discovery. Allow me to share my personal advice and then to provide methodological framework for initiating palliative care.

Box 15.3 MOVE from cure to healing

- Meaning
- Origin of suffering
- Validate meaning
- Envision an end

Some personal advice

Since I don't own their space, I ask for permission to come aboard. Don't stand over the bed, sit at the side of the bed where eye contact is on the same level. If you have residents that accompany you, introduce them, but if you forget that they are there, the patient will also.

Not everyone wants to be touched, but don't be afraid to hold an old man's hand. I am sincere about my presence. I am non-judgemental and accept the patients for who they are at that point in time.

Allow for silence. Silence is uncomfortable for physicians, especially surgeons. Let the hard conversation go forward; don't change the subject. Avoid clichés. Conversation about the person that died or who is dying helps to bring closure.

Listen to feelings as well as thoughts. Angry accusatory outbursts are feelings, which must be heard and acknowledged. Sometimes the best that you have to offer is to echo the patient's words, e.g. 'You sound angry, and this place stinks!' 'I know just how you feel' just doesn't cut it. Being supportive, but not condescending, is part of reflecting a positive outlook.

A framework for palliation

1 Develop spiritual history: what is important to the patient. *What has meaning to the patient?* Life at any cost, physical functions, cognitive functions? What defines the limits of life? What are the patient's priorities? God, family, children, job, community, self, a dog or cat, birds in the garden? Vanity, athleticism?

2 Explore experimental, hypothetical, and standard palliative management options. Non-traditional options may have a place.

3 Explain the emotional and physical costs of treatment in terms of the patient's experience.

4 Estimate minimum, mean, and maximum life expectancy with and without treatment.

5 Make best recommendation to patient and family based on point 1 above.

6 Manage the symptoms and complications of treatment.

7 The team members most essential to providing the best outcome and an enduring care plan are a social worker and a nurse coordinator. Regularly planned conferences with the family, patient, and care-givers are key in coordinating care. A single meeting seldom solves conflicts.

8 Anticipate grief and have a mechanism for bereavement follow-up.

Criteria for referral or consultation

Physicians often wait to refer the patient until the clinical problem becomes insufferable.

- *Hospitalization longer than 7 days.* Prolonged hospitalization raises the spectre of futile treatment or that disposition is problematic. Enduring dispositions reduce the rate of hospital readmission.

- *Anticipated morbidity of ≥50%.* If complications do occur, coordination of care becomes problematic, and communication with the family is all the more important.

- *Anticipated mortality of ≥20%.* Developing a 'Plan B' ahead of time lays the groundwork for a timely transition to the appropriate level of care.

- *Problematic family communication.* Although too many cooks spoil the stew, two heads are often better than one.

- *Dysfunctional family or high level of anxiety.* Communication can be a quagmire, and usually requires more time.

- *Subarachnoid haemorrhage,* Hunt–Hess grades III and IV because of the high morbidity and mortality.

- *Patient age ≥80%; minority race.* The pain and suffering of older folks, minorities, and women tend to be neglected.

- *Return to surgical intensive care unit or transfer to medical intensive care unit.* The flag of medical or surgical futility – in not wanting to fail despite the poor prognosis and the abysmal quality of life projected.

- *Major morbidity projected*:

  – meningitis

  – impaired level of consciousness

  – stroke

  – Glasgow coma score ≤4

  – grade IV subarachnoid haemorrhage.

- *Suboptimal pain management.*

- *Malignant brain tumours.* These patients inevitably die or have major morbidity. Early recognition and acceptance of 'Plan B' facilitates care.

- *Neurofibromatosis.* This is a disease complex which does not deserve an aggressive surgical approach, but many aspects of the condition deserve better palliation.

- *Brain or spine metastases.* The emotional impact and prognostic significance of intracranial metastases is immense and a source of profound emotional and cognitive suffering. Spinal metastases and the prospect of incontinence and/or paraplegia present all the dimensions of suffering – physical, emotional, cognitive, spiritual, and existential.

- *Intractable nausea or vomiting.*

- *Cerebral palsy.* Beware the lessons of history.

- *Spina bifida.* These children become adults. There is no cure, but a great deal of palliation can be done.

- *Problematic disposition.*

Neurosurgical management of intractable pain

The patient's 'total' perception of pain is multidimensional: physical, emotional, spiritual, cognitive, and existential.[7,8] No doubt that the physical dimension of specific pain syndromes is amenable to surgical treatment. Entrapment neuropathies such as carpal tunnel syndrome can be released. Spinal nerves compressed by herniated discs and osteoarthritic spurs can be decompressed, and segmental instability of the spine can be stabilized by fusion. Causalgia and Raynaud's syndrome are relieved by sympathectomy, but sympathectomy does not reduce pain in atherosclerotic or vasculitic arterial occlusive disease. The treatment of choice for classic tic doloreux is microvascular decompression.

No doubt that the neurosurgeon can palliate the physical dimension and dull the cognitive and emotional aspects of intractable pain (through cingulotomy – see below) associated with cancer. With equal certainty, surgery can do little to palliate non-cancer pain, and the spiritual, cognitive, and 'existential dimensions of 'malignant' cancer pain and 'benign' non-cancer pain cannot be touched by the surgeon's pallet. The neurosurgical treatment of pain is not a delicate microscopic manipulation of the senses but rather a rough cut through known primitive neural pathways, like clear-cutting virgin timber, which can never be replaced.

Cancer pain

The vast majority of cancer pain can be palliated medically or with radiation therapy. For pain that is intractable to skillful medical management, a number of procedures are worthy of consideration (Figure 15.8). No neurodestructive or ablative procedure is curative, and each procedure adds an encumbrance to healing. This point was made especially poignant to me early in my career when I interviewed a patient following cingulotomy, which is the end-point (i.e. when all else fails) of all neurosurgical pain procedures. To my question, 'Do you still have pain?' she replied, 'Yes, but I just don't care anymore.'

Equipment availability and the skill and experience of the neurosurgeon often dictate the choice. Costs of these procedures are not inconsiderable.

Non-cancer pain

There are limited indications for neurodestructive or ablative surgical palliation of medically intractable non-cancer pain other than the specific, well-identified syndromes mentioned above. Nociceptive pain is often converted to neuropathic pain, which itself is not amenable

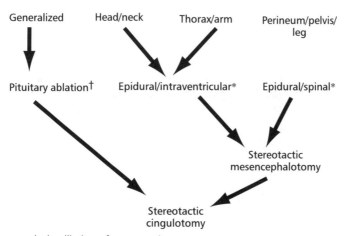

Fig. 15.8 Neurosurgical palliation of cancer pain.

*Continuous infusion or implantable pump

†Pituitary ablation

◆ Transphenoidal hypophysectomy is preferable to 'open' subfrontal hypophysectomy because the hair is not shaved and a scalp incision is not needed and spares the risk to the optic apparatus. However, postoperative nasal packing can be very uncomfortable, and CSF leakage with meningitis are potential complications of the transphenoidal approach.

◆ Stereotactic radiofrequency hypophysectomy is minimally invasive, does not endanger the visual apparatus, and avoids the risk of CSF leakage. Panhypopituitarism and diabetes insipidus are predictable.

◆ ^{60}Co Gamma Knife with 25 000 R to the pituitary fossa is perhaps the least invasive procedure but carries the same risk profile as radio-frequency pituitary ablation.

Box 15.4 Pain classification

Nociceptive (neurophysiological)

- Intermittent
- Cramping
- Aching
- Throbbing
- Sharp or shooting

Neuropathic (neuropathological)

- Steady and relentless
- Numbness
- Burning
- Crushing
- Ripping or tearing

Box 15.5 Neuropathic pain syndromes not responsive to ablative neurosurgery

- Peripheral nerve injuries
- Phantom limb
- Anaesthesia or hypaesthesia dolorosa
- Postherpetic neuralgia
- Postcordotomy dysaesthesias
- Spinal cord injury
- Thalamic pain syndrome
- Central poststroke pain

Box 15.6 Neurosurgical procedures seldom used for palliation of pain

- Dorsal spinal rhizotomy
- Ganglionectomy
- Cordotomy
- Thalamotomy

to further ablative procedures (Boxes 15.4 to 15.6). Transient improvement can be achieved by nerve root stimulation, cord stimulation, and deep brain stimulation. However, the benefit is cut short by glial proliferation around and insulation of the electrodes. The long-term benefit of most stimulation procedures is no better than the placebo effect.

Movement disorders

The first attempts to palliate movement disorders surgically date back to Victor Horsley in 1890, but enduring palliation has only been possible in the last 50 years.[9] In addition to

Box 15.7 Indications for ventrolateral thalamotomy

◆ Post-traumatic cerebellar tremor
◆ Intention tremor of multiple sclerosis
◆ Essential tremor
◆ Parkinson's disease

Box 15.8 Indications for ventroposterolateral pallidotomy

◆ Resting tremor
◆ Choreoathetosis
◆ Hemiballismus
◆ Parkinson's disease

Box 15.9 Cerebral palsy

Spasticity: pulvinotomy[14]
Athetosis: thalamotomy[15]
Choreoathetosis: pallidotomy[16]
Dystonia: thalamotomy[9]

effective palliation, stereotactic procedures have dramatically reduced both the morbidity and mortality of surgery. The principal contraindications to surgery are a life expectancy of less than six months and dementia.

The most common movement disorders are Parkinson's disease, essential tremor, and cerebral palsy, and the most effective stereotactic procedures are ventrolateral thalamotomy and ventroposterolateral pallidotomy (Boxes 15.7 and 15.8).

The tremor and rigor of Parkinson's disease are usually reduced by thalamotomy.[10–12] The rigidity, bradykinesia, dyskinesia (even when induced by levodopa), gait and balance difficulties, and myalgias of the disease are most effectively palliated by pallidotomy.[9] However, the symptoms and signs of 'Parkinson Plus' are not mitigated by pallidotomy.[13]

Essential tremor and other intention tremors are best assuaged with thalamotomy. The palliation of cerebral palsy varies according to the neurological manifestations (Box 15.9).

Thalamotomy should only be done unilaterally (stimulating electrodes can be placed in the opposite thalamus), but pallidotomy can be done either unilaterally or bilaterally. Pallidotomy can also be done following a thalamotomy.

Spasticity

The spasticity that accompanies cerebral palsy and spinal cord injury can be very disabling. Spastic diplegia can be palliated with a selective posterior rhizotomy or more simply with a 50% ablation of the posterior spinal roots which supply the legs. Intrathecal baclofen administered through an implanted pump is more versatile and can be titrated to effect. The

> ## Box 15.10 Procedures with limited expectations
>
> ◆ Bilateral anterior upper cervical rhizotomy
> ◆ Stereotactic thalamotomy
> ◆ Epidural cervical stimulation
> ◆ Microvascular lysis of the ascending root of the spinal accessory nerve and the dorsal roots of C1 and C2
> ◆ Selective neck muscle resection

downside of implantable pumps is the network of care (telemetric device, logistical network for filling and troubleshooting pumps) that is needed to back up the service and maintenance.

For disabling hemiplegic spasticity, contralateral pulvinotomy may be the most effective palliation.

Spasmotic torticollis

Spasmotic torticollis or torsion dystonia of the neck is a terribly disabling involuntary movement disorder characterized by a deformity of head and neck created by violent flexion and twisting of the head over one or the other shoulder. The disorder occurs in families, and a gene for torsion dystonia has been identified.[17]

Selective peripheral denervation of the spasmodic muscles is the technique of choice in the palliation of spasmotic torticollis (Box 15.10). The posterior primary divisions of C3, C4, C5, and C6 and the C1 and C2 roots are cut after being identified by stimualtion. The muscles involved in swallowing as well as the levator scapulae and trapezius muscles are spared to avoid swallowing difficulties and a dropped shoulder.[18]

Case studies

'Benign' non-cancer pain

A 51-year-old woman presents with severe, unremitting left leg pain which is only partially relieved by intravenous (IV) meperidine (100 mg every four hours IV). She is never without pain, but there is no back, pelvic, or buttock pain. The pain is worsened by walking and is least severe when she awakens in the morning. The left leg is swollen and sensation is dysaesthetic to touch in a stocking-glove distribution distally. Motor and reflex testing was antalgic. She was plaintive, and her affect flat.

She is trained as a nurse but now subsists on disability. She has suffered four myocardial infarctions and as many cardiac arrests. The diagnosis of ischaemic cardiomyopathy confounded by a ventricular aneurysm was substantiated, and she was considered for heart transplantation. Two months ago she was treated for deep vein thrombosis of the left leg. A recent evaluation for chest pain was inconclusive; during the same hospitalization she was treated for sepsis. Her only point of venous access was a right inguinal venous catheter, which was inserted at the time of her resuscitation. On coumadin, her INRs range from 1.5 to 5.0. Allergies include morphine, codeine, oxycodone, yellow dye, penicillin, and intravenous contrast media.

Low-dose, patient-controlled analgesia was started with hydromorphone at 0.05 mg/hour (equivalent to 0.25 mg morphine/hour or 1 mg of morphine every four hours) as a basal or continuous infusion rate. She was allowed to give herself an additional 0.05 mg every six minutes for a maximum of 0.55 mg/hour (equivalent to 3 mg morphine/hour).

She was discharged home to Visiting Nurse Association (VNA) care. Her pain was controlled and at home the frequency of patient-controlled boluses diminished.

The inguinal IV line became locally infected without sepsis; the erythema and induration subsided with IV vancomycin. The line was left in place, and she returned home where she lives alone. She was transferred back from another hospital two weeks later following a syncopal episode, which was initially interpreted as a pacemaker malfunction. She also complained of leg pain and asked for meperidine. The transfer summary conveyed a strong suspicion of drug addiction. Rapid postural change during a bingo game probably precipitated a vasovagal response and syncope. Oral hydromorphone was started and the inguinal IV line was removed, and she returned home to be seen biweekly in the office to check an INR.

Commentary

The picture of a nurse with end-stage cardiomyopathy, chronic pain, drug addiction, anticoagulation, multiple allergies, and poor venous access is ugly but challenging. The picture was confounded by repetitious work-ups performed by multiple care-givers, who changed with the call schedule month to month and night to night. The magnitude of her suffering was much larger than the left leg pain. The suffering had physical, emotional, spiritual, and existential dimensions. The physical reality of the pain was occlusion of the femoral vein and venous stasis which worsened when the leg was dependent or when she walked. She struggled emotionally because of a pervasive fear of dying – the painful leg not unlike the sore tooth of death. Her spiritual base had also eroded. Even though she is not a churchgoer, she believes in God but lacks the security and support of a church community. She felt isolated in a tough, hostile environment, and her human experience was not explainable. She was abused by her former husband, her two adopted children were given up to another family, her mother had recently died in her home of cancer, and her father was ill. Her nursing background heightened the cognitive dimension of suffering, e.g. syncope suggests yet another heart attack or ventricular arrhythmia.

By focusing first on the leg pain and by giving her back some control over her life with the patient-controlled analgesia (PCA), she gained confidence that she would survive. Concurrently we explored her hostile environment and gave her a sounding board to vent her frustrations. She was encouraged to reach out to the community and was involved with community bingo when she experienced her vasovagal attack. The cognitive, spiritual, and existential dimensions of her pain led to pseudo-addictive behaviour to obtain meperidine, 'because it makes me feel better'. The small dose of meperidine which relieved her pain on this occasion was 24 mg IV, and once the PCA was started she reduced the dose of hydromorphone by her own accord. With her renewed confidence, the inguinal line was removed and she regained her mobility. She returns to have her INR drawn every other week because of her difficult venous access and the labile blood level of coumadin. A dose reassurance is also given. She is now working part time as a private duty nurse, and her self-esteem has dramatically improved.

'Malignant' cancer pain

This 46-year-old woman presented to a neurosurgeon for cordotomy for the treatment of severe, unrelenting pain in her legs, back, and pelvis associated with metastatic and locally invasive colon cancer. She was free of pain following the procedure, but eight hours later had a series of three 'seizures'. When I first saw her in the early morning, she was suffering constant, incapacitating multi-focal myoclonus. Through the severe, painful spasms she stuttered, 'Please help me!' Preoperatively IV morphine had been escalated to 80 mg/hour, and postoperatively it had been reduced to 40 mg/hour. To stop the myoclonus she was pharmacologically paralysed and intubated. She did not wish to be resuscitated in the event of respiratory or cardiac arrest but agreed to be intubated temporarily. Rhabdomyolysis ensued, and acute renal failure developed. She then died of multi-system failure.

Commentary

This case bears stark testimony to the futility of ablative neurosurgery at the end of life. White and Sweet's biblical textbook, *Pain and the neurosurgeon*, deservedly gathers dust on library book shelves.[19] A hint of multi-focal myoclonus was present prior to surgery and presaged overt neurotoxicity. A palliative alternative to cordotomy is opioid rotation or changing to another narcotic (for example, hydromorphone). Epidural or intrathecal hydromorphone and/on bupivacaine would be workable options. More expeditious recognition of the myoclonus on our part may have aborted the rhabdomyolysis. The physical dimension of her suffering was overpowering.

Malignant brain tumour

This 13-year-old boy was diagnosed with anaplastic astrocytoma involving the right parietal and temporal lobes in 1996. The tumour was surgically debulked, and he received conventional radiotherapy and chemotherapy. He was densely hemiparetic. A large cyst developed with a deep solid tissue component. The cyst was evacuated and the deep solid component was biopsied to confirm the original pathology, anaplastic astrocytoma. He entered a nationally based experimental study, but the tumour progressed. Headaches and increasing gait instability were treated with ever-increasing doses of dexamethasone. Several months later he was admitted with severe Cushing's syndrome, seizures, pancreatitis, and haemorrhagic gastritis. The tumour recurrence appeared attached to the wall of the cyst but no further encroachment of deeper structures or spread of the tumour to the opposite side was apparent. To reduce his dependence on dexamethasone and to manage the gastritis and pancreatitis more directly, the cyst and all visible tumour were removed. He entered a new experimental protocol at NIH (National Institutes of Health), and he was weaned from steroids. Last year, he came of age to hunt deer and shot his first deer. The suspicion on imaging studies of persistent tumour remains stable and unchanged four years later.

Commentary

This boy and his brother live and breathe baseball, the outdoors, and hunting. They were known to shoot groundhogs from their bedroom window. During his treatment a discussion about deer rifles or shotguns would always brighten his day. Amidst the misery of his chemotherapy, a 12-guage over-and-under shotgun was smuggled onto the paediatric floor for his appraisal, much to his delight and to the chagrin of the paediatric staff. Palliative neurosurgery in this boy's case had a very specific goal in mind – not to cure him of disease but to reduce the physical suffering caused by palliative dexamethasone, which is clearly a double-edged sword. The additional improvement in quality of life has been his return to hunting, albeit with a gun prop to compensate for his paretic left arm.

Malignant brain tumour

This 46-year-old advertising executive became aphasic and was diagnosed with a left temporal glioblastoma by stereotactic brain biopsy. Increasing the dose of dexamethasone from 2 mg twice a day to 4 mg every six hours relieved her headaches but provoked disruptive paranoid agitation. The paranoia and agitation lessened when the dose of dexamethasone was reduced but did not disappear. After exploring options at New York University, Duke University, and Salt Lake City with the family, her husband opted for conventional radiation therapy. Radiation therapy was aborted after 10 treatments because of 'screaming' headaches. Global dysphasia added to her confusion and ability to cooperate for treatment. Sundowning or sleep–wake cycle reversal disrupted the sleep patterns of her care-givers, and her agitated paranoia forced away several attendants. Headaches were contained with an escalation of IV morphine to 25 mg/hour, and rectal chlorpromazine effectively reduced both her agitation and paranoia and let her sleep. A month after the radiation was stopped, her headaches subsided and the morphine was gradually discontinued. In the comfort of her own home with her mother as the primary care-giver, the paranoia eased and her ability to participate in conversation improved. Hospice nursing support was helpful in responding to day-to-day needs, but their role as spiritual counsellors was rejected. Four months after diagnosis, her speech approached normal. The family dismissed hospice and asked to revisit the issue of chemotherapy. Within weeks she developed a stiff neck, disruptive agitation, a right twelfth nerve palsy, urinary retention, and diminished hearing in the right ear. Despite the futility of further treatment, the family requested that other treatment options be explored and investigated. Leptomeningeal metastases were evident on MRI of brain and spine. She became less responsive and died at home three weeks later.

Commentary

Our effort to assuage this woman's suffering was inadequate. The physical pain was adequately managed, but the reason for her unremitting suffering is threefold: (1) global dysphasia, (2) paranoid agitation, and (3) existential anxiety. The inability to comprehend conversation and to speak were major barriers for communication and for lessening anxiety. On the one hand she did not seem to comprehend the full significance of her illness, but on the other hand she periodically vocalized her poorly articulated anger and fear of dying towards the end of her illness. Management of her paranoid agitation was also problematic. For example, any exposure of or contact with her perineum provoked an agitated, paranoid outburst. Her mother came from her home in Colorado to care for her daughter in Pennsylvania and did not wish her daughter to have 'mind-altering' drugs. She preferred instead to be constantly at the bedside, protecting her from climbing out of bed while reassuring her at the same time. The husband, patient, mother, and father were not religious, and they envisioned their lives pulled together in a circle, like a circle of wagons, separating and protecting them from a tough, hostile outside world. Their loved one's death was inexplicable, and her disappearance into a void of nothingness was very anxiety-provoking. Even in retrospect we did the best that we could.

Hydrocephalus

This four-year-old girl presented with acute shunt malfunction, and the shunt was revised emergently. The parents, however, had wished only that a diagnosis be made and that an easily manageable disorder such as an ear infection be discovered and the source of the child's irritability be taken care of. The child had been born premature, weighing less than 800 grams, and suffered an intraventricular haemorrhage, developed hydrocephalus, and a CSF shunt was performed. Feeding was problematic as an infant and a Nissen fundoplication was necessary to prevent gastroesophageal reflux. She was fed by mouth. At four years of age she could not roll over, sit, stand, or walk, but she smiled and recognized the individual members of her family. Though she seemed resilient to the usual childhood illnesses, in the six months prior to her shunt revision she suffered two major respiratory tract infections. After the second illness feeding became more difficult because of nasopharyngeal congestion and coughing. Despite anticholinergic medication, the child would cough during feeding. Feeding took about 40 minutes, and the child's input gradually diminished. Two previous shunt revisions had been performed, but the parents struck an accord with their paediatrician that if the shunt failed again, the child's irritability and discomfort would be assuaged, but no further surgical intervention would be done. When their child became increasingly irritable, uncomfortable, and lethargic, they took her to the paediatrician's office. Unfortunately, her paediatrician was not on call, and she was sent to the University hospital to rule out shunt malfunction. After the diagnosis was made, the parents were told that if they did not consent to revision of the shunt that they would be referred to Children's Protective Services and be prosecuted for neglect. The shunt was revised. Since I was the original surgeon, the angry parents came to me to vent their frustration. The threat of prosecution for child abuse was discounted, and the issue of medical and surgical futility clarified. The child was referred to a paediatric hospice. Because of discomfort associated with feeding, oral feeding was eventually stopped and the discomfort subsided. Discomfort was assuaged with small doses of oral morphine, and irritability managed with lorazepam and physical contact. The child died in the home one month later free of pain and smiling to the end.

Commentary

This child lived unnaturally until she died naturally. Repeated shunt malfunction is a form of physical suffering, and the spectre of shunt infection would add to her suffering and prolong death. An alternative to revising the shunt is pharmacologically managing the apparent headaches and irritability and allowing the child to die in a dry, clean bed. Allowing a child to die, especially at home, is difficult for her parents and requires a great deal of care-giver time and grief preparation. The dying process is not a drive-through lane at a fast food restaurant. Repeated explanations and reassurance are helpful in guiding the family through the process. Anticipating the grieving process long before the death and continuing the process after death are keys to enduring satisfaction and closure. Families with no religious base or a shaky spiritual base suffer the most.

Head injury

This 82-year-old woman was struck by a car as she was crossing the street of a college town. She was briefly conscious at the scene but had suffered a subarachnoid haemorrhage, a small left subdural haemorrhage, a cerebral contusion, and a right tibial fracture. She had been an avid reader and walked daily for exercise, but now responded semi-purposefully to voice and touch, and her Glasgow coma score was 8. After conferring with a son in Maine and a daughter in Montana, IV fluids were minimized and she was offered food and drink. Initially she refused both food and drink. Three days after her injury, she took a sip of water but then was comforted just by moistening her lips. The tibial fracture was splinted. Because of grimacing and shrugging, as well as writhing movements of her shoulders and pelvis, a continuous infusion of morphine at 1 mg/hour was administered. She was able to acknowledge her children but did not respond verbally to them. She died in a dry, clean bed five days later and was free of pain.

Commentary

By all accounts this woman had lived a full life and had no wish to be encumbered by disability. Neither nutrition nor hydration would have improved the quality of outcome. Hydration may have worsened her cerebral oedema and hastened her death. Nasogastric tubes for feeding are uncomfortable and increase the risk of aspiration. Timely nutrition would, however, prolong the dying process. The heroic frontal decompressions of Kjellburg to relieve intracranial pressure and posterior fossa decompressions to prevent tonsillar compression of the brainstem are broken lessons of history.

Intracerebral haemorrhage

This 78-year-old woman lived independently but was found 'down' at home by the mailman. A large, deep, left thalamic haemorrhage was identified which rendered her unconscious and hemiplegic. Her hypertension had been managed with two different drugs, and she was hypertensive on admission. She had made it very clear to her daughters that in the event of a stroke or disabling injury, she did not wish to be resuscitated or have her life prolonged unnaturally. Most of all she did not wish to be placed in a nursing home. Hypertension was treated, she was turned regularly in bed, and a Foley catheter drained her bladder. No enteral feeds were given, and 1400 ml of IV fluids were administered daily. Purposeful movements in the left arm and hand became evident, and she awakened to voice and vigorous tactile stimulation. Because periodic grimacing and writhing movements of the left shoulder and arm were interpreted as pain, IV morphine at 1 mg/hour was given. She refused food and water but was comforted by sponging her lips. On the fourth day following admission, IV fluids were stopped. Five days after her stroke she slowly began taking some ice chips, sips of water, then soft foods. The patient remained hemiplegic and unable to talk. She comprehended simple conversation but could only respond with grunts and 'yells'. Intravenous morphine was changed to oral morphine to be taken as needed. At her daughters' direction, she was discharged to a nursing home. When informed of her disposition, she reacted angrily and reduced her daughters to tears with speechless daggers of guilt. Twelve hours later, however, she had accepted her fate, and the relationship with her daughters returned to normal. The close relationship with her granddaughter was rekindled in the sharing of a story of a young lost bat who was befriended by another animal family until she could be returned to her mother. When released to the ambulance en route to the nursing home she was clutching a stuffed bat 'Stella Luna' to her chest. She died three weeks later in the nursing home.

Commentary

This elderly woman was not abandoned on the 'back ward' with her major stroke syndrome, nor was a natural means for her recovery withheld. Surgery to remove a deep thalamic haemorrhage does not reduce the neurological deficit or improve the quality of life. Water and food were offered but refused until thirst and hunger intervened and she began to eat. In contrast to the previous case her stroke was survivable. Not uncommonly, a barrier to discharging patients from an acute care hospital is their premorbid aversion to placement in a nursing home and the family's intent to honour those verbal directives. Not infrequently, the practical circumstances don't allow their wishes to be honoured. A fear of or bias against nursing homes often dissolves if the family visits the home ahead of time. The patient offers some resistance until she witnesses the appropriateness and quality of care. Firm direction and a disposition which includes hospice surveillance and back-up reduces unnecessary readmissions and is more enduring.

Summary: when all is said and done

The passion of young physicians and surgeons is to 'push the envelope' and never to say 'never'. We sacrifice our nights, our health, and often our families to the name of our profession. Our education, training, and research charge us to study and cure human disease. Many diseases in surgery, especially neurosurgery, are not curable and yet the patients continue to suffer. The diseases that we try to treat are inseparable from the patients' suffering. In palliative medicine and surgery we are called to confront this suffering.

Physical pain is but one dimension of suffering. The emotional, cognitive, and spiritual dimensions of suffering are just as disabling. Existential suffering presents the greatest challenge of all.

To come to grips with suffering we must be willing to listen to our patients and discover what meaning and values contribute to the quality of their lives in order to maximize the quality of their life which remains.

When it is all said and done, the mitigation of suffering is the enduring goal of medicine and surgery and the true measure of our continuing success.

References

1. Cassell, E. (1991). Recognizing suffering. *Hastings Center Report* (May–June 1991), 24–31.
2. Soelle, D. (1975). *Suffering.* Fortress Press, Philadelphia.
3. Prochnik, L. (1980). *Endings: death, glorious and otherwise, as faced by ten outstanding figures of our time.* Crown Publishers, Inc., New York.
4. Borg, M. (1994). *Meeting Jesus again for the first time.* Harper, San Francisco.
5. Bonhoeffer, D. (1971). *Letters and papers from prison.* Simon & Schuster, New York.
6. Buber, M. (1970). *I and thou.* Simon & Schuster, New York.
7. Saunders, C. and Sykes, N. (ed.) (1933). *The management of terminal malignant disease.* Edward Arnold, London.
8. Coffey, R. (1996). Neurosurgical management of intractable pain. In: J. Youmans(ed.) *Youmans' neurological Surgery.* Saunders, New York.
9. Laitinen, L., and Hariz, M. (1996). Movement disorders. In: J. Youmans(ed.) *Youmans' neurological Surgery.* Saunders, New York.
10. Kelly, P.J., and Gillingham, F. (1980). The long-term results of steriotaxic surgery and levodopa therapy in patients with Parkinson's disease: a 10-year follow-up study. *J. Neurosurg.,* **53**, 332–7.
11. Tasker, R., Siqueira, J., *et al.* (1983). What happened to Vm thalamotomy for Parkinson's disease? *Appl. Neurophysiol.,* **46**, 68–83.
12. Matsumoto, K., Shichijo, F., Fukami, T. (1984). Long-term follow-up review of cases of Parkinson's disease after unilateral or bilateral thalamotomy. *J. Neurosurg.,* **60**, 1033–44.
13. Fazzini, E., Dogali, M., Berich, A., Chin, L., Eidelberg, D., Stereo, G., Samelson, D., *et al.* (1993). Ventral pallidotomy operations in patients with Parkinson's Plus syndromes. *Ann. Neurol.,* **34**, 266.
14. Martin-Rodriguez, J., and Obrador, S. (1975). Evaluation of stereotaxic pulvinar lesions. *Confin. Neurol.,* **37**, 56–62.
15. Krayenbuhl, H., and Siegfried, J. (1972). Dentatotomies or thalamontomies in the treatment of hyperkinesias. *Confin. Neurol.* **34**, 29–33.
16. Shima, F., Iancono, R., Sakata, S. (1993). *Posteroventral pallidotomy in treatment of dystonia.* Eleventh Meeting of the World Society for Stereotactic and Functional Neurosurgery, Ixtapa, Mexico.
17. Fahn, S. (1992). Idiopathic torsion dystonia. In: *Movement disorders in neurology and neuropsychiatry* (ed. A. Joseph and R. Young), pp. 569–74. Blackwell Scientific Publications, Oxford.
18. Bertrand, C. (1993). Selective peripheral denervation for spasmodic torticollis: surgical technique, results, and observations in 260 cases. *Surg. Neurol.,* **40**, 96–103.
19. White, J., and Sweet, W. (1969). *Pain and the neurosurgeon: a forty-year experience.* Charles C. Thomas, Springfield, ILL.

Chapter 16

The role of the ophthalmologist in advanced disease

David Yorston

Happily there are few eye diseases that are likely to have a fatal outcome. However, this does not mean that palliative care is irrelevant to ophthalmology. The eye is exquisitely sensitive. Diseases or inflammation of the eye may be associated with severe pain. Our eyes are also important for social interaction, and disfigurement can lead to a significant handicap. Ophthalmologists are primarily concerned with treatment to restore or preserve sight. However, there will be occasions when the eye's vision has been irretrievably lost, yet the patient remains symptomatic because of pain, disfigurement, or both. In this situation palliative treatment to reduce the pain, and improve the appearance, can lead to a greatly enhanced quality of life for the patient.

Although ocular malignancy is uncommon, and frequently can be controlled by local radiotherapy or excision, occasionally patients will present with tumours that are too advanced for curative treatment. Without any treatment, the patients will succumb with a disfiguring, painful, malodorous mass in their orbit. The aim of palliation in this situation is to achieve local control – if necessary by radical surgery – while accepting that distant metastases will limit long-term survival.

Finally, ophthalmic problems can occur in patients who are terminally ill from other conditions, and palliative measures may be valuable to prevent symptoms of ocular pain or discomfort.

Management of blind painful eye

Causes of blind painful eye

Blind painful eyes may be caused by glaucoma (particularly neovascular glaucoma), trauma, intraocular inflammation or infection, chronic retinal detachment, and an intraocular tumour. Before considering an eye for palliative treatment alone, it is essential to ensure that there is no possibility of restoring useful vision.

Cyclodestruction

Moderate rises in intraocular pressure are usually asymptomatic. However, as the pressure rises above 40 mmHg, the eye is more likely to become painful. If the pressure can be reduced, the pain may be controlled. In severe neovascular glaucoma, which is most frequently caused by proliferative diabetic retinopathy, or an ischaemic central retinal vein occlusion (Fig 16.1), topical treatment is rarely adequate to lower the intraocular pressure sufficiently, and surgery is required. The most commonly performed operation to reduce intraocular pressure is trabeculectomy. However, this is an invasive intraocular procedure, and has a poor success rate in neovascular glaucoma. An alternative is to use an aqueous shunt implant, such as a Molteno tube. However this is a complex procedure, and there is a substantial risk of postoperative complications, such

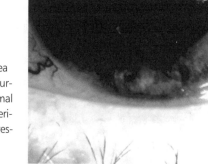

Fig. 16.1 Rubeosis. The cornea is oedematous, leading to blurring of the iris detail. Abnormal vessels are visible on the anterior surface of the iris. These vessels are responsible for the severe secondary glaucoma.

as a flat anterior chamber. In a situation in which vision has already been lost, the use of an aqueous shunt is not justified as there are other, simpler means of lowering intraocular pressure. If the priority is to lower the intraocular pressure without preserving vision, then reducing the production of aqueous humour, by destruction of the ciliary body, is effective.

The ciliary body is very sensitive, and it is essential to have good analgesia before attempting any cyclodestructive procedure. All cyclodestructive procedures suffer from the drawback that insufficient treatment will not lower the pressure enough, but excessive treatment will cause the eye to become phthisical. In neovascular glaucoma, the effect of treatment is particularly unpredictable.

Damage to the ciliary body will inevitably lead to a brisk uveitis. This should be controlled with mydriatics and topical steroids postoperatively.

The reduction in intraocular pressure usually becomes apparent after about one or two weeks.

Cyclocryotherapy

Cyclocryotherapy requires a cryoprobe. The probe is applied to the sclera 2 mm posterior to the limbus, and the tissue is frozen to −80° Celsius. Two quadrants are treated at any one time; each quadrant normally requires four applications of the cryoprobe. Cyclocryotherapy is effective at reducing the intraocular pressure, but causes severe inflammation, and may even be associated with a hypopyon.

Trans-scleral cyclophotocoagulation

An alternative is to use a contact diode laser. This solid state laser emits light in the infrared range. This passes freely through the conjunctiva and sclera, and is absorbed by the pigment of the ciliary body. A specially designed probe is used, the edge of which is aligned with the limbus. The laser delivery fibre optic should then be directed at the ciliary body. This can be verified by using a bright source to transilluminate the sclera and demonstrate the position of the ciliary body. Approximately 40 burns are applied to the entire circumference of the ciliary body at a power of 1500–2000 mW, with each application lasting one to two seconds. The ciliary body in the horizontal meridian – at 3 o'clock and 9 o'clock – should be avoided in order to prevent damage to the long ciliary nerves.

This treatment may also cause a marked uveitis, but it is thought to be less severe than the inflammatory response after cyclocryotherapy. Postoperatively the patient should be treated with topical steroid drops for at least one month. If the reduction in intraocular pressure is insufficient, the treatment can be repeated. Approximately half of all patients will require more than one treatment to reduce the pressure to near normal levels.[1-3] In patients who still have vision in the eye, approximately 30% will lose some visual acuity;[1] however, this may be due more to the progression of disease in an already severely damaged eye rather than to an adverse effect of the laser treatment.[2] Hypotony and phthisis are uncommon following diode laser cyclophotocoagulation.

Trans-scleral diode laser cyclophotocoagulation is very effective at relieving the pain caused by raised intraocular pressure. In one study, 73% of patients had relief of their pain after one treatment, and this improved to 97% after repeat treatment of eyes that were still symptomatic.[4]

A continuous-wave Nd:YAG laser may be used as it also emits light in the infrared range. It can be employed in contact or non-contact modes. The available evidence suggests that both Nd:YAG and diode lasers are equally effective at lowering intraocular pressure, with a similar incidence of adverse effects.[5]

Retrobulbar injections

Some patients may refuse to have a blind painful eye removed, particularly if it has a normal appearance. If controlling the intraocular pressure does not relieve their symptoms, injection of a neurolytic chemical into the retrobulbar space may provide good analgesia.

Both alcohol and phenol have been used. Injection of absolute is very painful, so it is important to obtain complete analgesia by injecting local anaesthetic first.[6] Phenol is itself a local anaesthetic, and may be less painful on injection.[7]

Retrobulbar neurolytics work by causing precipitation of proteins in the nerve sheaths. They have been used for many years for the treatment of spasticity, and for chemical sympathectomy. The drug will damage all the nerves with which it comes into contact, not only the pain fibres. Its effect will be temporary as the peripheral nerves will regenerate.

Injection of retrobulbar alcohol or phenol is similar to a retrobulbar injection of local anaesthetic for intraocular surgery. The injection is given through the skin of the lower lid, in the infero-temporal quadrant of the orbit, while the patient looks infero-temporally (in order to move the optic nerve supero-nasally, away from the advancing needle). Initially, lignocaine 2% is injected into the intraconal space. After this has had time to take effect, 1.5–2 ml of absolute alcohol, or 1:15(6.7%) aqueous phenol, is injected through the same needle.

Retrobulbar phenol successfully relieved pain in eight out of 10 eyes.[7] The analgesia is usually apparent within one day of the injection. The average duration of the pain relief was 15 months, with a range of 4–48 months. Retrobulbar alcohol provided analgesia for a mean of seven months.[6] The injections may be repeated if the eye pain recurs.

Because all the orbital nerves may be affected, transient oculomotor problems are common. Ptosis occurs most frequently, followed by abducens weakness. Because the eye is blind, the patient will not experience diplopia. However, a squint may be a significant cosmetic problem. Marked chemosis and lid swelling are common, but usually resolve within a week.

More importantly, destruction of the sensory nerves may lead to neuroparalytic keratitis, and persistent corneal epithelial defects. These are chronic, painful corneal ulcers, and they may lead to enucleation or evisceration.[7] They can be treated by a conjunctival flap (p. 00) or a central tarsorrhaphy.

Corneal and ocular surface disease

Occasionally a chronically painful eye may be caused by corneal disease. This is usually treatable by a corneal transplant. However, if the eye has no visual potential – because of secondary glaucoma, for example – a less complex procedure may be indicated.

The corneal epithelium is densely innervated and exquisitely sensitive. Any epithelial defect is likely to be very painful. Most epithelial defects will heal within a few days at most. However, some conditions, such as bullous keratopathy, lead to recurrent epithelial defects and a chronically painful eye. If some form of corneal protection can be achieved, the eye will be much less painful.

A variety of different corneal treatments have been shown to be effective. These include conjunctival flaps,[8] amniotic membrane grafts,[9] and excimer laser treatment of the corneal surface.[10]

The key to successful conjunctival flap surgery is to raise a very thin flap of conjunctiva, free of any underlying Tenon's capsule. The flap is raised in the superior fornix, at least 12 mm from the limbus. After the flap has been fashioned, the corneal epithelium is removed and the flap is sutured to the cornea with 10/0 nylon sutures. Initially the flap will be thickened and vascular. With time the flap becomes thin and less vascular (Fig 16.2) and it may be possible to insert a cosmetic shell which will improve the appearance still further.

Patients with severe ocular surface disease not only suffer from pain, but they must also instil drops frequently and attend an eye clinic regularly. Covering the cornea with a conjunctival flap not only provides excellent pain relief, but also reduces the requirement for medication and frequent review.[8]

Amniotic membrane has been shown to promote corneal epithelial healing and minimize conjunctival inflammation and scarring. Following removal of the corneal epithelium, suitably processed amniotic membrane is placed in the epithelial defect and sutured to the cornea.

Following this procedure, 90% of eyes experienced pain relief within one day of the graft.[9] The epithelial defect heals within three weeks in most cases, although the epithelium may break down again in the future. The vision is usually stable.

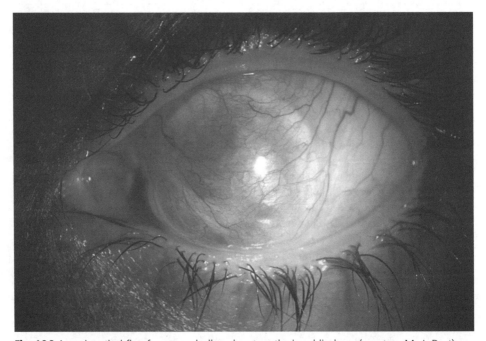

Fig. 16.2 A conjunctival flap for severe bullous keratopathy in a blind eye (courtesy Mr J. Dart).

Amniotic membrane transplantation is technically easier than raising a large and thin conjunctival flap. However, it is very expensive and is unavailable in most of the world.

The sensory nerves of the cornea lie in the anterior stroma, deep to Bowman's membrane. It has been suggested that excimer laser photoablation of the superficial stroma would destroy the nerve plexus, and reduce pain from any ocular surface disease. Deep ablation of up to 25% of the corneal stroma provided pain relief in 83% of eyes in Australia.[10] Some of these patients suffered from recurrent epithelial defect following manual removal of the epithelium. Phototherapeutic keratectomy can be performed under topical anaesthesia as an office procedure. However, the excimer laser is very expensive and treatment is costly.

Removal of the eye

If reduction of intraocular pressure and medical therapy to control inflammation are insufficient to relieve pain, then it may be necessary to remove the eye in order to achieve symptomatic relief. Removal of the eye has been shown to be highly effective at relieving ocular pain.[11,12] In one study, 94% of patients said they would recommend the operation to other people with blind painful eyes.[12]

The goals of removing an eye are to achieve the therapeutic objective, and, at the same time, minimize deformity and achieve the best possible cosmetic result. Different treatment strategies will be required for different situations, and there is no clear consensus that any single procedure is ideal for all circumstances.

There are three operations that are used to remove the eye (Table 16.1):

◆ evisceration – the ocular contents are removed, leaving the scleral shell intact

◆ enucleation – the entire globe is excised

◆ exenteration – the globe and orbital contents, including the periorbita, are removed en bloc.

Table 16.1 Operations used to remove the eye

	Evisceration	Enucleation	Exenteration
Definition	Removal of all ocular contents	Removal of entire globe	Removal of all orbital contents
Anaesthesia	L/A or G/A	G/A	G/A
Risk of sympathetic ophthalmia	Small	None	None
Prosthesis mobility	Fair	Fair with implant; poor without implant	None
Tissue available for histology	No	Yes	Yes
Orbital implant required	Possibly	Yes	No
Prosthesis fitting	Simple	Simple	Complex
Ophthalmic malignancy	Unsuitable	Suitable if confined to globe	Suitable for advanced extraocular malignancy

Counselling and preoperative preparation

Before any operation to remove the eye, it is essential to provide the patient with a very clear explanation of what is intended and the likely outcome. In particular, it should be made absolutely clear that the operation will lead to permanent and irreversible loss of sight in the eye. Some patients may opt for surgery in the belief that sight may be restored later by an 'eye transplant'. Many people will be extremely concerned about postoperative pain and will need reassurance that this will be controlled. Every patient will be worried about their appearance following removal of the eye. It is important to explain what steps will be taken to minimize deformity, while being realistic about the outcome. Many blind, painful eyes are unsightly to start with, and the cosmetic appearance may even be improved by removal of the eye and insertion of a prosthesis.

Prior to any operation to remove the eye, the eye should be marked indelibly. Removal of the wrong eye has occurred, and is the most catastrophic complication in ophthalmology.

Although evisceration can be performed under local anaesthesia, it is far kinder to perform all operations to remove the eye under general anaesthesia if possible.

Regardless of the final cosmetic result, removal of an eye is a very traumatic event for any patient. Little has been published regarding the psychological sequelae of enucleation, and the Collaborative Ocular Melanoma Study will address this deficit.[13] However, the removal of a blind painful eye is likely to be less disturbing than the sudden loss of a previously healthy eye from trauma or malignancy. All patients who have had an eye removed should be offered every opportunity to discuss their fears and concerns. In some cases, removal of the eye can lead to long-term psychiatric morbidity.[14] It is not unusual for loss of the eye to be followed by a grieving reaction. Eventually most patients will overcome this and adapt to their loss. However, this process can be facilitated by respecting the patient's anxieties and emotions, and discussing them openly and sympathetically. Meeting other patients who have had an eye removed, with a good outcome, may also be helpful.

Evisceration

This is the least invasive means of removing an eye. The cornea is excised, and the contents of the scleral shell (the retina, uveal tract, vitreous, and lens) are then scraped out by inserting a spatula into the potential space between the sclera and the uveal tract. There is usually some haemorrhage from the vortex veins and central retinal artery. This can be controlled by diathermy, or pressure. The interior of the sclera should be cleaned with a swab in order to remove any remaining uveal tissue. Some surgeons suggest doing this with a swab soaked in alcohol to kill any viable uveal cells. Following removal of the contents of the scleral shell, it is possible to insert an implant – usually a plastic sphere – which will help to maintain the orbital volume. If an implant is used, the scleral remnant must be closed over the anterior surface, in two layers, in order to stop the implant being extruded as the scleral shell contracts.

The advantages of evisceration are that it is a quick and simple procedure. It is a less traumatic method of removing the eye as it does not disturb any of the orbital tissues outside the eye. As the extraocular muscles are not disturbed, the scleral remnant will move normally, and some of this movement will be transmitted to a prosthesis. It is easy to insert an orbital implant and the extrusion rate is low, provided the sclera is closed in two layers anteriorly. Because the orbit is not disturbed, this procedure may be valuable when there is intraocular infection as it prevents the dissemination of micro-organisms into the orbit and subarachnoid space.

Unfortunately evisceration may be complicated by sympathetic ophthalmia, a severe uveitis which affects the normal eye following an injury to the other eye. This is thought to be due to retained uveal tissue following evisceration. The incidence of sympathetic ophthalmia following evisceration is extremely low, and one recent survey failed to find any proven cases.[15] Evisceration is also unsuitable for eyes suspected of harbouring a malignancy as it is difficult to obtain a good specimen for histopathology. Because the scleral shell is left *in situ*, it can be affected by scleritis, and this is one cause of persistent socket pain following evisceration.[16] In this case, removal of the scleral remnant by enucleation will abolish the pain.

Enucleation

Enucleation is a more radical procedure than evisceration. The conjunctiva and Tenon's capsule are incised around the limbus. The extraocular muscles are then identified and divided. The optic nerve is divided using a snare, or large curved scissors, and the globe is removed. Bleeding from the optic nerve can be controlled by pressure or diathermy. The conjunctiva and Tenon's capsule are then closed in layers.

Removal of the globe leads to an immediate reduction in the volume of the orbital contents. This in turn leads to ptosis, and a 'hollow-eyed' appearance. This can be reduced by inserting an implant to replace the lost volume. An orbital implant can be inserted into the muscle cone, and the muscles sutured to the implant. This gives near normal mobility. Many implants are made of porous materials, such as hydroxyapatite or polypropylene mesh. These implants become vascularized and have a low extrusion rate. When they are fully vascularized, a socket may be drilled in the implant to receive a peg on the posterior surface of the artificial eye. This provides good motility of the prosthesis and an improved cosmetic result. However, these implants are costly. An acrylic sphere, covered in Dacron mesh, is much less expensive and also has a low extrusion rate. The extraocular muscles can be sutured to the mesh to provide some motility. Although orbital implants can become exposed, leading to recurrent pain and infection, complications are rare.

Because enucleation removes the entire globe in one piece, there is no risk of leaving uveal tissue behind and sympathetic ophthalmia should not occur. The excised globe is also much more accessible for histopathological examination than the scrapings from an evisceration specimen. For this reason enucleation is always used if there is a suspicion of intraocular malignancy.

However, enucleation is a more complex procedure than evisceration. For the treatment of a blind painful eye due to non-malignant disease, its only advantage is the lower risk of sympathetic ophthalmia. Since this is a very rare complication, evisceration is probably the better operation for most blind painful eyes.

Management of advanced periocular disease

Occasionally ophthalmic malignancies will present at such an advanced stage that surgical cure is impossible. In this case the surgeon's aim is to achieve local control of the disease to avoid the distress caused by a fungating mass in the orbit. This may require radical surgery, such as exenteration. The indications for exenteration include the following:

◆ lid and conjunctival tumours extending into the orbit, e.g. basal cell carcinoma, squamous cell carcinoma of the skin or conjunctiva (see Figure 16.3 & 16.4), conjunctival melanoma

◆ intraocular tumours extending beyond the sclera, e.g. retinoblastoma, choroidal melanoma

◆ primary or secondary orbital tumours, e.g. lacrimal gland adenocarcinoma

◆ benign conditions causing severe deformity or pain, e.g. teratoma, orbital pseudotumour.[17] These conditions are usually amenable to more conservative treatments. However, rarely, all other treatments may be ineffective. When orbital disease causes intractable pain, exenteration is an effective means of providing symptomatic relief.[17]

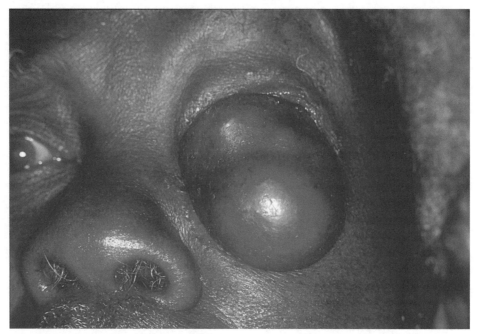

Fig. 16.3 Squamous cell carcinoma of the conjunctiva. This patient has an advanced conjunctival malignancy filling the lower orbit and invading the globe.

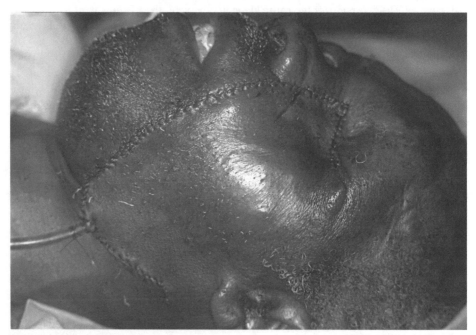

Fig. 16.4 Postoperative following exenteration. The same partient as in Figure 16.3 immediately after exenteration and reconstruction with a cervico-facial flap. The risk of a local fungating tumour has been greatly reduced, although distant metastases remain probable. Cosmetically, the appearance is improved.

Lid and conjunctival tumours are usually managed by local excision. However, these tumours may recur and invade the orbit. Rarely, patients may present late with an advanced lesion which has already destroyed the globe.

Some tumours, such as rhabdomyosarcoma, which used to be treated by exenteration are now managed by a combination of radical radiotherapy and chemotherapy. Advanced retinoblastoma is rarely seen in the industrialized countries, but remains common in poorer countries where delayed presentation may mean than the child has massive orbital involvement when first examined (Fig 16.5). In this situation, exenteration alone may achieve local control, although it probably does not affect survival.[18]

There is little evidence that such radical surgery improves survival in cases of advanced malignancy, particularly choroidal melanoma with extrascleral extension.[19,20] However, achieving local control of a fungating tumour is a worthwhile goal, and exenteration may well achieve this.[20]

Exenteration may be carried out in two ways. The eyelids may be spared if the lesion arises in the globe or the orbit. This may allow direct closure of the lids to cover the defect. If the lesion involves the lids, they must be removed as well. This leaves a large defect. A variety of strategies have been used to close the defect. They include:

◆ *Laissez-faire* granulation. This is simple and produces a relatively shallow cavity. Unfortunately, it is slow and the patient may need regular dressings for months before the cavity is completely healed.

◆ Split-skin graft. The split skin is applied directly to the bone of the orbit. This heals rapidly but produces a very deep cavity, and can be associated with an offensive discharge.

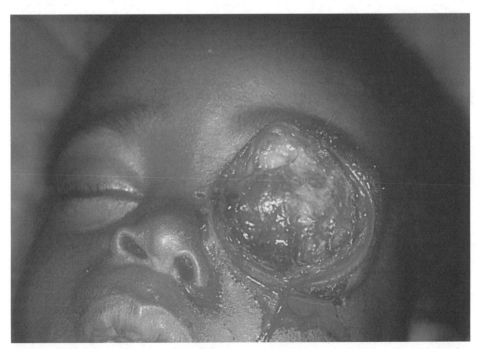

Fig. 16.5 Advanced retinoblastoma. Late-presenting retinoblastoma manifests itself as a fungating tumour replacing the globe. In this case an exenteration can spare the eyelid skin, making primary closure much simpler.

◆ Flap repairs (see Figure 16.4). Many different flap repairs have been described. They may be local flaps – from the forehead or the cheek – or free flaps. These are technically more difficult but result in rapid healing, without leaving a deep cavity. The disadvantage of flaps is that they may mask locally recurrent disease.

A prosthesis may be constructed which can be attached to spectacles, or can be inserted into the orbit and attached to osseous integrated implants.[17] These prostheses are unsatisfactory. Not only is the eye unnaturaly immobile, but the lids do not move either. The skin colour of the lids can change, making it very difficult to achieve a convincing colour match. Many patients prefer not to use a prosthesis and simply wear a black patch instead.

Eye care in critically and terminally ill patients

Patients who are critically ill as a result of life-threatening disease may also develop eye problems. Some of these are easily avoidable. It has been shown that 40% of patients in intensive care units have a superficial keratopathy.[21,22] This is linked to the use of artificial ventilation and to reduced levels of consciousness. In most cases the keratopathy is relatively mild, and, while producing some discomfort, does not threaten vision. However, it may predispose to the development of bacterial keratitis, which is far more severe, painful, and likely to lead to permanent loss of vision.[23] Conjuctival oedema (chemosis) is common in critically ill patients, and this too can increase the risk of corneal ulceration.

Many of these problems can be prevented by simple measures to prevent corneal and conjunctival exposure. Examination with a torch should reveal whether or not the lids are completely apposed in a comatose patient. If only the conjunctiva is exposed, then ocular lubricants should be used every four hours. If the cornea is exposed as well, the lids should be taped. This is best done by closing the eye lids and placing Micropore tape horizontally along the lid margins.[24]

Most patients who are terminally ill will be elderly. Many of them will have potentially blinding eye problems, the most common being cataract, glaucoma, age-related macular degeneration, and diabetic retinopathy. The management of glaucoma and diabetic retinopathy is usually secondary prevention; that is, the prevention of further visual loss from an established disease. In most cases little can be done to improve vision. In a patient whose life expectancy is only a few months, active treatment to prevent visual loss in five years is probably best avoided, particularly if the treatment is either uncomfortable or associated with a risk of immediate loss of vision, e.g. panretinal laser photocoagulation for proliferative diabetic retinopathy, surgical trabeculectomy for chronic open angle glaucoma. Obviously each case has to be considered individually, and ophthalmologists should remember that they are treating the whole person and not just the eyes!

On the other hand, small-incision cataract surgery usually produces significant visual improvement within one month.[25] If a terminally ill patient has symptoms of visual impairment due to cataract, there is no reason to withhold surgery, providing the patient can lie still and flat. The ability to see clearly leads to a huge improvement in the quality of life, regardless of other concurrent illnesses.

Conclusion

Surgery has a lot to offer people with intractably painful or unsightly eyes. Pain should initially be managed by controlling intraocular pressure and treating any ocular surface disease. If these measures fail, then removal of the eye, with an implant, and later prosthesis, will abolish the pain in almost all patients. Modern implants and prostheses have a low complication rate and provide a good cosmetic result. In advanced disease of the orbit and eye lids, exenteration may offer the best palliation. Although the cosmetic results are mediocre, they are invariably better than the appearance of advanced disease and the surgery produces rapid relief from pain.

Nobody should have to endure the pain and shame of a chronically painful and unsightly eye.

Further reading

1. Easty, D.L., and Sparrow, J. (ed.) (1999). *Oxford textbook of ophthalmology*. Oxford University Press, Oxford.

2. Migliori, M.E. (ed.) (1999). *Enucleation, evisceration, and exenteration of the eye*. Butterworth Heineman, Oxford.

3. Moshfeghi, D.M., Moshfeghi, A.A., and Finger, P.T. (2000). Enucleation. *Surv. Ophthalmol.*, **44**, 277–301.

References

1. Bloom, P.A., Tsai, J.C., Sharma, K., Miller, M.H., Rice, N.S., Hitchings, R.A., *et al.* (1997). 'Cyclodiode'. Trans-scleral diode laser cyclophotocoagulation in the treatment of advanced refractory glaucoma. *Ophthalmology*, **104** (9), 1508–19.

2. Spencer, A.F., and Vernon, S.A. (1999). 'Cyclodiode': results of a standard protocol. *Br. J. Ophthalmol.*, **83** (3), 311–16.

3. Walland, M.J. (2000). Diode laser cyclophotocoagulation: longer-term follow-up of a standardized treatment protocol. *Clin. Experiment Ophthalmol.*, **28** (4), 263–7.

4. Martin, K.R., and Broadway, D.C. (2001). Cyclodiode laser therapy for painful, blind glaucomatous eyes. *Br. J. Ophthalmol.*, **85** (4), 474–6.

5. Youn, J., Cox, T.A., Herndon, L.W., Allingham, R.R., and Shields, M.B. (1998). A clinical comparison of trans-scleral cyclophotocoagulation with neodymium: YAG and semiconductor diode lasers. *Am. J. Ophthalmol.*, **126** (5), 640–7.

6. al Faran, M.F., and al Omar, O.M. (1990). Retrobulbar alcohol injection in blind painful eyes. *Ann. Ophthalmol.*, **22** (12), 460–2.

7. Birch, M., Strong, N., Brittain, P., and Sandford-Smith, J. (1993). Retrobulbar phenol injection in blind painful eyes. *Ann. Ophthalmol.*, **25** (7), 267–70.

8. Alino, A.M., Perry, H.D., Kanellopoulos, A.J., Donnenfeld, E.D., and Rahn, E.K. (1998). Conjunctival flaps. *Opthalmology*, **105** (6), 1120–3.

9. Pires, R.T., Tseng, S.C., Prabhasawat, P., Puangsricharern, V., Maskin, S.L., Kim, J.C. *et al.* (1999). Amniotic membrane transplantation for symptomatic bullous keratopathy. *Arch. Ophthalmol.*, **117** (10), 1291–7.

10. Maini, R., Sullivan, L., Snibson, G.R., Taylor, H.R., and Loughnan, M.S. (2001). A comparison of different depth ablations in the treatment of painful bullous keratopathy with phototherapeutic keratectomy. *Br. J. Ophthalmol.*, **85** (8), 912–15.

11. Shah-Desai, S.D., Tyers, A.G., and Manners, R.M. (2000). Painful blind eye: efficacy of enucleation and evisceration in resolving ocular pain. *Br. J. Ophthalmol.*, **84** (4), 437–8.

12. Custer, P.L., and Reistad, C.E. Enucleation of blind, painful eyes. *Ophthal. Plast. Reconstr. Surg.*, **16** (5), 326–9.

13. COMS Quality of Life Study Group. (1999). Quality of life assessment in the Collaborative Ocular Melanoma Study: design and methods. COMS-QOLS Report No. 1. *Ophthalmic Epidemiol.*, **6** (1), 5–17.

14. Lubkin, V., and Sloan, S. (1990). Enucleation and psychic trauma. *Adv. Ophthalmic Plast. Reconstr. Surg.*, **8**, 259–62.

15. Levine, M.R., Pou, C.R., and Lash, R.H. (1999). The 1998 Wendell Hughes Lecture. Evisceration: is sympathetic ophthalmia a concern in the new millennium? *Ophthal. Plast. Reconstr. Surg.*, **15** (1), 4–8.

16. Glatt, H.J., Googe, P.B., Powers, T., and Apple, D.J. (1993). Anophthalmic socket pain. *Am. J. Ophthalmol.*, **116** (3), 357–62.

17. Rose, G.E., and Wright, J.E. (1994). Exenteration for benign orbital disease. *Br. J. Ophthalmol.*, **78** (1), 14–18.

18. Kiratli, H., Bilgic, S., and Ozerdem, U. (1998). Management of massive orbital involvement of intraocular retinoblastoma. *Ophthalmology*, **105** (2), 322–6.

19. Kersten, R.C., Tse, D.T., Anderson, R.L., and Blodi, F.C. (1985). The role of orbital exenteration in choroidal melanoma with extrascleral extension. *Ophthalmology*, **92** (3), 436–43.

20. Mouriaux, F., Martinot, V., Pellerin, P., Patenotre, P., Rouland, J.F., and Constantinides, G. (1999). Survival after malignant tumors of the orbit and periorbit treated by exenteration. *Acta Ophthalmol. Scand.*, **77** (3), 326–30.

21. Mercieca, F., Suresh, P., Morton, A., and Tullo, A. (1999). Ocular surface disease in intensive care unit patients. *Eye*, **13** (Pt. 2), 231–6.

22. Hernandez, E.V., and Mannis, M.J. (1997). Superficial keratopathy in intensive care unit patients. *Am. J. Ophthalmol.*, **124** (2), 212–16.

23. Dua, H.S. (1998). Bacterial keratitis in the critically ill and comatose patient. *Lancet*, **351** (9100), 387–8.

24. Suresh, P., Mercieca, F., Morton, A., and Tullo, A.B. (2000). Eye care for the critically ill. *Inten. Care Med.*, **26** (2), 162–6.

25. Minassian, D.C., Rosen, P., Dart, J.K., Reidy, A., Desai, P., and Sidhu, M. (2001). Extracapsular cataract extraction compared with small-incision surgery by phacoemulsification: a randomised trial. *Br. J. Ophthalmol.*, **85** (7), 822–9.

Chapter 17

Perspectives from the developing world and diverse societies

A. Aluwihare

Introduction

Palliation refers to the relief of symptoms, discomfort, and anxiety, and the provision of enjoyable and worthwhile activity with the retention of the patient's contact with family and place in society to as great an extent as possible, so that quality of life improves in the context of any illness that is terminal. In developing countries some illness is incurable (e.g. some malignancies) and in some instances the illness will last till death and may hasten death because the facilities may not be available for better management (e.g. paraplegia). The terminal or potential terminal nature of an illness may be because of very late presentation or inadequate facilities to treat it, and many who might have been cured need palliative care (e.g. a pneumonia, or severe diarrhoea with undernutrition and cachexia, Madura foot, tuberculosis, some leukaemias and lymphomas, nephroblastoma, acute surgical illness, burns, trauma including paraplegia)[1]; or may be terminal by the very nature of the disease itself in that it has a very low remission or cure rate (e.g. glioblastoma, rabies, AIDS and its consequences). Sadly, infections, infestations, trauma, and surgical illness are included because sometimes patients come very late and moribund, and cure is not possible within the time and resources available at the place of presentation and moving them is not feasible. This situation and the problems of palliation when cancer patients present late[2] cannot easily be visualized in the industrialized world. Even in texts that attempt to deal with issues outside the economic 'North', the 'on the ground' situations in the developing world are underemphasized.[3] The 'malignant' effect on matters pertaining to palliation that poverty and negative attitudes sadly can and do have, pervade much of this chapter.

Death, cancer, and different religious systems

In the developing world, generally human beings do not consider themselves to be immortal. Different religious systems have an impact on the views of death and incurable illness. Attitudes to cancer and terminal illness also vary widely in different societies.[4–6] It is important for people who are unfamiliar with the different religious systems not to categorize people but to treat them as individuals. In different environments there is a series of viewpoints to be considered with respect to each individual. They include the attitude to death, washing, modesty, fasting, food preparation, conventions, hair, weapons, underclothes, festivals, and rituals.[7] In Christianity of all hues, death is a matter for relatives to grieve about, but can represent a triumph and liberation of the soul as far as the patient is concerned. This aspect is often forgotten.[8] On a personal note, after this author's recovery from a life-threatening illness, a clergyman thanked God for the fact that the treatment was 'successful'. On being challenged as to what was success, in that it might have been better to leave this life and go on to a better one, he agreed that recovery could not necessarily be equated with success! Buddhists are very active in philanthropy and social work but are very fatalistic about life and death, believing that many things are preordained in a cycle of repeated rebirths progressing to triumph over bodily feelings and cravings and leading to nothingness. Death and the incurability of some illness are inevitable. In Islam, the believer is convinced of being better off after death. In Hinduism there is fatalism about illness and death. Judaism invokes in its followers a hostile attitude to death. Confucianism encourages acceptance and fatalism. In sub-Saharan Africa[9,10] and indigenous communities in Australia, many of which remain cut off from the twenty-first century,[11] there are indigenous practitioners and practices and the lack of access to modern methods that complicate palliative management. In most of these situations the concept of not striving assiduously to preserve life is accepted. Quality of life is considered more important than pure longevity. In none of these situations is euthanasia accepted. It is understood that measures to relieve pain may sometimes hasten death and in some communities the philosophy of enduring pain makes analgesia difficult but necessary. Clear communication to patients and relatives about what can and should be done and the conflict that sometimes exists between these two is accepted; but there are subtle variations in different cultures[12] about informing a patient of the truth about an illness.

Non-interference and palliation

Acceptance of death and suffering by the patient and family is sometimes used by doctors and others who treat and look after patients to give themselves the licence to be careless about palliative care. Carers (medical or other) have no right to allow others to suffer when pain and anguish can be relieved. One of the very few multicentre studies comparing the 'North' and 'South' has shown a similar need for pain relief in the inpatient setting.[13] Carers have no right to withhold information either on the grounds of fatalism in the patient's religious system or the belief that life after death is better, or for any other reasons as already discussed (e.g. patient of different social and economic class, different cultural group).

Communication with patients

The communication difficulties created by socio-economic problems are a crucial matter. In industrialized countries there are differences between rich and poor and persons of different social standing. However, their lifestyles and dress, and the goods they can command, are not as different as social status might lead one to expect; the language(s) they speak are the same. Amongst professionals there is an acceptance that the patients' demands for information, pain relief, and palliation are similar. The legal system and the rights of patients as described in hospital documents reinforce the view that patients' needs are the same, irrespective of social or financial status. In the developing world this equality is not respected: because patients are poorer, dress differently, speak only the national language, and feel or are made to feel inferior, there is an insidious and incorrect perception that their needs for good communication, pain relief, and proper palliation are less than those from different backgrounds. This has serious implications for all situations in which patient–doctor communication is needed. Any failure in palliation is partly a reflection of poor communication with patient and parents and applies whether the patient is an adult or a child.[14] The best place in which to realize the inadequacy of pain relief is outside the labour rooms of hospitals; the noise made by patients is indirectly proportional to their social and financial status. Poor, socially deprived patients may be considered a nuisance and the question of spending time and resources on proper palliative care is felt to be a waste; such patients are thought not to need, expect, or appreciate proper care – which is even worse. These terrible attitudes have to be recognized if the palliative care that patients with terminal illness receive is to improve. They limit the procurement of necessary drugs and other facilities for what is thought to be low-priority care, and the general scarcity of resources compounds the problem! Where funding agencies and physicians are more enlightened, better services do develop in poorer countries[15–21] and richer developing ones.[22] Sadly, most of these deal only with cancer and not the vast range of other terminal surgical diseases, referred to in the introduction to this chapter. Changes of attitude in medical school and postgraduate programmes need to develop and will have to run counter to the attitudes displayed in other sectors of the countries concerned. The services of the indigenous practitioners and medical systems in the developing world are hardly utilized at all in palliative care, and very few studies of their value exist. One of the few shows the help given by a Japanese massage system in London[23] and another, in India, the effective management of morphine-induced constipation.[24] Other communication problems relate to the lack of telephone facilities and the physical distance between a patient's home and the hospital in which the diagnosis and initial management takes place. This latter problem also makes home-based palliation difficult as access to supervision and medications is complicated and costly. However, it is important not to underestimate the capabilities of a well-informed, poor, rural family to help with the care of a patient with a terminal illness. Even when telephones are good there may be nobody ready to take the calls and be troubled about the needs of distant and poorer people. Attitudes may remain the biggest obstacle.

Paternalism

In the management of particularly advanced cancers, the multidisciplinary team should include those with an understanding of palliation[25] in the context of the patient's society, and not just cure-oriented oncologists and surgeons. This ensures that a positive and holistic approach is adopted to both palliation and cure; a recognition of the risks of killing a patient in a too aggressive attempt to cure (possibly for the satisfaction of the doctor or because early consideration of palliation is often regarded as a sign of failure by a very 'cure targeted' clinician!) is part of the balanced approach needed.[26] This balance is very difficult to achieve if the palliative personnel are either non-medical or thought to be doctors of lower 'standing' than the 'curing' ones (e.g. surgeons). In many developing countries the paternalistic attitude of doctors hinders this holistic approach. An example of how paternalism might be responsible for making physicians feel their patients do not need to know about the true nature of an illness comes from a comparison between South America and developed country experiences.[27] It also hinders the idea of allowing a patient and family some true degree of autonomy[28] in the choice of management of advanced disease (whether it be malignancy or other advanced disease needing palliation). Choice is vital, particularly when considering the preferred place of death,[29] which depends on the patient's medical, social, psychological, religious, and cultural environment.

The extended family

The situation is much better where the family is intact with children/parents in or near the patient's house and there is other support readily available. The value of being at home in familiar surroundings and with loved ones in attendance can then be realized. The family members can and do actively help in the care of the patient, provided they are given clear instructions in words and idiom they understand. Simple medication for pain is often available, though many countries still make oral opiates difficult to obtain.[8,30] Where pain is recognized as meriting relief and resources are provided, the World Health Organization (WHO) analgesia ladder system is operable in the developing world.[31,32] Feeding, positioning, cleaning, and other nursing measures are important, while mental activity – entertainment – and the stimulus of having family around are invaluable. It is possible for short visits to be arranged if some procedure has to be done in an institution. The usual problem is that the hospital-to-family communication is not good. A lot is possible because of the integrity of the family network, and the hospital-based services need to be very careful not to take over what can be done at home and by doing so add an extra burden. Whatever the financial condition of the family, most developing country families and patients prefer death of the terminally ill to occur at home even when, as they may be in Japan,[33] they are hostile to the idea of death. Australian indigenous people are almost the only exception to this.[11]

Home/institution-based palliation

Family cohesion is greater in developing countries than in the West. This is so mainly in rural areas. Unplanned and uncontrolled urbanization in search of employment and associated with the decline in income from agriculture have led to not only extended but even nuclear family disintegration. Home-based palliative care has to be considered in both situations. When the family has broken up then it is very difficult as the State does not provide help (a generalization, but most often true). The private sector (for profit or non-profit) is slow to enter this field and certainly does not cater for the huge mass of people who cannot pay. Non-government organizations are better but very limited in number. This problem is one of the consequences of urban drift that does not receive mention in discourse on that subject.

Home-based care is, however, possible with visiting services in poorer countries.[34] With imagination, more hospital-linked, home-based palliation is possible.[35]

The effect of poverty

Poverty can make a patient present late and affect support systems after presentation.[2] The facilities available to the State for palliation suffer in any resource crisis. Poverty in the family can have even more adverse effects. Washing and the provision of clean clothes and linen are a problem. Temperature control (heating, cooling, ventilation) may not be adequate. Smell often persists around the patient. Hunger and thirst, and general nutrition, are neglected. The provision of clean drinking water and appropriate toilet facilities are difficult. Light to read (if the person can) and measures to relieve the monotony of living are often neglected. Pain and other symptom relief may be considered unimportant as they are necessary 'parts' of the dying process and the available resources should go to the living. In all these areas there are money problems and attitude problems and hardly any public education about palliation.

Costs

The priority given to palliative care is lower than that to prevention and cure. Costs compound this problem, although this is not to say that costs have more influence than the attitudes of the health provider. Many drugs are produced in industrialized countries though this situation is rapidly changing. India, China, Pakistan, Brazil, and several countries in sub-Saharan Africa are increasingly manufacturing drugs either under licence or by flouting copyright laws. The percentage of gross domestic product (GDP) spent on health care is relatively low (often under 3%) and this is a percentage of a developing country's wealth. Anything needed from wealthy countries is therefore even more inaccessible when one considers the exchange rates and the costs of labour in those areas. This problem affects drugs, intravenous fluids, prepared semi-digested or elemental diets, stents, and the mechanisms for non-invasive diagnostic and stent-insertion mechanisms. Hospice work is more likely to develop with innovative funding from non-State subsidies.[36] The role in the economy of many developing countries of the private sector is increasing as far as decision making and financial power are concerned. This stronger private sector is only slowly realizing the obligation to carry an increasing social responsibility as well.

Psychological and emotional support

Apart from counselling it is important to provide entertainment and work as a part of palliative care, to keep active and occupied whatever part of the body and mind are available to function. Examples include, reading (in the few places where levels of literacy permit), radio and other audiovisual activity (available to very few), the chance to chat and be listened to, a handicraft of whatever kind, the chance to move functioning limbs and muscles, and the chance to see trees and the sky. In the tropical developing countries it is possible to be outdoors most of the year in the shade. The problem is often not the lack of something positive, but the belief that it is not necessary or not worth doing for the patient. This aspect is also often forgotten in the fight that the fit have to survive. However, it is attitudes and a willingness to try that can bring the biggest improvement. Many in the Industrial North cannot envisage this scenario. The role of religious and spiritual counsellors who will listen to the terminally ill is very important; the two may not be the same person, and both patients and carers may need help.[37]

Vulnerable groups

Women, children, the old, and the disabled are particularly vulnerable groups in many developing countries. When any of these groups are dying this disadvantage may be compounded. Women in particular may have to do housework that can tax them greatly, even though some domestic activity may be good. There is resentment that some other arrangement has to be made to look after children and the house.

Children

In the developing countries, childhood malignancies form 4–5% of all malignancies, unlike the 1% in the developed world. All are not terminal and the improvement in the well-being of the child after resuscitation from the acute presentation may be remarkable. However, with any serious or advanced disease, children and parents have psychosocial problems. These have to be dealt with in context and although the classical Western norms often cannot be applied,[14] the need for proper palliation remains vital. Children over ten years old, and often younger, have concerns about survival. Parents may not allow or like children to express their feelings, and it may be thought to be improper. Many children thus have to mask their concerns, which makes them tired and 'weak; and leads to somatization of anxiety'. It is important for children to lead as normal a life as possible, and the fact that play and education have an important role in palliation of anxiety is either forgotten or resources are not available.

The psychological requirements of children[14] are often left entirely to the family, recognizing perhaps by default the existence of a family support system. Medical professionals deal only with the 'technical medical' aspects. This leaves children and their families without the support from knowledge that is available. A multidisciplinary approach is needed to fill this vacuum. Poverty, ignorance, illiteracy, and significant hierarchical difference between doctor and client contribute to the 'vacuum'.

Parents feel they have failed a child when terminal illness is recognized and this has many repercussions. The family may fragment or sometimes become more united. In either event, special support is needed but usually not available within the 'health system'. Parents are desperate when a child is ill and want to do 'everything', but may not be able to afford it. In the developing world the State support systems for this are very variable, and in many countries the result of the macroeconomic policies advocated by the major international lending institutions (insisting on cost recovery in health systems) combined with local corruption and bad governance mean that the needs for palliation in vulnerable groups cannot be met. In the inpatient environment and in the community there is a willingness of relatives, friends, and even the parents of other children with similar problems to help with money, medicines, food, companionship, and other forms of support.[14] Whether these informal systems to help in the financial and psychosocial aspects of palliation will disappear as countries 'advance' is uncertain.

There is also often conflict between what an astrologer has said and what the doctors may think important for potential cure or palliation. An attempt to understand the value system of the parents is important, and even a willingness to meet an astrologer or indigenous physician may be needed.

Communication of the child's problem to parents and child is painful.[14] In the developing world it is rare for any empathy between doctor and family to be evident and for doctors to show an understanding of the distress of the parents or to even reveal their own distress. This is perhaps part of the felt or unconscious need to preserve the 'god-like' status of doctors. Proper privacy for discussion is rare. In the South Indian situation, parents' preferences were for the doctor to show caring (97%), to allow parents to talk (95%), to allow parents to show their own feelings (93%), to share information (90%), to be highly confident (89%), and to have parent-to-parent referral (87%).[14] To meet these needs in the developing world, where familiarity with terminology may be poor and literacy low, innovative ways of imparting information do work and are appreciated.[14]

It is sad to have to care for curable children who are dying slowly because there are no facilities to treat them. Examples abound of congenital and acquired cardiac disease, renal failure, and liver failure. Many of the palliative measures needed in the more dramatic situations of malignancy are pertinent but forgotten. The late presentation of children with malignancies, chronic infections, and infestations (e.g. Madura foot) mean that many who might have been cured need palliative care. The late presentation is another consequence of poverty, difficulty of access (fear, finance, distance, etc.), and poor public education.

The place of home care for dying children in the developing world is important. Evidence shows[4] that where it is attempted, it is successful. Even in very deprived environments the most important element is pain relief. The vital factor in home care in any situation is the presence of loved parents and siblings – difficult for them but good for the dying child. The religious systems often help parents to cushion their loss and this may have a fatalistic element. In the developing world it is important to maximize what homes can offer and not to take children away into overcrowded and terrifying hospitals with no privacy. Non-government organizations will have to step in, and are doing so, to help in this very particular way with home-visiting personnel, analgesics, and suitable nourishment. Those who have been to poor villages all over the world will have no illusions about the difficult situation faced by children and their parents when the child is dying – no formal palliation, but at least loving parents.

Training

The training systems of medical and other health professionals neglect the matter of communication, and of communication in the palliative situation in particular. This is not unique to the developing world, but is worse and reflects both ignorance, pressure from other priorities, and a feeling that the family system will help. Special training is needed, with a multidisciplinary emphasis,[38] in dealing with the social issues and diseases of developing countries and the Tropics and those of the developed world, and ageing, a double burden of disease;[8,39] learning in the developing country environment.[40]

Evaluation of success of palliation

If palliation aims at quality of life rather than quantity, as measured by longevity alone, measures of quality are needed to assess progress in palliation or compare methods. It is crucial that patient-centred systems are employed. There are various patient consultation questionnaires in use for illnesses as diverse as hernia and large bowel symptoms that show patients can cooperate, but these are developed and used in industrialized countries (Cade and Selvachandran, personal communication 2000). The same applies to postal questionnaires[41] and to Functional Living Index for Cancer (FLIC) measures used in palliation. Goh *et al.* [42] have shown well the care needed to translate the words and meanings of such questionnaires into the cultural context of mixed populations and to validate them. They have shown that this is possible and lay stress on many factors rather than the mainly physiological ones that health professional questionnaires might use. They have shown that as malignancy advances, FLIC scores decrease, as expected, and are developing the method to assess success of palliation. Very few countries in the non-industrialized world have evaluated the success of palliative medicine, an example from a country – still considered to be only 'almost industrialized' – being provided by Singapore.[43]

Conclusions

There are many challenges in developing countries and only a few are listed here. Data on the need for palliative care, even for malignant disease, are lacking. Carers are in short supply. Medical and nursing schools have very little in their curricula on this subject. The information, medications, appliances, and strategies available in the economic 'North' are not used, with suitable modification, as much as they could be. The attitudes of hospital personnel do not help good communication with patients and families. The overwhelming majority of the patients in the world who need palliative care are in developing countries, and fortunately much can be done to help just by improving staff attitudes and communication with patients and families.

References

1. Dhar, A., and Aluwihare, A.P.R. (2000). The surgery of late presentation and delayed diagnosis. In: *Oxford textbook of surgery* (ed. P.J. Morris and W.C. Wood). Oxford University Press, Oxford.

2. Sureshkumar, K., and Rajagopal, M.R. (1996). Palliative care in Kerala. Problems at presentaion in 440 patients with advanced cancer in a south Indian state: *Pall. Med.*, **10**, 293–8.

3. Doyle, D. Hanks, G.W.C., and MacDonald, N. (ed.) (1998). *Oxford textbook of palliative medicine.* Oxford University Press, Oxford.

4. Navon, L. (1999). Cultural views of cancer around the world. *Cancer Nurs.*, **22**, 39–45.

5. Granda-Cameron, C. (1999). The experience of having cancer in Latin America. *Cancer Nurs.*, **22**, 51–7.

6. Delbar, V. (1999). From the desert: transcultural aspects of cancer nursing care in Israel. *Cancer Nurs.*, **22**, 45–51.

7. Neuberger, J. (1998). Introduction to cultural issues in palliative care. In: *Oxford textbook of palliative medicine* (ed. D. Doyle, G.W.C. Hanks, and N. MacDonald), pp. 777–86. Oxford University Press, Oxford.

8. Stjernsward, J., and Pampallona, S. (1998). Palliative medicine – a global perspective. In: *Oxford textbook of palliative medicine* (ed. D. Doyle, G.W.C. Hanks, and N. MacDonald), pp. 1227–45. Oxford University Press, Oxford.

9. Olweny, C.L.M. (1998). Cultural issues in sub-Saharan Africa. In: *Oxford textbook of palliative medicine* (ed. D. Doyle, G.W.C. Hanks, and N. MacDonald), pp. 787–92. Oxford University Press, Oxford.

10. Defilippi, K. (2000). Palliative care issues in sub-Saharan Africa. *Int. J. Pall. Nurs.*, **6**, 108.

11. Blackwell, N. (1998). Cultural issues in indigenous Australian peoples. In: *Oxford textbook of palliative medicine* (ed. D. Doyle, G.W.C. Hanks, and N. MacDonald), pp. 799–804. Oxford University Press, Oxford.

12. Chan, K.S., Lam, Z.C.L., Chun, R.P.K., Dai, D.L.K., and Leung, A.C.K. (1998). Chinese patients with terminal cancer. In: *Oxford textbook of palliative medicine* (ed. D. Doyle, G.W.C. Hanks, and N. MacDonald), pp. 793–6. Oxford University Press, Oxford.

13. Fainsinger, R.L., Waller, A., Bercovici, M., Bengtson, K., Landman, W., Hosking, M., *et al.* (2000). A multicentre international study of sedation for uncontrolled symptoms in terminally ill patients. *Pall. Med.*, **14**, 257–65.

14. Bharath, S. (ed.) (1999). Psychosocial aspects of children who are terminally ill. Proceedings of Symposium NIHMANS, Bangalore. National Institute of Mental Health and Neurosciences, Bangalore.

15. Sadovska, O. (1997) Department of palliative care in Bratislava and the development of the palliative care movement in Slovakia. *Support. Care Cancer*, **5**, 430–4.

16. Sun, W.Z., Hou, W.Y., and Li, J.H. (1996). Republic of China: status of cancer pain and palliative care. *J. Pain Sympt. Manage.*, **12**, 127–9.

17. Zhang, H., Gu, W.P., Joranson, D.E., and Cleeland, C. (1996). People's Republic of China: status of cancer pain and palliative care. *J. Pain Sympt. Manage.*, **12**, 124–6.

18. Chaturvedi, S.K., and Chandra, P.S. (1998). Palliative care in India. *Support. Care Cancer*, **6**, 81–4.

19. Beck, S.L. (1999). Health policy, health services, and cancer pain management in the New South Africa. *J. Pain Sympt. Manage.*, **17**, 16–26.

20. Seamark, D., Ajithakumari, K., Burn, G., Saraswalthi Devi, P., Koshy, R., and Seamark, C. (2000). Palliative care in India. *J. Roy. Soc. Med.*, **93**, 292–5.

21. Burn, G. (2001). A personal initiative to improve palliative care in India: 10 years on. *Pall. Med.*, **15**, 159–62.

22. Almuzaini, A.S., Salek, M.S., Nicholls, P.J., and Alomar, B.A. (1998). The attitude of health care professionals toward the availability of hospice services for cancer patients and their carers in Saudi Arabia. *Pall. Med.*, **12**, 365–73.

23. Stevensen, C. (1995). The role of shiatsu in palliative care. *Complement. Ther. Nurs. Midwif.*, **1**, 51–8.

24. Ramesh, P.R., Kumar, K.S., Rajagopal, M.R., Balachandran, P., and Warrier, P.K. (1998). Managing morphine-induced constipation: a controlled comparison of an Ayurvedic formulation and senna *J. Pain Sympt. Manage.*, **16**, 240–4.

25. Goh, C., O'Sullivan, B., Warde, P., Groome, P., and Gullane, P. (1996). Multidisciplinary management controversies in laryngeal cancer *Ann. Acad. Med. Singapore*, **25**, 405–12.

26. Schipper, H., Goh, C.R., and Wang, T.L. (1995). Shifting the cancer paradigm: must we kill to cure? *J. Clin. Oncol.*, **13**, 801–7.

27. Bruera, E., Neumann, C.M., Mazzocato, C., Stiefel, F., and Sala, R. (2000). Attitudes and beliefs of palliative care physicians regarding communication with terminally ill cancer patients. *Pall. Med.*, **14**, 287–98.

28. Ng, L.F., Shumacher, A., and Goh, C.B. (2000). Autonomy for whom? A perspective from the Orient. *Pall. Med.*, **14**, 163–4.

29. Goh, C. (1998). Preferred place of death. *Singapore Med. J.*, **39** (10), 430–1.

30. Takeda, F. (1996). Japan: status of cancer pain and palliative care. *J. Pain Sympt. Manage.*, **12**, 118–20.

31. Soebadi, R.D., and Tejawinata, S. (1996). Indonesia: status of cancer pain and palliative care. *J. Pain Sympt. Manage.*, **12**, 112–15.

32. Isbister, W.H., and Bonifant, J. (2001). Implementation of the World Health Organization 'analgesic ladder' in Saudi Arabia. *Pall. Med.*, **15**, 135–40.

33. Kashiwagi, T. (1998). Palliative care in Japan. In: *Oxford textbook of palliative medicine* (ed. D. Doyle, G.W.C. Hanks, and N. MacDonald), pp. 797–8. Oxford University Press, Oxford.

34. Ajithakumari, K., Sureshkumar, K., and Rajagopal, M.R. (1997). Palliative home care: the Calicut experience. *Pall. Med.*, **11**, 451–4.

35. Tanneberger, S., and Pannuti, F. (1998). The Bologna Hospital-at-Home: a model for cost-effective care of advanced cancer patients in developing countries. *Natl. Med. J. India*, **11**, 231–5.

36. Carter, H., MacLeod, R., Hicks, E., and Carter, J. (1999). The development of funding policies for hospices: is casemix-based funding an option? *N.Z. Med. J.*, **25**, 236–9.

37. Speck, P. (1998). Spiritual issues in palliative care. In: *Oxford textbook of palliative medicine* (ed. D. Doyle, G.W.C. Hanks, and N. MacDonald), pp. 805–14. Oxford University Press, Oxford.

38. Suhatno, S. (2000). Palliative care in cervical cancer. *Gan To Kagaku Ryoho*, **27**, (Suppl.2), 440–8.

39. Maddocks, I. (2000).Teaching palliative care in east Asia. *Pall. Med.*, **14**, 535–7.

40. Weir, E. (1996). A summer in India. *Car. Med. Assoc. J.*, **55**, 785–7.

41. Jacoby, A., Lecouturier, J., Bradshaw, C., Lovel, T., and Eccles, M. (1999). Feasibility of using postal questionnaries to examine carer satisfaction with palliative care: a methodological assessment. South Tyneside MAAG Palliative Care Study Group. *Pall. Med.*, **13**, 285–98.

42. Goh, C.R., Lee, K.S., Tan, T.C., Wang, T.L., Tan, C.H., Wong. J., *et al.* (1996). Measuring quality of life in different cultures: translation of the Functional Living Index for Cancer (FLIC) into Chinese and Malay in Singapore. *Ann. Acad. Med. Singapore*, **25**, 323–34.

43. Goh, C.R. (1996). Singapore: status of cancer pain and palliative care. *J. Pain. Sympt. Manage.*, **12**, 130–2.

Chapter 18

Epilogue: a message to all surgeons

Geoffrey P. Dunn and Alan G. Johnson

Surgical palliative care: a new sub-speciality or a new fundamental basis for all surgery?

Following a presentation on surgical palliative care, a cardiovascular surgeon expressed his concern that an emphasis on symptom control would undermine efforts to cure, which he felt was the primary mission of the surgeon. He added, 'Don't worry, I palliate patients every day!' Depending upon which surgeon is asked, palliation may be seen as synonymous with their daily work or it may be a remote province of expertise by others. The future of the definition and practice of palliation by surgeons and surgical means will depend on the balance of these two positions. Only time will tell to what extent a comprehensive philosophy of palliation whose origins can be identified in post-World War II Britain will influence the practice of surgery worldwide in the current millenium. The result of these influences may be as radical as a shift in perspective in all surgical sub-specialities brought about by the abandonment of a disease-based model of care in exchange for patient-defined outcomes; or the future may see a much more limited change in surgical thinking in which the task of palliation becomes an occasional exercise of the surgeon under the supervision of a small cadre of specialists with palliative care expertise. The most lamentable outcome would be that all 'palliative' surgical patients would be identified and referred outside the orbit of surgical care altogether.

Surgical palliative care in the future is what the practice of surgery, itself, might have looked like if Dame Cicely Saunders had become a surgeon! Despite this optimistic thinking (encouraged by recent increased attention to palliative care in surgery in a number of countries), surgical palliative care runs the risk of becoming relegated to sub-speciality status. The alternative is that all surgical practice will be guided by the principles of palliative care that have evolved globally during the last quarter of a century.

This same battle has already been fought in the medical arena, resulting in fully-fledged speciality status for palliative medicine in some countries; but in other countries palliative care has grudgingly been added to the credentials of the primary speciality. In the US, expertise in some areas such as critical care is recognized as 'added credentials' to a surgeon's basic board certification in surgery. Should palliative medicine not achieve fully-fledged medical speciality status in the US as it has in the UK, the 'added credentials' approach would be the most likely way to incorporate palliative care into the existing specialities, including surgery.

Although the initial writings by surgeons were confined to the operative management of symptoms related to advanced oncological disease,[1] we can foresee an expansion beyond technical procedures in trauma, vascular, and transplant surgery as well as cancer. Much of the theory and practice presented in this book has been the experience of surgeons not specializing in oncology, but who have used cancer as a reference point for developing principles and techniques of palliative care, just as their medical colleagues have done.

At the time of writing, the necessary pieces of this new vision of surgery are already coming into sharper focus. An ethical framework has been proposed by Little[2] that could incorporate palliative principles without departing from traditional surgical values. Newer techniques of surgery such as laparoscopy are increasingly influenced by quality-of-life considerations while the measurement of quality of life in patients undergoing surgical procedures has an increasingly firm scientific basis.[3]

As always, there is a hidden danger during the current rapid technical innovation of the 'how' outpacing the 'why?'. One of the authors recalls during a recent Clinical Congress of the American College of Surgeons when a well-attended symposium on physician-assisted suicide was held alongside an enormous technical exhibit. As the panelists looked over this vast sea of technology during lunch someone half-jokingly remarked, 'This is probably one of the reasons we are in such a hell of a mess with end-of-life care!' Principle-based medical ethics has emphasized the point that there is nothing intrinsically wrong or right with treatments or the agents for carrying them out. Their danger grows in proportion to their degree of isolation from the context of meaning to a given patient living in a social context.

Surgery must change its traditional views or perish!

One hundred years ago, a surgeon could function as primary physician, anaesthetist, surgeon, pathologist, guidance counsellor, and provider of the care of patients. This was due to the nature of the social contract and the limited scientific knowledge and operative capabilities of that time. Few vestiges of this portrait of individual authority remain, though many of the surgeon's instincts or character traits do. Krizek, in his address at the 11th Ethics and Philosophy Lecture given at the 87th Clinical Congress of the American College of Surgeons,[4] offered a darker view when he described surgery as an impaired and impairing profession with the seeds of impairment – which were planted during medical school and residency education – bearing fruit later in high rates of job dissatisfaction, substance abuse, and suicide. He further noted that the fragmentation of vision of the profession, concurrent with surgical fragmentation, are results and causes of impairment of the surgeon and the profession as a whole.

For those whom perceive dying as a natural process necessary for renewal, the comparison should be reassuring! The arrival of genetic engineering and the full impact of information technology can either be seen as a crisis or as a new opportunity for the surgical community to redefine itself, just as it did following all the basic science discoveries in the nineteenth century. We are now living in an era when the craft of surgery could actually be replaced by mechanized surgery performed by robots. Should such a transition take place, the remaining role of the surgeon would consist primarily that of communicator, educator, and guide.

Without the ability to interpret a patient's experience and provide a perspective on the new therapies which are emerging almost daily, the surgeon could quickly become irrelevant – an admirable historical curiosity along with the village blacksmith.

During the previous 'crisis' of the late nineteenth century, surgeons assimilated the new knowledge derived from the basic sciences with the result that surgeons reached a new position of influence in the promotion of health and opened vast new frontiers of shared experience with patients, not possible in their brief, traumatic encounters for blood letting or amputation.

In the sixteenth century, the French surgeon Ambroise Parè described the duties of surgery as 'to remove what is superfluous, to restore what has been dislocated, to separate what has grown together, to reunite what has been divided and to redress the defects of nature'. Surgery

> ## Box 18.1 The transient place of surgery in the history of the management of tuberculosis
>
> 1. Fresh air and hope
> 2. Gross surgery – thoracoplasty
> 3. Refined surgery – phrenic crush
> 4. Antibiotics
> 5. Immunization
> 6. Elimination of source

is good at dealing with structural abnormalities but not nearly so good at treating metabolic, neoplastic, or infectious disease. The history of the management of tuberculosis provides an excellent illustration of the rise and fall of surgery in the treatment of infection (Box 18.1). This is a pattern we would expect to see with many other common diseases. For example, over the last 20 years we have seen elective surgery for peptic ulcer give way first to acid-blocking drugs and then to antibiotics.

Appropriately, the management of trauma that provided the first opportunity for surgery may also be the last when other disorders are pre-emptively managed at a molecular level without the contact of a surgeon's hand. This development would not undermine the validity of a palliative philosophy in the future practice of surgery; indeed it would enhances it because care for the traumatized patient has historically been the most compelling expression of palliative care in surgical experience. In trauma, an individual's restoration to wholeness is only possible when his suffering is relieved first. Think of that writhing, burnt patient who can not keep still for dressings and grafting until his pain is controlled. The great test awaiting surgeons is their willingness to adjust their capabilities to respond effectively to more diverse forms of suffering in addition to physical suffering.

Surgery is once again ready to assimilate a new body of knowledge in addition to the ongoing discoveries of the basic sciences. This new body of knowledge includes the insights of psychological, social, and spiritual disciplines. We are also less timid in acknowledging the sacred knowledge acquired from experiences of life and death shared with our patients, such as recounted in general surgeon Sherwin Nuland's *How we die*[5] and neurosurgeon Marc Flitter's *Judith's pavilion*.[6] If we are not afraid of these gifts, surgeons should have no trouble finding a meaningful place at the bedside in the future, no matter how microscopic or galactic the scale of intervention.

There will always be a surgeon as long as there is someone willing to use tools to touch someone in order to restore health. Defining those tools and how to use them is the surgeon's job. Only by viewing their efforts in the greater context of the patient's and society's vision of health can the surgeon reverse the trend towards the status of a technician back to that of a craftsman and healer. Fortunately, attention is now being directed to the cognitive, social, and psychological preparation necessary to enable surgeons to participate more broadly and profoundly in the treatment of suffering, whether based on elimination of disease or conditioning the patient to co-exist with illness. If Krizek is right about the 'writing on the wall' for surgeons and surgery, this preparation could not come too soon.

Barriers to a comprehensive philosophy and practice of surgical palliative care

If surgeons and the practice of surgery have shortcomings in providing satisfactory palliative care, it reflects a lack of a comprehensive vision, not a lack of effective techniques, motivated individuals, or experience. The barriers can be conveniently classified into categories reminiscent of the four dimensions of 'total pain' described by Cicely Saunders.[7] The barriers can be classified into cognitive, psychological, social, and spiritual categories (Box 18.2).

Cognitive barriers

Cognitive barriers to a comprehensive philosophy and practice of surgical palliative care consist of gaps in surgical education, training, textbooks, and articles. In a survey of the Society of Surgical Oncology,[8] McCahill *et al.* determined that only a small percentage of those surveyed

---

Box 18.2 Barriers to surgeons' effective participation in palliative care

Cognitive

- Confusion concerning the definition of 'palliative'
- Limitations in training:
  - symptom control
  - communication skills
  - ethics
- Lack of validated quality-of-life measurement instruments for many surgical problems

Psychological

- Fear of failure – the need to 'do something'
- Fear of loss of control and facing ambiguity
- Fear of introspection
- Pre-existing psychological barriers due to 'burn-out' and/or previous psychological disorder

Social

- Prevailing hierarchical structure of surgery (surgeon as 'captain of the ship')
- Mortality and morbidity as outcome measurements
- Economic concerns:
  - fears concerning loss of referrals from fellow physicians
  - surgeon reimbursement concerns related to low reimbursement for services such as family conferences, home visits

Box 18.2 Barriers to surgeons' effective participation in palliative care *(continued)*

    – loss of income by not doing procedures on patients

    – fear of attracting 'problem' patients who require much time and energy

  ◆ Legal concerns:

    – fear of 'killing the patient' when withdrawing life support or not offering surgery

    – fears related to scrutiny of prescribing practices (narcotics)

    – fear of litigation if perceived as 'giving up' by patient and family

    – general fears related to litigation eroding trust in patients and their families

Spiritual

◆ Inherent conflict between spiritual and physical reality in Western culture

◆ Surgeon's own spiritual or religious bias.

◆ Inability to differentiate spiritual from religious matters

◆ Individual surgeon's or speciality's own spiritual crisis

received more than 10 hours of training in palliative care. A study by Rappaport and Witzke[9] found that 84% of junior and 50% of senior residents reported never having heard an attending surgeon discuss how to manage a terminally ill patient. Not surprisingly, reviews[10,11] of surgical textbooks and articles found little attention to death and dying or palliation as the result of a systematic, interdisciplinary approach.

Adding to the cognitive barriers to surgeon's understanding of palliation as a core principle and practice is the inconsistent use of the word 'palliation' itself in the surgical literature. Many surgeons when asked to define palliation will respond as when asked how great art or pornography are defined: 'I can't define it, but I know it when I see it.' In the survey mentioned above by McCahill *et al.*, 43% defined palliative surgery on the preoperative intent, 27% defined it on the basis of postoperative findings, and 30% defined it based on the patient's prognosis. Other definitions of 'palliative' include resection for recurrent or persistent disease after primary treatment failure.[12] Some[13] have included diagnostic procedures as a part of the palliative surgery repertoire. They argue that they are part of a supportive strategy even though they provide no direct symptom relief.

Palliative surgery and surgical palliative care

These varied definitions reveal several profound differences in perspective from the operational definition of palliation familiar to practitioners of palliative medicine and hospice care: the relief of distressing symptoms and suffering as perceived by a patient. Only after the accumulated experience in palliative medical care has it been possible to see a clear distinction between palliative surgery and surgical palliative care. Palliative surgery consists of procedures for the relief of burdensome symptoms and suffering with the intention of enhancing the quality of life of a patient as defined by the patient, regardless of its impact on the underlying disease process. Surgical palliative care is palliative care by surgeons and their colleagues (nursing, anaesthesia, etc.) using operative (palliative surgery) and non-operative means. 'Palliative surgery' describes a specific means of palliation at the disposal of the surgeon, while 'surgical palliative or supportive care' reflects the broader context in which these operations are done. The language of surgery offers metaphors useful to all palliative care practitioners.

Quality of life

The definition of palliation is closely linked with measurement of quality of life outcomes. Its measurement, a relatively new science in the field of palliative medicine, is an even more recent arrival to the field of surgery. There was, however, a prescient surgical paper[14] reporting QOL outcomes as the primary focus of a clinical trial as far back as 1982, measuring QOL outcomes in advanced sarcoma trials. The investigators made an observation which is now widely accepted: 'Because of the quality of life data generated and shared with all members of the staff, personnel became more aware and consequently more sensitive to quality of life issues experienced by the patient population . . . The project improved patient care by raising the sensitivity of those delivering care . . . this research tended to improve the doctor–patient relationship. Patients were glad to know that physicians, nurses, and other members of the oncology team were interested in the non-medical consequences of treatment.'

Since the mid 1990s there has been a marked increase in the number of surgical papers using QOL measures, though scarcity and deficiencies in QOL data still exist in surgical and surgical oncology literature.[15,16] An indication of the growing acceptance of QOL outcomes as a primary focus for surgical outcomes is the recommendation by Langenhoff *et al.*[17] that QOL measurement based on appropriate selection of validated QOL instruments should be an integral part of outcomes assessment in cancer surgery.

Improved QOL data collection and analysis will resolve a common debate over the role of the 'pre-emptive surgical strike', i.e. palliative procedures designed to *prevent* symptoms anticipated in asymptomatic patients. This debate is still active in cases of malignant biliary and gastric obstruction[18] among many others. For major palliative resections, one authority[19] argues that resection should be done only in symptomatic patients, assuming other criteria (the right surgeon, the right disease, the right operation, and the right patient psychology) are met.

Psychologic barriers

Sherwin Nuland, a surgeon, wrote in *A surgeon's reflections on the care of the dying*[20] that surgeons take pride in decisiveness and this is demonstrated in the surgeon's capacity to effectively act, do, and take charge. The language of surgery reflects this action-prone temperament and uneasiness with ambiguity: 'do', 'cut', 'close', 'mobilize', and 'resect'. Even though they often have to take these important decisions on inadequate data, surgeons are nervous about 'watching' and can't stand 'waiting', but they definitely like 'closure'. Unfortunately these very same characteristics can make relationships difficult, especially in circumstances calling for an introspective and expectant mind when little *active* treatment should be given. Palliative care practice may be anathema to those who demand a high degree of control and sense of certainty.

Social barriers

There is some danger that the social aloofness of surgeons that has traditionally characterized their clinical relationships with non-surgeons will express itself once again as they develop a comprehensive philosophy of palliation. There is a danger that surgical palliative care could develop parallel but independently of others. To prevent this from happening it is critical at this juncture that surgeons receive as much encouragement and direction as possible from their non-surgical colleagues in all disciplines at all levels.

A major disincentive for surgeons doing surgery for palliation of symptoms alone is the prevailing system of accountability for morbidity and mortality because any death within 30 days of an operation has traditionally been considered a postoperative death. The rate of complications (morbidity) of all types is higher in a group of patients with advanced illness likely to select procedures solely for symptom relief. The surgeon is understandably fearful of statistics that may invite increased scrutiny and discourage referrals from those not aware of the particular circumstances. Another social barrier to effective participation of surgeons in palliative care is the fear that a surgeon who sees himself as acting on behalf of a patient may put himself at odds with referring non-surgical colleagues. For example, the surgeon may recognize the futility of abdominal exploration for malignant bowel obstruction due to diffuse carcinomatosis, yet there may be considerable pressure from the referring physician to 'do something'. Or, conversely, the surgeon may recognize that pinning a pathological fracture would be a far more effective technique for pain control (even in a patient with probably only a few weeks to live) than the pharmacotherapy alone recommended by the attending and referring physician.

Overexaggerated or misfounded fears of running foul of the law due to withdrawal of care, the prescription of controlled substances (narcotics) on a chronic basis, and fear of litigation for not 'saving' the patient are all reasons why a surgeon may feel reluctant to embrace some of the principles and practices of palliative care. Adding to the surgeon's anxiety and frustration in the United States is the increasing number of lawsuits because these measures were *not* done or done well.

Long hours in the operating theatre may prevent the surgeon from participating in many group or family meetings that occur during the 'prime time' of day. Lack of sleep from excessive emergency calls does little to foster patience or sympathy for fatigued and sleep-deprived patients.

Spiritual barriers

Despite recent interest of surgeons in spiritual matters related to their professional work[21,22] and increasing attention to the concept that the world of the mind, body, and spirit are in a continuum, the chasm between the highly physical world of surgery and the spiritual world is still a wide one for many surgeons. Krizek, writing about the spiritual dimensions of surgical palliative care, summarized this chasm: 'Surgery is not a spiritual or religious enterprise. Surgeons may be devoutly religious and the performance of surgery may seem transcendent and spiritual at times. Surgeons seem deeply reflective about many issues and should be expected to be among the most ethical, moral, and honorable physicians. What we do is life and death . . . But the spiritual, moral, and societal challenges [of suicide as a part] of palliative care are not part of surgery.'[23] Due to public pressure and increased transparency of the conduct of medical affairs, the spiritual, moral, and societal challenges to which he refers are becoming part of the surgical landscape whether welcome or not. This may offer surgeons an opportunity to bridge the chasm between spiritual matters and the physical world with which they are so intimate.

How involved should surgeons be in palliative care?

Although most surgeons will readily acknowledge the value of good palliative care for their patients, they may not necessarily believe that they should personally be active in providing it. Some surgeons will say outright that they have no interest or qualifications in palliative care, even though their operative skills may greatly enhance the quality of life of their patients, their patient's families, and even their colleagues. A recent survey of surgeons in Australia gives an added sense of urgency to educating all surgeons about definitions of palliative care that have achieved cross-cultural consensus. In this study of 992 eligible general surgeons, more than a third of the 247 who responded reported giving drugs with the intent of hastening death, often in the absence of an explicit request.[24] Assuming it is advantageous to patients for surgeons to develop a consistent and comprehensive philosophy of palliation, we propose a classification of the levels of involvement which recognizes a wide range of ability and interest. This will help to plan future educational and research initiatives. A secondary reason for this classification is to signal to surgeons that their interest is needed and appreciated, no matter what the depth of their involvement (Box 18.3). Each level of involvement has implications for non-surgeons active in palliative care, education, research, and clinical practice. In this classification, the more sophisticated and research-oriented a surgeon's approach to palliative care, the more critical the free exchange of ideas between them and the non-surgical disciplines.

Surgeons deeply involved in palliative care should first concentrate on educating their colleagues at the first level, in order to overcome the scepticism some may have towards a philosophy that appears to run counter to traditional ideas of clinical success. Since July 2001, the American Board of Surgery requires that 'the surgeon must be familiar with the unique requirements of the geriatric surgical patient and must have knowledge and skills in palliative care, including operative care, counselling patients and families, and management of pain, cachexia, and weight loss.'[25] The Surgical Royal Colleges in Great Britain and Ireland have similar expectations outlined in their general examination syllabus[26] and are introducing end-of-life issues in their higher training syllabus. These expectations for certifying exams represent only a minimum basis of knowledge for the conduct of palliative care. Much more difficult will be the uniform assessment of the necessary attitudes and skills, such as communication. The presence of these requirements is encouraging since the content of certifying exams drives the curriculum taught at the postgraduate level (residency). Currently there is a cohort of 32 surgical residency programmes in the United States enrolled in an End-of-Life training programme, which had been extensively used in Internal Medicine residencies.[27] The importance of this type of educational initiative is highlighted by the findings in a survey[28] of surgeons in which nearly a third reported being not competent in encouraging patients to express anxieties about their condition and an even higher percentage reported lack of competence in providing bereavement counselling. More studies such as this will be invaluable in making palliative care relevant to surgical education.

Box 18.3 Fours levels of surgeons' involvement in palliative care

1. Surgeons in active practice familiar with the basic principles of palliative care and subject to the competency requirements of their certifying boards.

2. Surgeons active and not active in the practice of surgery who participate in hospice and palliative care teams or as a volunteer for hospice services.

3. Surgeons still in practice who participate in palliative care indirectly by membership on ethics committees, patient care committees, critical care, etc.

4. Surgeons active in the practice of surgery whose primary focus is palliative care education, research, or surgery (the surgical palliative care specialist).

The second level of palliative care education for surgeons is more amenable to education by non-surgeons. The third and fourth level would need direction from specialists in the field of surgery as well as palliative care specialists outside the domain of surgery.

In order to focus educational initiatives for surgeons, definition of core competencies in palliative care will need to be identified and adjusted for some of the unique aspects of the surgical encounter. Familiarity with symptom control procedures, such as coeliac plexus block,[29] that have proven temporary efficacy based on prospective studies would be an expectation of surgeons in addition to those competencies previously proposed for end-of-life care education for non-surgeons. Additional competencies would address communication issues related to operative complications and a revision of the informed consent process that would place these discussions in a broader context than an appraisal of immediate physical risk and benefit.

Surgical institutions and the promotion of palliative care

Surgeons have participated in some of the earliest hospice programmes in Great Britain, Canada, and the United States and in supportive (palliative) care whether in a burn unit in the United States, a leprosy hospital in India, a cancer programme in London, or an aid station in a war zone; but only in the past few years has the concept of palliation as a comprehensive philosophy of patient care been defined and endorsed by leading surgical institutions and societies of the world. As already mentioned, both the Surgical Royal Colleges of Great Britain and Ireland, the American College of Surgeons (which has membership chapters in over 30 countries of the world[30]), the Royal College of Physicians and Surgeons of Canada, and the

Box 18.4 American College of Surgeons' *Statement of principles guiding care at end of life*[31]

1. Respect the dignity of both patient and care-givers.
2. Be sensitive to and respectful of the patient's and family's wishes.
3. Use the most appropriate measures that are consistent with the choices of the patient or the patient's legal surrogate.
4. Ensure alleviation of pain and management of other physical symptoms.
5. Recognize, assess, and address psychological, social, and spiritual problems.
6. Ensure appropriate continuity of care by the patient's primary and/or specialist physician.
7. Provide access to therapies that may realistically be expected to improve the patient's quality of life.
8. Provide access to appropriate palliative care and hospice care.
9. Respect the patient's right to refuse treatment.
10. Recognize the physician's responsibility to forego treatments that are futile.

The principles were developed by the American College of Surgeons Committee on Ethics and were adopted by the Board of Regents in February 1998.

American Board of Surgery have all taken steps during the past decade to promote competence in palliative and end-of-life care, and to include it in their examinations.

In 1998, the Board of Regents of the American College of Surgeons adopted the *Statement of principles guiding care at end of life* (Box 18.4). [31] These were recommended by the College's Committee on Ethics, though at the time the College had no educational programmes for its membership that specifically addressed care at end of life by surgeons or surgical means. The Statement was issued several months after the College had held a well-attended symposium that debated physician-assisted suicide. Similar guidance has been issued by the Senate of Surgery of Great Britain and Ireland in its publication *The surgeon's duty of care*.[32] The ethical debate on physician-assisted suicide certainly brought attention to end-of-life care and palliative care in general; but it risked distracting surgeons as well as non-surgeons from the clinical tasks of first, identifying ways to introduce palliation for all forms of suffering in the care of all patients, and secondly, developing skill in palliative care. Familiarity with ethical dilemmas, however relevant, is a poor substitute for the competent provision of palliative care. Representatives of the American College of Surgeons met with a self-organized group of surgeons from several speciality backgrounds with previous experience in hospice care or palliative care research; these combined with physician leaders in palliative medicine to form a work group under a grant from the Robert Wood Johnson Foundation, a private, non-profit, philanthropic organization.

The primary goal of this group was to facilitate introduction of the precepts and techniques of palliative care to surgical practice and education in the United States and Canada through a shared surgical society that over the years has had credibility in scientific, socio-economic, and spiritual matters related to surgery. During the following year and a half it became incorporated into the American College of Surgeons within its Division of Education. The *Journal of the American College of Surgeons* published a series of articles on palliative care[33] which address such topics as chronic pain control, hydration and feeding at end of life, management of malignant bowel obstruction, and spiritual assessment. Continuing medical education credits were awarded for those answering questions about material from selected articles. The palliative care series has become an ongoing feature of the *Journal*.

A secondary goal of the work group emerged which was to lay the foundation for a systematic philosophy of palliation that would incorporate the College's *Statement of principles guiding care at end of life*. There was a consensus of the work group that the language of the *Statement* should get away from the term 'end of life' and focus more on the concept of palliation and supportive care as a means of reducing suffering and affirmation of the individual's integrity and purpose, regardless of the point in the trajectory of an illness. In October 2002, the work group became incorporated into the administrative structure of the American College of Surgeons when it became designated as a task force in the College's Division of Education.

The surgical society is the largest unit of surgical culture and therefore has a major role in bringing the principles and practice of palliation to the daily life of the surgical patient and the surgeon. Box 18.5 suggests a phased plan for palliative care initiatives by surgical societies. They are particularly well placed to survey the level of understanding of palliative and supportive care within the surgical community. Date[34] are emerging about families' perceptions of surgical critical care for both survivors and non-survivors that will be useful in designing future educational programmes for surgeons in training. Similar information about end-of-life issues will be crucial when planning the palliative care programmes.

Box 18.5 Phased plan for palliative care initiatives by surgical societies

1. *Introductory phase*

- ◆ Publications (articles, etc.) by interested surgeons in society publications
- ◆ Symposia, lectures, courses by surgical and non-surgical experts in palliative care at society meetings

2. *Organizing phase*

- ◆ Formation of a committee specifically addressing palliative care
- ◆ Creation of a bureau of speakers approved by the society to lecture on palliative care topics
- ◆ Creation of a society-sponsored website for distribution of information, information resource links, and consultation
- ◆ Funding of fellowships for the study of palliative care by surgeons and others interested in surgical palliative care
- ◆ Grant funding for surgical palliative care research

3. *Operational phase*

- ◆ Surveys of the field
- ◆ Data banking
- ◆ Recognition awards for achievement
- ◆ Outreach to other medical organizations and societies
- ◆ Developing standards for palliative care by surgeons, i.e. identifying competencies, participation in certification process
- ◆ Initiating a process of certification for competency in surgical palliative care
- ◆ Support function for surgeons

4. *Outreach phase*

- ◆ Participation in government policy decision making
- ◆ Public education

Surgical societies must also give social and psychological support to those working in this field because good palliative care is costly to the carer. Care that reduces suffering of a patient at the expense of the care-giver is martyrdom, not palliation. Contact with others who are part of the interdisciplinary team is the safest way to diminish adverse effects of our own suffering and ideal palliation occurs when both the patient and care-giver are relieved or uplifted.

Conclusion

Merging of the great traditions of surgery and palliative care holds great promise for the supportive care of all patients at all stages of their illnesses. However, the personal and professional characteristics of each discipline can be a barrier to this merger and the union will be complete when these differences are recognized and accepted. Surgical palliative care certainly has a busy future!

References

1. Ball, A.B.S., Baum, M., Breach, N.M., Shepherd, J.H., Shearer, R.J., Thomas, J.M., *et al.* (1998). Surgical palliation. In: *Oxford textbook of palliative medicine* (ed. D. Doyle, G. Hanks, and N. Mac Donald), pp. 282–97. Oxford University Press, Oxford.

2. Little, M. (2001). Invited commentary: is there a distinctively surgical ethics? *Surgery*, **129** (6), 668–71.

3. Wood-Dauphinee, S. (1996). Quality of life assessment: recent trends in surgery. *Can. J. Surg.*, **36**, 368–72.

4. Krizek, T.J. (2002). Ethics and philosophy lecture: surgery – is it an impairing profession? *J. Am. Coll. Surg.*, **194** (3), 352–66.

5. Nuland, S.B. (1994). *How we die, Reflections on life's final chapter*. Alfred A. Knopf, New York.

6. Flitter, M. (1997). *Judith's pavilion. The haunting memories of a neurosurgeon*. Warner Books, New York, New York

7. Saunders, C., and Sykes, N. (1993). *The management of terminal malignant disease* (3rd edn). Edward Arnold, London.

8. McCahill, L.E, Krouse, R.S., Chu, D.Z.J., Juarez, G., Uman, G.C., Ferrell, B., and Wagman, L.D. (2002). Indications and utilization of palliative surgery – results of Society of Surgical Oncology Survey. *Ann. Surg. Oncol.*, **9**, 104–12.

9. Rappaport, W., and Witzke, D. (1993). Education about death and dying during the clinical years of medical school. *Surgery*, **113** (2), 163–5.

10. Easson, A.M., Crosby, J.A., and Librach, S.L. (2001). Discussion of death and dying in surgical textbooks. *Am. J. Surg.*, **182**, 34–9.

11. Dunn, G.P. (1998). Surgery and palliative medicine: new horizons. *J. Pall. Med.*, **1** (3), 214–19.

12. Finlayson C.A., and Eisenberg, B.L. (1996). Palliative pelvic exenteration: patient selection and results. *Oncology*, **10**, 479–84.

13. Easson, A.M., Asch, M., and Swallow, C.J. (2001). Palliative general surgical procedures. *Surg. Oncol. Clin. North Am.*, **10** (1), 161–84.

14. Sugarbaker, P.H., Barofsky, I., Rosenberg, S.A., and Gianola, F.J. (1982). Quality-of-life assessment in extremity sarcoma trials. *Surgery*, **91**, 17–23.

15. Miner, T.J., Jacgues, D.P., Tavaf-Motamen, H., and Shriver, C.D. (1999). Decision making on surgical palliation based on patient outcome data. *Am. J. Surg.*, **177**, 150–4.

16. Velanovich, V. (2001). The quality-of-life studies in general surgical journals. *J. Am. Coll. Surg.*, **193** (3), 288–96.

17. Langenhoff, B.S., Krabbe, P.F.M., and Ruers, T.J.M., (2001). Quality of life as an outcome measure in surgical oncology. *Br. J. Surg.*, **88**, 643–52.

18. Dunn, G.P. (2002). Surgical palliation in advanced disease: recent developments. *Curr. Oncol. Reports*, **4**, 233–41.

19. Cady, B. (2001). 'Major palliative resections. Are they justified?' Lecture given at the 54th Annual Cancer Symposium, Society of Surgical Oncology, March 15–18, 2001.

20. Nuland, S.B. (2001). A surgeon's reflections on the care of the dying. *Surg. Oncol. Clin. North Am.*, **10** (1), 1–5.

21. Hinshaw, D.B. (2002). The spiritual needs of the dying patient. *J. Am. Coll. Surg.*, **195** (4), 565–8.

22. Tarpley, J.L. (2002). Spirituality in surgical practice. *J. Am. Coll. Surg.*, **194** (6), 642–7.

23. Krizek, T. (2001). Spiritual dimensions in surgical palliative care. *Surg. Oncol. Clin. North Am.*, **10** (1), 39–55.

24. Douglas, C.D., Kerridge, I.H., Rainbird, K.J., McPhee, J.R., Hancock, L., and Spigelman, A.D (2001). The intention to hasten death: a survey of attitudes and practices of surgeons in Australia. *med. J. Australia*, **175**, 511–5

25. American Board of Surgery, Inc. (2001). Booklet of information. July 2001–June 2002. Philadelphia.

26. Kirk, R.M., Mansfield, A.O., and Cochrane, J.P.S. (ed.) (1999). *Clinical surgery in general. Royal College of Surgeons* (3rd edn), pp. 370–84. Churchill-Livingstone, London.

27. Surgeons Palliative Care Work Group (2003). Report from the field. Executive summary. *J. Am. Coll. Surg.*, **196** (5).

28. Rappaport, W., and Witzke, D. (1993). Education about death and dying during the clinical years of medical school. *Surgery*, **113**, 163–5.

29. Lillemoe, K.D., Cameron, J.L., Kaufman, H.S., Yeo C.J., Pitt, H. A., and Sauter, P. K. (1993). Chemical splanchnicectomy in patients with unresectable pancreatic cancer. A prospective randomized trial. *Ann. Surg.*, **217**, 447–55.

30. American College of Surgeons (1998). Yearbook, p. 1281. American College of Surgeons, Chicago.

31. Committee on Ethics, American College of Surgeons (1998). Statement of principles guiding care at end of life. *Bull. Am. Coll. Surg.*, **83** (4), 46.

32. The Surgeon's duty of care: Guidance for surgeons on ethical and legal issues (1997). Senate of Surgery of Great Britain and Ireland. 35–43. Lincoln's Inn Fields, London WC2A2PS.

33. Dunn, G.P., and Milch, R.A. (2001). Introduction and historical background of palliative care: where does the surgeon fit in? *J. Am. Coll. Surg.*, **193** (3), 325–8.

34. Buchman, T.G., Ray, S., Wax, M., Cassell, J., Rich, D., and Niemczycki, A. (2003). Family matters: perceptions of surgical intensive care. *J. Am. Coll. Surg.*, **196** (6).

Index

abdominal symptoms 159–72
  ascites 165–6
  decision making 159
  gastrointestinal obstruction 159–63
  haemorrhage 163–5
  jaundice 166–8
  pain 168
  reduction of tumour bulk 169–70
  resection of metastases 169–70
acupuncture 128
acute phase protein response 42, 44
adequate palliation 35
adrenocorticotrophic hormone (ACTH) 42
advance directives 25–6, 117, 118, 153, 154
alkylating agents 117
amniotic membrane transplantation 230
anabolism 39, 45, 48
anaesthesia 4, 24, 112–20
  and age 112
  and ASA grade 112
  balanced 120
  and cardiovascular disease 115
  and chemotherapy 117
  and diabetes mellitus 116
  and DNR orders 117–18
  fasting and gastric contents 119
  general 119–20
  management of co-existing disease 115–17
  and metabolic response to surgery 46, 47, 48
  and neurological impairment 116–17
  optimisation 113
  pre-anaesthetic assessment 113
  and pulmonary disease 115–16
  and radiotherapy 117
  regional/local 47, 118–19, 120, 122, 127–8
  and renal disease 116
  risks 112–13
  routine investigations 113–15
  and sepsis 117
  spinal 120, 127–8
  techniques 118–20
  and urgency of surgery 112
analgesia, see pain management
analgesic drugs 48, 121, 123–7
Andy Gump operation 200
angiodysplasia of colon 164
angiotensin II 42
anorexia 20, 43
antegrade ureteric stenting 177
antibacterials, topical 195, 196, 202
antibiotics, systemic 195, 201–2
anticonvulsants 126
antidepressants 126, 173–4
antidiuretic hormone (ADH) 41–2

appropriate death 57
argon beam coagulator 164–5
ascites 18, 165–6
aspirin 124
asthenia 20

baclofen 219
bacterial keratitis 236
beneficence principle 86
bladder cancer 175, 178, 181, 182–3, 186–7
bladder outflow obstruction 178–80
bleomycin 117
blind painful eye 227–33
  causes 227
  corneal and ocular surface disease 229–30
  counselling and preoperative
    preparation before eye removal 230–1
  cyclocryotherapy 228
  cyclodestruction 227–9
  enucleation 232–3
  evisceration 231–2
  retrobulbar injections 229
  trans-scleral cyclophotocoagulation 228–9
body image 61
bone pain 184–5, 187
bone-seeking radionuclides 185
brain metastases 116, 216
brain tumours, malignant 216, 222–3
breakthrough pain 121
breast cancer 5, 73–4
Budd–Chiari syndrome 180
burn care 9, 199, 203
  intubation 204–5
  management 203–4
  as metaphor for palliative care 7–8
  pain relief 205
  resuscitation 205
  surgical procedures 205
  unprecedented survival 204

cachexia 20, 27–8
Calman–Hine Report (1995) 153, 154
carbohydrate metabolism 43–4
carcinoid syndrome 169
cardiac surgery 5–6
cardiopulmonary rescuscitation (CPR) 35, 36
cardiovascular disease 115
carotid blow-out 145, 147
catabolism 40, 45, 49
cataract surgery 236
catheterization 175, 178–9
cerebral palsy 219
'channel' TURP 179
chaplains 80–1

chemotherapy 117, 183, 186–7
children 223–4, 243–5
cingulotomy 217
classic scientific model 9
clonidine 126
codeine 124
coeliac plexus blockade 20, 128, 168
cognitive dimension of suffering 209
colorectal cancer 74, 169–70
colostomy 161
communication difficulties 62
conjunctival flap surgery 229–30
conjunctival oedema 236
consent 46–7, 59
corneal disease 229–30
costs of care 243
counter-reaction 56–7
counter-transference 56–7
coxibs 124–5, 127
cryosurgery 145, 169, 228
cultural conflict 3, 85
curative model 34
cyclocryotherapy 228
cystectomy 175, 177, 181, 182–3
cytokines 42, 44, 48, 184

defence mechanisms 55, 57, 58–9
denial 55, 58, 59, 105
dental issues 142–3, 147
dependency 55, 69
depression 69, 213–14
developing world and diverse societies 239–47
    children 243–5
    communication with patients 240–1
    costs 243
    death, cancer and religious systems 239–40
    evaluation of success of palliation 245
    extended family 242
    home-based palliation 241, 242, 244–5
    late presentation 239, 244
    non-interference and palliation 240
    paternalism 241
    poverty 242
    psychological/emotional support 243
    social inequalities 240–1
    training 245
    vulnerable groups 243
dexamethasone 222
dextropropoxyphene 123–4
diabetes
    and anaesthesia 116
    retinopathy 227, 236
    wound healing 192, 194
diamorphine 125
diclofenac 124, 125
dihydrocodeine 124
disfigurement/deformity 62, 63, 197, 198, 199,
    200, 230–1
distortion 58
diverticular disease 164, 165
do not resuscitate (DNR) orders 36, 117–18
double effect principle 5

doxorubicin 117
dry mouth 147
dying
    moving towards death 212
    and religious systems in developing world 239–40
    spiritual journey in 68–9
    three-stage model of process 60

Eaton–Lambert syndrome 117
effusions 18–19
ego 57–8
embolization 143, 165, 169, 174–5, 181
emotional dimension of suffering 209
endoscopic retrograde
    cholangiopancreatography (ERCP) 24, 166–8
energy metabolism 43
enucleation of eye 230, 232–3
epidural blockade 47, 120, 122, 127, 128
eschar 205
ethics 6, 249
    curative vs. palliative operation 34–5
    and interdisciplinary care 86–7
    of interventional care 33–8
    limits to palliative surgery 36
    patients 'too sick for surgery' 35–6
    philosophical basis of surgical
        intervention 33–4
    and reconstructive surgery 198–9
    redefinition in advanced illness 14
    and spirituality/religion 74–5
    surgical interventions differ
        from others 36–7
etomidate 119
European Organization for Research and
    Treatment of Cancer (EORTC) QOL
    questionnaire C30: 98, 99, 100, 101
evisceration of eye 230, 231–2, 233
exenteration of eye 230, 233–5
existential dimension of suffering 209
expectations 105
eye problems, see opthalmic problems

family members 59, 60, 63, 215–16, 242, 244
fat metabolism 44
feeding gastrostomy 163
feeding jejunostomy 163
fentanyl 125, 126
fibroplasia 192, 193
fish oil 49
fluid resuscitation 47, 205
formalin intravesical irrigation 174
free tissue transfer 145–7
Functional Assessment of Cancer Treatment
    (FACT) questionnaire 98, 99, 100
Functional Living Index for Cancer (FLIC) 245

gastrectomy 5
gastrointestinal haemorrhage 163–5
    embolization 165
    endoscopic techniques 164–5
    exclusion and bypass 165
    resection 165

gastrointestinal obstruction 159–63
  bypass with side-to-side anastomosis 160–1
  feeding 162–3
  laser destruction of tumours 161–2
  prophylactic resection 160
  proximal stoma 161
  reduction of secretions 162
  resection 160
  stenting 162
gastrojejunostomy 161
glaucoma 227–8, 236
gluconeogenesis 44
goals of care 25–6, 33, 34
granulation tissue (proud flesh) 195
growth hormone 48–9
gynaecological cancer 74

haematuria 174–5, 176, 186
haemobilia 164
haemoglobin 114
haemorrhage, control of 19, 147, 163–5, 181
head and neck cancer 135–51
  airway patency 142
  and anaesthesia 117
  arrest of haemorrhage 147
  cryosurgery 145
  dental issues 142–3, 147
  embolization and image-guided
    ablation 143
  fistulae 143
  heroic surgery 145
  loco-regional control 142–7
  microvascular free tissue transfer 145–7
  morbidity and quality of life 138–9
  myocutaneous pedicle 145
  natural history 137–8
  nutritional support 142
  pain control 142–3
  photodynamic therapy 143
  previous treatment 140
  psychological response to surgery
    62–3
  reconstructive surgery 145–7, 197, 200
  squamous cell carcinoma 135, 138
  surgical procedures 141–7
  surgical rehabilitation 139
  symptoms 141
  tarsorrhaphy 143
  tumour ablation 145
  tumour debulking 143–5
head injury 224–5
health-related quality of life, see quality of life
historical background 4–7
home-based palliation 241, 242, 244–5
hope 79–80, 210–11
hopelessness 69
HOPE questions 72
hospice care 7
hydrocephalus 223–4
hydromorphone 220–1, 222
hypercoagulability 45
hypertension 115

ibuprofen 124, 125
ileal conduit 177
ileostomy 161
imaging 23–4
immune deficiency 194
immunotherapy 180, 181, 182
incident pain 121
inflammatory response 42, 44, 48, 192, 195
inflammatory response syndrome 43
innovations, history of 4–7
insulin 49
insulin resistance 44, 47
intellectualization 58
interdisciplinary care 85–93
  definition of interdisciplinary team 87–9
  ethical and clinical foundation 86–7
  models 89–92
intermittent self-catheterization (ISC) 175, 178–9
interstitial tumour therapy (ITT) 143
interventional care, ethics of 33–8
intracerebral haemorrhage 225
intraocular pressure, raised 227–9
intrathecal blockade 120

jaundice 166–8
  itching 168
  stents 166–8
  surgical bypass 166

Karnofsky Performance Scale 21
ketamine 119, 126
ketorolac 124, 125

laparoscopic surgery 48
laser therapy 143, 161–2, 228–9, 230
leg oedema 175
liver tumours 169–70
living wills 25–6, 153
loss of control, fears of 55
lung cancer 152, 153

marital relationships 63
meaning 79–80, 214, 215
melanoma 74
metabolic response to cancer 41, 46, 49
metabolic response to surgery 9, 39–53
  acute phase protein response 44
  anabolic phase 45
  and anaesthesia and drugs 46, 47, 48
  appropriateness 45
  and appropriate surgery 48
  blood coagulation changes 45
  carbohydrate metabolism 43–4
  changes in vital signs and symptoms 42–3
  characteristics 42–5
  and co-existing disease 46
  and early mobilization 49
  ebb and flow phases 39–40, 42–3
  energy metabolism and substrate cycling 43
  fat metabolism 44
  and fluid resuscitation 47
  gastrointestinal effects 43

metabolic response to surgery (*continued*)
  and infection 46
  initiation 40
  and magnitude of surgery 46
  mediators 41–2
  and minimal access surgery 48
  modulation 47–9
  and nutritional status 46
  perioperative modifying factors 46
  planning surgery, patient understanding
    and consent 46–7
  and postoperative nutrition 49
  and preoperative carbohydrate loading 47
  protein metabolism 44
  specific pharmacological intervention 48–9
  and surgical complications 46
  and thromboembolic prophylaxis 47
  water and salt retention 43
methadone 125
mithramycin 117
mitoxantrone 186
mobilization 49
morphine 120, 125, 205, 223
mortality and morbidity rounds 10–11
movement disorders 218–19
multidisciplinary teams 87, 88
MVAC (methotrexate, vinblastine, adriamycin,
  cisplatin) 186–7
myocardial infarction 115

nasogastric tubes 163
natural killer (NK) cells 121
neovascular glaucoma 227–8
nephrectomy 180–2
nerve blocks 127, 142
neuroendocrine response to injury 41–2
neurofibromatosis 216
neurological impairment 116–17
neurolytic blocks 128
neuropathic pain 121, 126, 173, 210,
  217–18
neurosurgical palliation 207–26
  cancer pain 129, 217, 221–2
  case studies 220–5
  criteria for referral/consultation 215–16
  head injury 224–5
  hydrocephalus 223–4
  intracerebral haemorrhage 225
  malignant brain tumours 222–3
  management of intractable pain 216–18
  movement disorders 218–19
  non-cancer pain 217–18, 220–1
  spasmotic torticollis 220
  spasticity 219–20
nociceptive pain 121, 209–10, 217–18
non-steroidal anti-inflammatory drugs
  (NSAIDs) 48, 124–5, 127, 173–4
nutritional status 46, 193
nutritional support 27–8
  and gastrointestinal obstruction 162–3
  in head and neck cancer 142
  and metabolic response to surgery 44, 48–9

obstruction 19, 159–63, 176–80
ocular malignancy 227, 233–5
ocular surface disease 229–30
oesophageal tumours 162
operative mortality 20, 24, 112, 113, 254
opioids 119, 120, 122, 123–4, 125–6, 127–8
opthalmic problems 227–38
  advanced periocular disease 233–5
  blind painful eye 227–33
  eye care in critical/terminal illness 235–6
  eye removal 230–5
  tarsorrhaphy 143
orbital implants 231–3, 235
outcome movement 96

pain management 19–20, 120–9
  abdominal pain 168
  acupuncture 128
  acute pain 122
  adjuvant analgesics 126
  assessment 104, 121
  bone pain 184–5, 187
  and burn care 7–8, 205
  chronic pain 123
  in developing world 240
  drug side-effects 127
  drug treatments 123–7
  education 122
  effects of cancer pain on outcomes 121
  in head and neck cancer 142–3
  incidence and causes of cancer pain 120–1
  local and regional analgesia 127–8
  neurosurgical 129, 216–18, 220–2
  non-cancer pain 217–18, 220–1
  opthalmic problems 227–33, 234
  pain and suffering 213–14
  physical methods 128
  pre-emptive analgesia 122
  recommendations 129
  routes of drug delivery 125–6
  specific issues in cancer pain 121
  teams 122
  transcutaneous electrical nerve
    stimulation 128
  in urological malignancy 173–4, 184–5, 186, 187
palliative care
  and active treatment 94–5
  definitions 198, 208
  framework 215
  guiding principles 213–14
  methodology 214
palliative model 13, 34
palliative surgery
  definitions 12–13, 16, 34, 252
  history 4–7
  limits to 36
  skill sets 208
  vs. surgical palliative care 252–3
pancreatic carcinoma 20, 128, 161, 163, 165, 168
pancreatitis, chronic 168
paracentesis 165–6
paracetamol 123–4

paralytic ileus 43, 47
paraneoplastic symptoms 176
Parkinson's disease 219
pastoral care workers 80–1
patient-controlled analgesia (PCA) 126, 127, 220–1
pedicled flaps 145
peptic ulceration 164
percutaneous direct puncture therapeutic embolization (DPTE) 143
percutaneous endoscopic gastrostomy (PEG) 142, 163
percutaneous fluid drainage 18
percutaneous nephrostomy tube insertion 176–7, 178
performance status 20–1
peritoneo-venous shunt 166
personal dignity 69
personality and character formation 57–8
photodynamic therapy 143, 162
physical dimension of suffering 209
physiological response to surgical trauma 39–53
plastic surgery 191, 196–203
PLC questionnaire 98, 99, 100
portal hypertension 165, 166
poverty 242
prayer 75–7
pre-emptive analgesia 122
pre-emptive surgery 160, 253
preoperative carbohydrate loading 47
preoperative imaging 23–4
preparation of patients 26–8
presence 14, 37
pressure sores/bed sores 192, 200–2
projection 58, 59
propofol 119
prostate cancer 183–6
    adjuvant prostatectomy 183
    bone pain 184–5
    'channel' TURP 179
    chemotherapy 186
    external beam radiotherapy 184
    hemi-body irradiation 185
    prostatic stents 179–80
    unsealed source radiotherapy 185
prosthetic devices 200, 231, 232, 235
protein metabolism 44
proton pump inhibitors 127, 162, 164
proximity 37
psychological response to surgery 54–64
    counter-reaction 56–7
    counter-transference 56–7
    defence mechanisms 58–9
    discussion of body image 61
    feelings of aloneness and physician's role 63–4
    in head and neck cancer 62–3
    personality and character formation 57–8
    postperative period 60
    preoperative period 59–60
    speaking the unspeakable 57
    surgeon's difficult role 54–6
    transference 56–7

psycho-spiritual distress 65–6, 69
pulmonary disease 115–16, 152–8

quality of life (QOL) 25, 94–111
    concepts of palliative care, outcome and QOL 94–7
    and enhancement of care 106–8
    evaluation in developing world 245
    in head and neck cancer 138–9
    implementation 107
    and interdisciplinary care 86
    lack of measures as barrier 253
    maximization 214
    measurement issues 97–101
    measurement problems in palliative/terminal situation 101–5
    proxy measures 101–4
    psychological issues 105
    QOL profiles 106–7
    qualitative approach to assessment 104–5
    questionnaire development 97–8
    and redefinition of surgical success 11
    and spirituality/religion 67–8
    well-being paradox 105

radical palliative surgery with curative intent 145
radiofrequency ablation 169
radiotherapy
    and abdominal symptoms 169
    and anaesthesia 117
    and urological malignancy 175, 181, 183, 184–5, 186, 187
    and wounds 194
rationalization 58
reconstructive surgery 191, 196–203
    in head and neck cancer 145–7, 197, 200
    mental/emotional/psychological issues 199–200
    as palliative care 198
    physical issues 200
    reconstructive ladder 196
    special procedures 200–3
regression 58
religion, see spirituality and religion
renal cell carcinoma (RCC) 175–6, 180–1, 187
renal disease, and anaesthesia 116
repression 58
requests to die 69
retinoblastoma 234
retrobulbar injections 229
retrograde ureteric stenting 176, 177
rhenium-186: 185
risk–benefit analysis 20, 28, 33–4, 35, 36
rofecoxib 125

safe surgery concept 5
salt retention 43
samarium-153: 185
scarring 200
selection of patients 17–26
    defining goals of care 25–6
    disease factors 17, 18–20
    local and regional symptoms 18–20

selection of patients (*continued*)
  medical factors 20–2
  natural history of disease 18
  patient factors 17, 20–2
  prognosis 20–2
  psychosocial factors 22
  societal factors 17, 24
  systemic symptoms 20
  technical factors 17, 22–4
sepsis 117
serum potassium 115
sexual issues 59–60
SF-36 questionnaire 98, 99, 100
silver sulfadiazine 195, 202
skeletal muscle breakdown 44
skin grafts 145–7, 194, 198, 204, 235
soft tissue tumour growth 19
somatization 58, 59
somatostatin analogues 162
spasmotic torticollis 220
spasticity 219–20
spinal anaesthesia/analgesia 120, 127–8
spinal metastases 216
spirituality and religion 65–84
  in clinical context 71–7
  and clinical outcomes 73–4
  in developing world 239–40
  distinction between 65–6
  ethical issues 74–5
  extrinsic and intrinsic religiosity 70
  fostering of hope and meaning 79–80
  and health 65, 66, 70–1, 73
  history in clinical setting 66–7
  management of issues in surgical unit 77–81
  measurement 67–8
  negative aspects 70
  place of pastoral care workers and chaplains 80–1
  positive aspects 70–1
  potential for conflict 80
  praying with patients 75–6
  psycho-spiritual distress 65–6
  public prayer for patients 76–7
  spiritual assessment 71–3
  spiritual barriers to surgical palliative care 254
  spiritual dimension of suffering 209
  spiritual journey in dying 68–9, 153
  studies in medical literature 73
splanchnicectomy 168
splitting 57
Stauffer's syndrome 175
stents 24, 162, 166–8, 176–7, 179–80
steroids 193
strontium-89: 185
subarachnoid haemorrhage 216
sublimation 58
success, redefinition in advanced illness 11–13
suffering
  dimensions 209–10
  origin 214

  relief of 213–14
  and surgical character 8–10
superficial keratopathy 235–6
supportive group therapy 63
surgeon–patient relationship 14, 37, 56–7, 71, 210
surgeons
  captain of ship metaphor 10–11
  character and problem of suffering 8–10
  and cultural differences 3
  decisiveness 11
  defence mechanisms 58–9
  difficult role 54–6
  distancing behaviours 10
  innovations and personalities 4–7
  levels of involvement in palliative care 254–6
  need to change traditional views 249–50
  and patients' feelings of aloneness 63–4
  roles in cancer palliation 13
  and spiritual practice 77–8
surgical institutions 256–8
surgical intensive care units 89–91
surgical palliative care 3–15
  cognitive barriers 251–3
  new sub-speciality or basis for all surgery 248–9
  psychological barriers 253
  social barriers 253–4
  spiritual barriers 254
  vs. palliative surgery 252–3
surgical trauma, physiological response to 39–53
sympathetic opthalmia 232

tarsorrhaphy 143
testis cancer 187
thoracic conditions 115–16, 152–8
thromboembolic prophylaxis 47, 120
'too sick for surgery' patients 35–6
total pain 7, 104
trabeculectomy 227–8
tracheostomy 139, 142
training and education 245, 251–2, 255–6, 257
tramadol 124
transcendence 68
transcutaneous electrical nerve stimulation (TENS) 128
trans-femoral percutaneous internal iliac embolization 174–5
transference 56–7
transplantation 6
trans-scleral cyclophotocoagulation 228–9
transurethral resection of prostate (TURP) 178, 179

ureteric obstruction 176–8
ureteric stents 176–7
urinary diversion 175, 176–8
urinary incontinence 175
urological malignancy 173–90
  adjunctive nephrectomy 181–2
  adjuvant cystectomy 182–3
  adjuvant prostatectomy 183
  catheterization 178–9

'channel' TURP 179
diversion for metastatic ureteric obstruction 176–8
haematuria 174–5
interventional radiology 181
leg oedema 175
lower urinary tract symptoms 175
malignant bladder outflow obstruction 178–80
multimodality procedures 181–3
nephrectomy/excision of renal bed recurrence 180–1
oncological interventions for palliation 183–7
pain 173–4
palliative cystectomy 181
prostatic stents 179–80
symptoms from renal cell carcinoma 175–6
symptoms of advanced malignancy 173–6
urinary incontinence and fistulae 175

ventrolateral thalamotomy 219
ventroposterolateral pallidotomy 219
visual analogue scales 104

vitamins 193
volatile anaesthetic agents 119

water retention 43
wounds 191–6
    acute 192–5
    and bacteria 194–5, 201–2
    burns 203–5
    chronic 192, 194–5
    closure 192–3, 196, 202–3, 204
    debridement 196
    healing 192–5
    and immune deficiency 194
    infiltration 127
    management 191–2
    and nutrition 193
    pressure sores 192, 200–2
    and quantitative microbiology 195
    and radiation 194
    scope of problem 192
    and steroids 193
    ulcerations from tumours 202–3
    and vascularity 194
    and vitamins 193